**NURSING
SERVICE ADMINISTRATION**
managing the enterprise

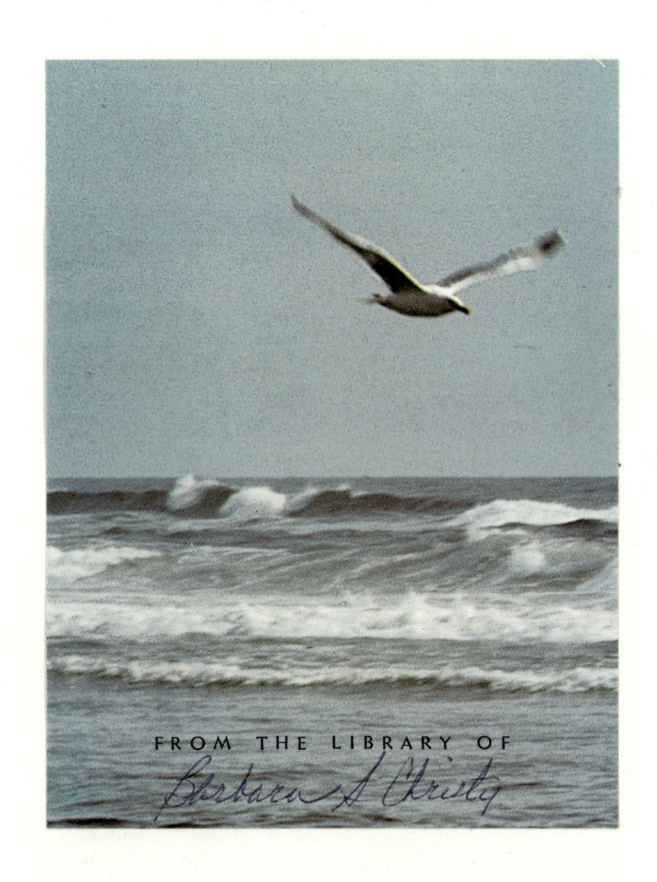

FROM THE LIBRARY OF
Barbara S Christy

NURSING SERVICE ADMINISTRATION
managing the enterprise

HELEN M. DONOVAN, R.N., M.A.

SAINT LOUIS

The C. V. Mosby Company

1975

Copyright © 1975 by The C. V. Mosby Company

All rights reserved. No part of this book may be reproduced in any manner without written permission of the publisher.

Printed in the United States of America

Distributed in Great Britain by Henry Kimpton, London

Library of Congress Cataloging in Publication Data

Donovan, Helen Murphy, 1916-
    Nursing service administration.

    Bibliography: p.
    Includes index.
    1. Nursing service administration. I. Title.
[DNLM: 1. Nursing, Supervisory. WY105 D687n]
RT89.D66   658'.91'36216   75-26845
ISBN 0-8016-1423-6

TS/M/M   9 8 7 6 5 4 3 2 1

TO
KATHARINE E. FAVILLE
DEAN EMERITUS WAYNE STATE UNIVERSITY

through whose wisdom and spirit
so many are enriched

FOREWORD

This book reflects the author's many years of concern for improvement in the management of patient care services. As hospital nursing assistant director, medical and surgical nursing, later instructor of nursing services administration, and more recently consultant and instructor in nursing service administration, her exposure to the problems faced by nursing services administrators has been extensive, and her interest in their solution has made her a student of the field for more than two decades. That interest culminates in this book.

Health care services are confronted by pressures from every side for more effective and more economical operations. Increased demand for services has brought increasing costs, and increasing costs have led to public insistence on greater accountability for both costs and quality of services rendered. Public accountability takes many different forms: review for accreditation, meeting criteria of licensing or regulatory bodies, certification for reimbursement from government funds, and PSRO and other audit mechanisms. Each of these reinforces the urgency for more systematic planning and operation of health care services. When one realizes that the nursing department accounts for just about one half of a hospital's annual operating expenditures, it becomes obvious that efforts to improve the effectiveness and efficiency of hospital operations will be required of the nursing department very quickly. Effectiveness and efficiency require administrators to be very knowledgeable about and skilled in the art and science of management.

The nursing profession has an uneven history in the emphasis it has placed on the management of nursing services. For the first four decades of this century, nurses were educated to administer nursing education programs. Because students constituted the staff of the nursing service, administrators were occupied with the organization and conduct of the educational program. Staffing the nursing service required a plan for rotating students through the various services and units of the institution and assigning them to the day or night shifts. Budgets were rare in hospitals; fiscal controls were almost unknown. Times and methods were simpler. Patient needs were met, and patients and community philanthropy met the costs.

The quickening of medical science spurred by World War II continues unabated. Advances in science in general and in medicine in particular have brought miracles of cure and amelioration to diseases once thought impervious to medical treatment. Such advances rapidly increased the technical capability required of physicians. It required greater skill in nursing care than nursing students in training possessed and led promptly to the employment of ever-larger numbers of professional nurses and eventually to the incorporation of trained practical nurses into the nursing staff. The problems of directing a staff of graduate professional and practical nurses in providing highly technical nursing care required a different kind of management philosophy and skill than did a corps of student nurses. The W. K. Kellogg Foundation understood the problem and supported a program for nursing service administrators in fourteen universities in the early 1950s (see Chapter 1). This effort prospered but could not expand as it should have, because of the need to attend to the education of nurse clinicians to meet the urgent requirements of developing medical technology. Universities have never adequately supported their nursing programs, and even with federal funds for nursing education, appropriations were not enough to support sophisticated training in both advanced clinical nursing and management at the same time. Because the numbers needed for more sophisticated practice far exceeded the numbers of administrators required, a very hard choice had to be made. Efforts at training nurse clinicians have been successful, but it has become obvious that their success in improving patient care requires the creation and maintenance of an environment in which their skills can be effectively used. The greater weakness in nursing service today is in its management.

This book signals a revived interest in nursing service administration. The beginning era of cost and quality consciousness must lead to the professionalization of management of nursing services. Only that can serve the needs of institutions and patients in the years ahead.

Mary Kelly Mullane, R.N., Ph.D.
Chicago, Illinois
March 1, 1975

PREFACE

This book is addressed to nurses at all levels who are responsible for the work of others. Administration cuts across the work of all nurses so engaged. Associate and assistant directors, supervisors, head nurses, charge nurses, and team leaders all share responsibility for carrying forward the goals of the nursing service. They are all administrators; the difference between them is one of degree, not of kind.

Administration is a body of knowledge. Along with the practice of nursing, administration holds the enterprise together. It gives cohesiveness, coherence, and order to the great task of providing nursing services. It encourages efficiency, comprehensiveness, and economy in carrying forward the purpose and goals of nursing service. It illumines the enterprise so that the parts may be seen in relationship to each other and sights may be continuously raised in fulfilling the purpose. It synthesizes the parts so that they become a whole committed to achievement of the purpose.

This book is designed to provide the fundamental structure, which can be examined for rudiments. Though it lays no claim to ultimacy, it does aspire to definitiveness. It is intended to provide a knowledgeable base line from which strengths and weaknesses can be identified and dealt with appropriately. It is rooted in classical administrative theory, thereby providing a useful parallel to other texts in the field.

It is my hope that the effect on nursing service of the pervasive complexity of our times, institutions, and practices can be reckoned with more fruitfully as a result of this work. If one sees where one is, where one wishes (and ought) to go, and what the alternative directions are, the complexity is rendered less threatening and frustrating. No matter how innovative and helpful an alternative or idea is, the degree of effectiveness will depend on the soundness of the base, that is, the quality of the nursing care and the administration that supports it. Rather than our being tossed about by the social and technological revolutions, the soundness of our base will put us in the position to use those revolutions wisely and well.

It is also my hope that the material will be assimilable. If it cannot be integrated into performance—or rejected on reasonable, deliberated grounds—the purpose of the book has been lessened. Though addressed primarily to institutional nurses, there should be common applicability to other settings such as health departments and health maintenance organizations.

Finer's statement that "administration begins with the self in relationship to the fulfillment of a purpose"* is basic to the book too, because thinking, analytical, self-administered nurses are required to carry forward the monumental goal of meeting the nursing needs of people.

The aim, essentially, is to increase our ability to perceive and provide comprehensive nursing care in the most congenial, productive, and economical ways possible.

I am very aware of the derivative nature of my work; there is much recapitulation of other peoples' thoughts. The literature, which is rich, and its generous providers have been tremendous assets. Colleagues, both in and out of nursing, and friends have been generous in sharing experiences, ideas, and materials.

Mr. John Watkins of the *Journal of Nursing Administration* encouraged this work at its inception. The Fort Vancouver Library and the Wilson W. Clark Library of the University of Portland provided invaluable services. Four typists, Lola Downs, Melody Pietila, Ruth Hannula, and Dolores Gill, worked graciously.

My husband, Thomas, and our children, Joseph, Teresa, Marcella, and Elizabeth, have given unstinting support throughout the project.

To all I am indebted and grateful, while remaining personally responsible for the content of and any error in the book.

Helen M. Donovan

---

*Finer, H.: Administration and the nursing services, New York, 1952, Macmillan, Inc., p. 53.

CONTENTS

PART I **Administration in nursing**

    1 Status of nursing service administration, 3
    2 What is administration? 7
    3 Examination of nursing care, 17
    4 Humanizing the enterprise, 27

PART II **Framework for study of nursing service administration**

    5 Planning, 50
    6 Organizing, 65
    7 Staffing, 84
    8 Directing, 128
    9 Controlling, 155
    10 Coordinating, 170
    11 Reporting, 185
    12 Budgeting, 193

PART III **Adjuncts to nursing service administration**

    13 In-service education, 201
    14 Personnel policies and contracts, 216
    15 Equipment, 227
    16 Legal aspects, 230
    17 Research and creativity, 235
    18 Public relations, 244

Appendix A Personnel evaluation forms, 253
          B Case studies and patient incidents, 259

PART I

ADMINISTRATION IN NURSING

CHAPTER 1
STATUS OF NURSING SERVICE ADMINISTRATION

Administration in nursing has been with us a long time, though often unrecognized as such and seldom subjected to thoughtful scrutiny either in relation to nursing or to administration in other areas.

Pressures of all kinds have always been exerted on nursing, creating a situation not conducive to an ordered, examined nursing service. "Getting the work done" has had high priority—a priority with which it is difficult to compete, for indeed patients must be cared for and physicians' orders must be carried out. However, this emphasis on work may have provided the very condition that insulates us from giving the work and *how* it is done the thought, analysis, and speculation necessary to the ordered and deliberate provision of nursing care. Instead, confusion and ceaseless activity have resulted.

Confusion in nursing service administration in general has been noted over the years. "The dominant note in nursing administration is not autocratic nor yet democratic order, but confusion."[1] Unfortunately, the confusion persists, as evidenced by the ambiguous position of the head nurse.

Burling and associates[1] made the following astounding statement: "We know of no other role in our society which quite compares in complexity with that of the head nurse of a hospital floor." Many note this complexity in terms of the great number of contacts the head nurse makes because she is at the pivotal point of a hospital—both internally with nursing service personnel of all kinds, other departments, and the medical staff, and externally with patients, their families, and the public. Clearly, the head nurse should be part of an ordered administration, yet she remains on the fringes of nursing service administration.

The head nurse is not eligible for membership in the nursing service administrators forum, now called Council of Nursing Service Facilitators. The American Nurses' Association did provide an occupational forum for head nurses, but this was insufficient because where sound management prevails the head nurse should be an integral and functional part of the management team. This role should carry over into the professional organization and the nurse's place in it. To the extent that the head nurse does not feel a part of nursing service administration, that administration is faulty and confused, whether in nursing services or professional associations.

In his monumental work on administration, Gross[2] is frank and clear on the point of inclusion of all levels of managerial personnel in professional societies: "[They] should include all levels of administrators. Thus a society for professional business administration should include foremen and supervisors instead of preserving the status-ridden, snob-appeal approach of the past. Top executives might gain every bit as much from interaction process as would the foremen." There is surely application here to nursing.

Separation of the head nurse from her administrative colleagues persists even when she is acknowledged as part of the administrative structure. Stevens[3] succumbs to this tendency when she says, "It is easy for a head nurse to continue with her institution's traditional delivery systems without even really evaluating them or even really seeing that they exist." Responsibility requires that the head nurse, in conjunction with others on the management team, question and evaluate the traditional delivery systems.

Donovan,[4] Pearsall,[5] and Hagen and Wolff[6] note confusion also in the position of the supervisor and the function of supervision; Shanks and Kennedy[7] corroborate that this confusion exists. Peterson[8] speaks to supervision realistically and clearly; she says that it is "a function of anyone who is responsible for the work of others." It should be practiced by all members of the nursing service administration.

The continuance of confusion demonstrates the newness of nursing service administration and the great need to bring purpose, order, and coherence to the mammoth task of providing nursing services of high quality.

DETERRENTS TO NURSING SERVICE ADMINISTRATION

There are many reasons why nursing service administration has not yet reached maturity. Ironically, one of the impediments to progress has been the emphasis placed on education. Often instructors have been prepared only in nursing education and have been afforded limited opportunity to study nursing service administration. The number of prepared nursing service administrators remains small as compared with the number of nursing educators.

Another deterrent has been the absence of trained hospital administrators. The competent doctor or nurse was the administrator until fairly recently, and they still leave their influence on nursing service. Through the growing field of hospital administration this situation is being corrected.

The historical inarticulateness of nurses is another curtailment to the development of nursing service administration. This is related to the long-standing authoritarianism of nursing, which allows little room for the consultative aspect of administration. Nurses have been largely "doers" rather than "thinkers," and as a result their analytical prowess has been impaired.

The economic condition that has prevailed in nursing until very recently is related to the underdevelopment of nursing service administration. Nowhere is this more evident than in the dissipation of nursing that derives from nurses doing the work of so many other departments of the hospital, without either identification or protest from nursing service administrators. Precision in pricing the service rendered has been absent in the same proportion as precision in defining the service. A profession that has fared so poorly in the economy is not one governed by sound administration, or the discrepancies, weaknesses, and other related factors would have been identified, exposed, and rectified.

Another deprivation linked with administration is the indifference with which nurses are held. Nurses have seldom had a voice in the conduct of affairs of the hospital, though they comprise such a large number of the employees and are crucial to the operation of the institution. Rarely are they involved in the planning of new construction or the introduction of new services. Likewise, nurses are conspicuously missing from national, state, and local health commissions and programs. As late as the 1971 National League for Nursing convention the question was raised regarding this lack of nurses in regional medical programs. Additionally, without consultation with the American Nurses' Association, the American Medical Association[9] has made a unilateral proposal to recruit doctors' assistants from the ranks of nursing.

These various privations have resulted in a powerlessness that keeps the profession from the forefront of health care issues. If the voice of nursing is to be heard, we must simultaneously increase competency in both administration and professional practice, for they are interdependent. In their masterful treatise on power and its use by nurses, Bowman and Culpepper[10] confirm the need for increased administrative competency when they speak of the crucial importance of specific goals around which a committed group can rally. The goals, however, must be refined, unequivocal, representative, and worthy of loyalty. We are witnessing probably the first use of power in the history of the profession in the Economic and General Welfare Program of the American Nurses' Association, which has had phenomenal success in raising salaries and removing other deprivations from nurses.

The careful and calculated use of power can dispel the indifference with which nurses are held. Only then will we be able to lead from strength as a profession and assume our proper position in the health care field.

BEGINNING OF FORMALIZATION

The first substantial impetus to nursing service administration was the 1950-51 Nursing Service Administration Project undertaken at the University of Chicago. Sponsored by the W. K. Kellogg Foundation, the project led to support for nursing service administration programs in fourteen universities. Finer,[11] the project director, wrote the first book on nursing service administration, and the project was also reported by Mullane[12] for the Foundation in *Education for Nursing Service Administration 1959*. There have been innumerable institutes, workshops, and so forth, sponsored by various nursing organizations and institutions, but the academic base remains small. Likewise, the literature is sparse though growing. In 1970-71 there appeared two new journals devoted exclusively to nursing service administration: *Supervisor Nurse* and *Journal of Nursing Administration*. It is noteworthy that the publication of these important journals coincided with the twentieth anniversary of the W. K. Kellogg Foundation project on nursing service administration. This project and the advent of the two journals are significant landmarks in the development of nursing service administration.

OBJECTIVES OF THIS TEXT

The administrative process in the conduct of nursing service will be viewed broadly. In principle, it should work for or be applicable to any enterprise. The application in this text will center on the hospital nursing service, but it should have equal application to public health care, nursing education, or any other facet of nursing.

The classical framework of administration and its constituent parts, as well as alterations that have occurred, will be identified and examined, both in relation to each other and to the whole. There are constants that appear in various parts in different forms, which alter the whole. Relationships are of great consequence in all aspects of administration. Accompanying relationships of theory and practice bind the whole.

An attempt will be made to conceptualize administrative principles that guide action and activities aimed at providing high-quality, economical nursing care. Such conceptualization should provide a firmer base from which to experiment and innovate, so that the experiments and innovations can be more controlled and cohesive.

The administrative process will be shown to cut across all levels of nursing service. It will be the same in kind for each level—top administrator and associates or assistants, supervisors, head nurses, charge nurses, and team leaders—though the degree will vary. The absence of uniform application of administrative principles and practices on each level has been strongly divisive and contributory to the confusion and conflict that often prevail. Unity and cohesiveness should be the objectives.

There will be clinical emphasis throughout. Clinical practice is at the core of nursing service administration and should not be separated from it.

There will also be an attempt to examine and determine difficulties and problems that militate against or render ineffective the efforts at building comprehensive nursing service administration.

This overall view of nursing service administration can contribute to integration of the parts, which in turn will lead to a better nursing service.

REFERENCES

1. Burling, T., Lentz, E., and Wilson, R.: The give and take in hospitals, New York, 1956, G. P. Putnam's Sons, pp. 101 and 124.
2. Gross, B. M.: The managing of organizations—the administrative struggle, vol. II, New York, 1964, The Free Press, p. 826.
3. Stevens, B.: The head nurse as manager, J. Nurs. Admin. **4**(1):39, 1974.
4. Donovan, H.: What is supervision? Nurs. Outlook **5**(6):371-374, 1957.
5. Pearsall, M.: Supervision—a nursing dilemma, Nurs. Outlook **9**(2):91-92, 1961.
6. Hagen, E., and Wolff, L.: Nursing leadership behavior, New York, 1961, Columbia University Press, p. 139.
7. Shanks, M., and Kennedy, D.: Administration in nursing, ed. 2, New York, 1970, McGraw-Hill Book Co., pp. 221-222.
8. Peterson, G.: Working with others for patient care, ed. 2, Dubuque, 1973, Wm. C. Brown Co., Publishers, p. 136.
9. American Medical Association urges major new role for nurses, Am. Med. News, February 9, 1970, p. 1.
10. Bowman, R., and Culpepper, R.: Power: Rx for change, Am. J. Nurs. **74**(6):1053-1056, 1974.
11. Finer, H.: Administration and the nursing services, New York, 1952, Macmillan, Inc.
12. Mullane, M. K.: Education for nursing service administration; an experience in program development by fourteen universities, Battle Creek, Mich., 1959, W. K. Kellogg Foundation.

CHAPTER 2
WHAT IS ADMINISTRATION?

Administration has been defined as "the attainment of a purpose: it is scientific when the purpose has been rationally defined and deliberately accepted, when the means of attainment have been rationally made appropriate to the object, with neither more nor less or other resources than those required to be successful" [p. 18] and "... the marshalling of resources to accomplish a purpose [p. 19]."[1]

Administration may be defined elaborately or succinctly, as above, or with variation. Multiple definitions serve to internalize the meaning so that it becomes more personal and therefore more useful to the administrator and to the enterprise that is administered. Essentially, however, administration is a combination of purpose and the means of achievement of that purpose. It is both something to be accomplished (purpose) and the whole range of persons and activities required to bring the purpose to fruition.

Nursing service administration is a complex of elements in interaction. It results in output of patients whose health is unavoidably deteriorating, maintained, or improved (purpose) through input of personal and material resources used in an orderly process of nursing services (means of achieving the purpose).

TERMINOLOGY ASSOCIATED WITH ADMINISTRATION
Management

For some, the term management has greater appeal because it seems to denote something more common to everybody and is less theoretical than the word administration. It is frequently used in industry, which adds to its appeal. Management is, however, essentially the same as administration in its twofold nature of purpose and the various means used to achieve that purpose. The terms will be used interchangeably.

Supervisory management. Those managers in the work situation called supervisors comprise supervisory management. The term most often refers to positions of middle management, but speaks as well to the work of upper management, such as directors, associates, and assistants, and to first-level managers, such as head nurses. Supervision is a part of the management function, not an alternative.

Office management. A mistaken idea of administration that should be mentioned is that of office management. Perhaps the position of administrative assistant gives rise to this point of view. Administrative assistants do much to keep the machinery working smoothly; but goals and purposes to which the *whole* operation is devoted and that the machinery serves constitutes administration. Control of paper work and office management are part of administration, but not synonymous with it.

The work of executives

Executives are administrators and shall be so considered. The act of execution is not so well circumscribed as management or administration, because it most often applies to a specific, discrete, or particularized plan or program; so the term is confined for the most part to the person who is the executor, or more commonly, the executive.

Bureaucracy

Bureaucracy is closely related to administration. While often connoted negatively as rigid adherence to rules, forms, and routines, it also suggests diffusion of authority. To the extent that rules, forms, and routines contribute to the smooth functioning of an organization in achieving its purpose, bureaucracy is desirable. Scrutiny and evaluation of all parts of a system are essential to maintain effectiveness and avoid stagnation and ineffectiveness. It is the absence of such scrutiny and periodic evaluation that produces the negative meaning found in bureaucracy.

Leadership

The relationship between leadership and administration is extremely close, if indeed the terms are not synonymous. Leadership has a strong natural component whereby certain persons, for various reasons such as possession of stamina, determination, imagination, and such, are capable of leading other people to achievement of a purpose. Physicians and nurses who have become hospital administrators, as well as the many strong and effective people in other fields, attest to a natural capacity for leadership. Capability for decision making, a strong reality orientation, complete acceptance of responsibility, or some other major strength supports the leadership role of such people.

In addressing the characteristics of supervisory leadership, Likert[2] speaks of four components: maintenance of a high level of both goal determination and commitment, support or concern with building up of people, attention to team building, and concern with facilitation of the work situation for the workers' benefit. Implied in these four characteristics are essential elements of sound administration. In a sense, they are virtually a summary of administration.

There are various styles of leadership. The autocrat makes decisions alone, and though they may be essentially correct, they lack the mobilizing power of decisions made with consultation. At the other end of the continuum, the democratic leader allows much leeway for discussion and deliberation with subordinates, which may result in dissipation of decision making. In general, the greater the professional preparation, the greater the use of the democratic style, as for example in the work of researchers. Where the team approach, concern for employee motivation and growth, and improvement of management decisions are important to the administrator, he or she will lean toward the democratic view. There are degrees along the continuum, such as crises where the individual decision of the leader is appropriate and other instances where wider representation of subordinates, especially those most knowledgeable and closely concerned, is in order.

Another pair of terms used to describe leadership that more or less parallel autocratic-democratic is strong-permissive.

There is an educational component of leadership (L. *ducere,* meaning to lead out, which provides the root for the word education, L. *educare*). This is demonstrated by those who coach, counsel, and encourage subordinates. There is little question that the more a leader can bring out and develop workers, the more effective he or she will be. This point of view implies technical knowledge for nurses: how else can they coach, guide, or direct the activities of workers? It suggests knowledge of human behavior, their own and others', because guiding and encouraging are limited without possession of behavioral knowledge. It also infers development of personnel for higher positions, even to replacing oneself in consideration of the ongoing and future good of the enterprise. Related to education too is the leadership derived from clinical competence or expertise. Intelligence is important, as are sensitivity and skill in the basic arts of writing and speaking.

Also relative to the educational point of view is the ability to conceptualize so that the whole enterprise and its parts can be seen for and in themselves, as well as the relationships surrounding them. Odiorne's admonition to look for outcomes, not activities, illustrates this requirement for conceptualization in the leader. Thoreau advises us to simplify everything, lest life be consumed by detail. This simplification is akin to conceptualization: both must control and use myriad details to arrive at a point of integration, synthesis, or wholeness in ideation. However, ability to perceive meaningfully the world around one precedes conceptualization. A leader must be a keen observer before he or she is able to imagine, abstract, theorize, or conceptualize. For example, nurse leaders must know or have observed a good deal about the care of patients in order to conceptualize the outcomes that are anticipated in nursing audit systems set up on outcomes rather than process. Knowing a situation is perceiving; knowing the possible effects of the situation is conceptualizing. They are complementary.

Leininger[3] speaks of crisis of leadership in nursing. She favors a current "confrontation-negotiation" style of leadership, as opposed to an earlier "establishment-maintenance" view. One might question whether this shift has taken place, is only beginning, or is yet to come. Leininger's own actions and those of other nurse leaders (notably those in state nurses's associations whose efforts have contributed to collective bargaining with hospitals) demonstrate that there are at least a few who have assumed the confrontation-negotiation style of leadership in redressing discrimination against women in the academic community. This stance also characterizes the latent potential of nurses to use professional power for their own aggrandizement and that of the public they serve.

Argyris[4] describes a confrontation as an open discussion of issues not usually discussed that are thought to be causing problems, rather than one in which persons and their opinions or positions are discussed or condemned or pent up feelings released. Depersonalization of the issues seems to be dominant.

The frequently heard lament that there are no leaders may be a result of increased general education and sophistication, which reduce the difference between leader and follower and foster more leadership qualities in subordinates than once was the case. If this is true, the practice of sound administrative skills by those in leadership positions is essential, especially for consultative management.

Finally, for those who strive for self-knowledge there comes the awful moment of truth when they realize that a leader is often a composite of strength and weakness, responding in different ways to various people, times, and places. This kind of knowledge, though painful, provides insights that can be used for growth. Character is indeed related to leadership. Leadership can be deliberately developed in people, using essentially the techniques and experiences as those utilized in preparing administrators.

• • •

For our purposes, then, administration shall be construed to be synonymous with management, the work of executives, bureaucracy in its nonpejorative sense, and leadership.

THEORIES OF ADMINISTRATION

There is a variety of themes in administration, some of which have developed into theories. They are excellent for freshening or sharpening a concept and providing a realigned structure. The danger lies in assuming that these theories are completely new, whereas in fact they are essentially traditional administration with a special emphasis or linear development of one part or another that the originator hopes or expects will hasten improved administration. They make an implicit traditional concept explicit; that is, they underline or illuminate traditional theory. It is important to understand their bases. Theories or variations on a theme can then be seen as insightful and valuable emphases with the expectation and often implementation of enriched administrative practice.

Management by objectives

The 1970s may be remembered as the decade of measurement. As hospitals become increasingly accountable to the public, both privately and to various levels of government, they are required to measure their practice more exactly. Nursing is affected also. This decade is witnessing the beginning of applications of standards to care given, certification of practitioners and the care they give, and greater specificity in the quantitative measure of nursing in staffing and the qualitative measure through audit. Measurement may speed us to good order and achievement of purpose. Management by objectives is conducive to measurement.

Odiorne,[5] a pioneer in furthering management by objectives, sees the concept as a logical and effective system wherein superior and subordinate managers together set up common goals, delegate major areas of responsibility to individuals, and define expected results, and use these in order to efficiently operate the unit and assess the contribution of each of its members.

In the traditional view of administration, goal setting is submerged in planning, though early theorists such as Fayol tied decision making and actions to plans or objectives. This submergence may have given rise to the deficiency in goal identification that proponents of management by objectives have tried to remedy. (For more specific discussion of goal setting, see Chapter 5.) Progress toward achievement of the goal is not made explicit in the traditional point of view. It is implied, however, in all parts of the administrative process, because simultaneous evaluation is essential to organization, staffing, budgeting, and reporting.

The architects of management by objectives have attempted to compensate for these common faults in enterprises. At a regional seminar for nursing service administrators, the speakers disparaged the traditional management structure of planning, organizing, controlling, and so forth, as manipulating the activities of subordinates. Management by objectives encompasses these traditional elements, but emphasizes rationally defined goals that are arrived at and accepted by all members of the organization. Trying to get everyone committed to a common set of goals is indeed a worthwhile aim and does not exclude the necessity of planning, organizing, and controlling. An energizing concept such as management by objectives must necessarily embrace or relate to the gamut of administrative elements if it is to achieve its purpose.

Thus management by objectives and the traditional view are complementary, rather than exclusive. Cohesiveness and unity of the two points of view will be more effective in providing high-quality nursing care than will the view of management by objectives alone. Major emphasis must be placed on the goal to be achieved. The achievement, however, will require the mobilization of personnel and material, in turn requiring planning, organizing, staffing, directing, and controlling.

Some essential features of management by objectives, as described by Odiorne,[6] are the need for top management support and participation, in-service education for orientation of staff to the concept and its parts, appraisal of current status of the organization, and delineation of the desired outcomes from activities during the process of goal identification and selection.

He also spells out the need for continuing dialogue and memoranda between superior and subordinates, or both discussing and consequent recording, so that goals can be isolated and followed through to achievement. There should be periodic review and elaboration in writing as plans are selected and their schedules are implemented.

Odiorne sees three types of goals or objectives. Ranging from low to high, these are routine goals related to stability of the enterprise; problem-solving goals, or correction of processes; and innovative goals leading to growth. When goals are produc-

Table 1. JCAH audit system in nursing services (Vancouver Memorial Hospital, 1974-76)

Objective	Jan.-Feb.	March-April	May-June	July-Aug.	Sept.-Oct.	Nov.-Dec.
Installation (1974)						
Director and assistant director of nursing attend JCAH workshop on nursing audit.	X					
Report to supervisory staff; preliminary orientation.		X				
Decision to combine establishment of nursing standards with audit procedure.* Development of standards for one clinical entity.			X			
Conference with colleagues in nursing and medical records department. Rework standards for one clinical entity to coordinate outcomes and complications with audit criteria. Streamline nursing audit forms with medical records personnel.						
Workshop for supervisory staff, including evening and night shifts. Eight clinical areas covered: medicine, surgery, obstetrics, gynecology, pediatrics, emergency room, critical and intensive care units, and operating room. Complete audit of 20 charts, including retrieval from medical records (for practice only). Plan and schedule remedial work for discrepancies found.				X		
Select eight representative clinical audit committees.				X		
Orient total staff to procedure by clinical areas and by supervisory staff.				✔		
Set up audit and standards of care schedules for 1975, using clinical entity frequency lists from medical records (assistant director of nursing).				✔		
Workshop for each clinical committee. Develop audit criteria and standards of care for two clinical entities, according to schedule. Conduct complete audit on 20 charts (as in workshop for supervisory group). (2 clinical entities × 20 charts × 8 clinical areas = 320 charts)					✔	✔
Annual report.						✔
First year of combined standards of nursing care—audit system (1975)						
Clinical audit and standards committees to establish criteria and standards for one clinical entity† each month per clinical area (with retrieval of medical records). (12 entities × 20 charts × 8 clinical areas = 1,920 charts)	✔	✔	✔	✔	✔	✔
Installation of standards of care on units corresponding to content and schedule of clinical audit committees for direction of care. (12 entities × 8 clinical areas + overlaps [surgery-obstetrics-gynecology, medicine-surgery-pediatrics])	✔	✔	✔	✔	✔	✔

X, completed; ✔, not completed.
*Because directing standards of care and controlling standards for audit are essentially the same, they can be developed simultaneously, thus integrating both aspects of nursing practice.
†Once outcomes and complications are identified, they form a pool from which they can be drawn for use in other clinical entities, thus shortening the process. If shortened, the schedule can be increased to number 50% of patients in last 6 months or increased in the number of clinical entities per month.

Continued

Table 1. JCAH audit system in nursing services (Vancouver Memorial Hospital, 1974-76)—cont'd

Objective	Jan.-Feb.	March-April	May-June	July-Aug.	Sept.-Oct.	Nov.-Dec.
Evaluate for effectiveness and utilization. Count frequency of use for each set of standards × number of patients with a particular diagnosis.	✔	✔	✔	✔	✔	✔
View of progress by combined supervisory staff for consolidation, expansion, committee replacements, and collaboration with other nursing committees or other departments.		✔		✔		✔
Annual report.						✔

Second year of combined standards of nursing care—audit system (1976)

Repeat schedule for 1975 until all clinical entities are worked up and operating.

Reset schedules.

---

tion oriented and quantifiable, the movement is from regular to innovative; when they are project- or program-type goals, the movement is from innovative to routine. Drucker[7] implies a preference for the third type of goal: "Results (or goals) are obtained by exploiting opportunities, not by solving problems. All one can hope to get by solving a problem is to restore normality."

Drucker[8] also argues that the factors in an enterprise that operate against management by objectives are specialization, hierarchical structure, or differences between and containment of the various levels of the organization. He points out the necessity of overcoming these difficulties by appropriate administrative elements such as organization and policy making.

In agreement with Drucker, Skarupa[9] makes the telling points that management by objectives must carry the enterprise forward, not simply maintain the status quo; look for and expand opportunities, not just solve problems; and be concerned with growth and improvement to bring the social and financial operations of a hospital to a higher and clearer measure of efficiency designed to meet the increasingly sophisticated needs of society.

Brady[10] described the introduction of the concept of management by objectives to the Department of Health, Education, and Welfare. He showed an operational layout for achievement of a family planning objective that would increase the number of patients served by a specific number in four stages of increase over 1 year. Specificity and numerical count dominate.

The installation of a retrospective audit system (following the procedure of the Joint Commission on Accreditation of Hospitals [JCAH]) in a 206-bed hospital is shown in Table 1. The characteristics of management by objectives that obtain in this example are that it is written and communicated appropriately and agreed on in specific ways such as clinical departmentalization, steps to be taken by specific dates, and specific persons to carry specific responsibilities; measurable data are obtained for evaluation; there is flexibility in interim changes, as demonstrated by the introduction of the nursing standards component; and it incorporates an intermediate stage covering the year following installation. The long-range element carries the objective into a third year, during which all clinical entities treated in the hospital will be developed similarly for total coverage using the same procedure. Such a project requires commitment to a projected plan in specified ways so that the objective of installing a retrospective clinical audit system can be combined with the determination of standards of care over a 3-year period. The project illustrates the importance of using or exploiting opportunities, rather than just solving problems. By capitalizing on JCAH workshops, its clearly elaborated audit system, and use of similarly prepared staff and medical records personnel, the nursing service can make the best use of available opportunities to enrich its quality control system. Likewise, the insightful decision to develop standards of care simultaneously with the project demonstrates good use of existing opportunities.

Management by exception

The origins of management by exception go back in traditional management to F. W. Taylor, one of the pioneers of modern administration. However, Maynard [in Bittle[11]] says that "it was not until comparatively recently that the more progressive managers made Taylor's early vision a reality by practicing management by exception on 'all of the elements entering into management.' The idea is so sound and so practical that one can only wonder why its full realization took so long."

> Management by exception, in its simplest form, is a system of identification and communication that signals the manager when his attention is needed; conversely, it remains silent when his attention is not required. The primary purpose of such a system is, of course, to simplify the management process itself—to permit a manager to find the problems that need his action and to avoid dealing with those that are better handled by his subordinates.*

The system of management by exception consists of measurement, projection, selection, observation, comparison, and action phases. Implied in this list is definition of goal or purpose, organization and staffing to achieve it, standards with which to observe the work of personnel involved, and evaluation.

In implementing the management by objectives project shown in Table 1, management by exception would apply at any point where the assistant director of nursing or the supervisors were unable to move the project forward. For example, if a clinical committee were unable to develop audit criteria and standards of care for two clinical entities according to schedule, that failure to meet the goal would alert the assistant director of nursing to the fact that something was interfering. Together they would review the situation, identify the cause of the problem, and correct it. Illness, unanticipated work load, staff turnover, or simply inertia may be possible deterrents to finishing work as scheduled. In management by exception, and by objectives, periodic review isolates trouble before the terminal date is reached.

Inherent in both management by objectives and management by exception is the need for personal involvement in the selection of goals and their consequent achievement, to whatever degree of success or failure. Also featured in both theories is the knowledgeable worker, whose performance can be measured against standards with which he or she is familiar.

Human relations theory in administration

The concept of administration was formalized in the first part of this century by Taylor, Fayol, and others. Since that time, personal and interpersonal components have been a growing dimension in development of administration, paralleling the growth of the behavioral sciences (psychology, sociology, social psychology, and so forth). Human relations in industry and elsewhere have relied heavily on findings in the behavioral sciences; Flippo brings them together with the theory and practice of administration.

It is not surprising that there is a theory that frankly treats the traditional and the behavioral elements as both separate and yet closely related components of adminis-

---
*From Bittel, L.: Management by exception, New York, © 1964, McGraw-Hill Book Co., p. 5.

tration, "an attempted integration of traditional and behavioral approaches to management."[12] There have been continuing efforts to reconcile or to better integrate the scientific school of Taylor and Fayol and the human relations points of view represented by social scientists such as Mayo, Lewin, and Rogers.

It has been assumed, somewhat grossly, that the traditional view represents supremacy of the organization, and the human relations approach represents supremacy of the worker. Bennis,[13] while holding that the important concern of leadership is to negotiate between the individual and the organization so that the needs of each can be met satisfactorily, reviews the work and thinking of other revisionists and those likewise devoted to the task of reconciliation of the two schools of thought. He discusses with considerable illumination the theories of McMurry (the "benevolent autocrat"), McGregor (the theory of X and Y, with X being the inhibited person and Y being one who is encouraged by the organization to develop his or her own potential), and Argyris (meeting human needs and achieving organizational aims). Argyris [p. xi][4] used McGregor's theory as a base, but added patterns A and B in an effort to provide organizational climate and action consistent with the theory of X and Y. Thus the formula $XA \longrightarrow XB$ denotes the desirable shift for manager and organization in concert.

That human relations is a very important aspect of administration is certain. Whether it is inherent in administration or a major collateral factor either in general or in working out individual theories and practice of management is not so important as the deliberation and deepening of appreciation of the importance of this factor.

Finer[1] [p. 154] offers some forthright observations in considering the management–human relations dichotomy. He points to such administrative structures as budget, recruitment, and departmentalization, among others, as well as to human relations: "Administration is purposeful structure no less than process; it is imposed procedures no less than behavior."

Davis[14] describes a stage between traditional and human relations management as one of expecting "niceness" to prevail: if people were nice enough to each other, all would be well. In fact, the niceness may just cover authoritarian behavior and arrangements. Related to this erroneous opinion is thinking that good attitudes come about by instructing people to have them. Both of these points of view are illusory because they overlook the necessity of assessing the organization for trouble spots that give rise to authoritarian arrangements and consequent poor attitudes on the part of workers. Davis does support the human relations point of view in general, because he believes organizational growth accompanies personnel growth.

Levitt,[15] a long-acknowledged authority in the field of administration, believes that the administrator's personality is the most important aspect of management. He warns that knowledge of administration does not guarantee the quality of the practice of administration, that teaching and learning are separate though related entities, and that "the most crucial factors are his (the manager's) personality and behavioral style, that is, how he influences and affects those he manages." Levitt's view substantiates the dual nature of administration of which we have spoken (purpose and means of achieving the purpose), as well as acknowledging that there are management styles growing out of the manager's personality and life that render him effective or ineffective in a given position. He seems to emphasize that, while the composite view of the manager is important, personality and behavioral style are paramount: that it is not man as man, but man as a specific person that makes the difference in managerial effectiveness.

Variations on theories of administration

In reviewing other theories of management, one can see that authors vary in the emphasis they place on the various parts of administration.

Barnard[16] speaks of synthesis in the work of the executive: "It is precisely the function of the executive to facilitate synthesis in concrete action of contradictory forces, to reconcile conflicting forces, instincts, interests, conditions, positions and ideals."

Torgersen[17] reviews and restates the position of Barnard, but incorporates communications and the role of the manager (perhaps because of growth and application of the behavioral sciences, though it should be noted that Barnard was strong on the individual for his time). Organization is the core, and other parts of management are arranged around it. Torgersen defines administration as "coordinated activities of people directed toward some common objective" served by "three prerequisite and necessary elements . . . communication, the willingness and ability of participants to serve in the organization, and the purpose." The traditional ingredients such as staffing, directing, coordinating, and so forth, are present but "placed on their sides." The selection of organization as the principal point around which other functions are articulated not only enriches the theory of administration but gives the practitioner another frame of reference for viewing the gamut of activities and persons required to carry the purpose forward in complex institutions. It would be interesting to see other parts of administration selected as the key around which companion parts pivot.

Sisk's[18] definition of management brings coordination, often found in definitions of administration, to the fore. For him, management is "the coordination of all resources through the processes of planning, organizing, directing and controlling in order to attain stated objectives."

Adams,[19] writing much earlier than Sisk, also focussed on the coordination component and at least suggested the administration–human relations relationship when he said "administration is the ability to coordinate various and even divergent social energies into a simple entity, so skillfully that they will operate as one."

Gross[20] refers to the elements of organizational purpose as a "global matrix" that includes "satisfaction of human interests, production of goods and services, efficiency in the use of scarce resources, investment in organizational viability (growth), resource mobilization, observance of codes and technical and administrative rationality." This is a departure from above descriptions. However, production of goods and services may be related to direction, whereas resource mobilization seems to be staffing, and technical and administrative rationality probably embraces planning, organizing, and controlling.

Brown's definition encompasses twelve functions for managing, as enumerated below (left), with a list of comparable functions from other descriptions:

1. Developing purposes and objectives	Planning
2. Setting frames of reference	Philosophy
3. Forecasting and planning	Planning
4. Arranging for financing	Budgeting
5. Organizing	Organizing
6. Obtaining and developing personnel	Staffing
7. Coordinating and informing	Coordinating
8. Guiding and leading	Directing
9. Surveying performance; auditing	Controlling
10. Testing and evaluation	Controlling
11. Adjusting and integrating	Direction
12. Insuring proper external relationships*	Coordinating

A summary and formulary statement of management (from Battelle Northwest Workshop, May 1974) is $P = F (A \times M)$. P stands for performance, productivity, proficiency, or profitability; F for fre-

---

*This listing is from the monograph *Understanding the Management Function*, by David S. Brown, and is a part of the Looking Into Leadership series published and copyrighted by Leadership Resources, Inc., 1750 Pennsylvania Avenue, N.W., Washington, D.C. 20006. It is reproduced here by special written permission of the publisher.

quency; A for subordinates' abilities; and M for subordinates' motivation.

* * *

All views of management must be kept in mind so that components and their relationships can be delineated and examined, comparisons made, emphases identified, weaknesses and strengths spotted. Only in this way can one's view of administration grow and develop, be reassessed, refined, and put into practice. Only in this way can one see his or her efforts on a growth continuum, make judgments and choices from a rational and comprehensive base, and see tangential enthusiasms for what they are. There is an ongoing, cumulative, and "growth upon growth" aspect of the study of administration. The global view of management helps the administrator to control his or her own destiny as a manager; see refinements, strengths, weaknesses, growth, and stagnation so that a dynamic practice is achieved; and surmount the complexities of modern institutions.

REFERENCES

1. Finer, H.: Administration and the nursing services, New York, 1952, Macmillan, Inc., pp. 18, 19, and 154.
2. Likert, R.: The human organization; its management and values, New York, 1967, McGraw-Hill Book Co., p. 51.
3. Leininger, M.: The leadership crisis in nursing; a critical problem and challenge, J. Nurs. Admin. **4**(2):28-34, 1974.
4. Argyris, C.: Management and organizational development, New York, 1971, McGraw-Hill Book Co., pp. xi and 39.
5. Odiorne, G.: Management by objectives, New York, 1965, Pitman Publishing Corp., pp. 55-56.
6. Odiorne, G.: Personnel administration by objectives, Homewood, Ill., 1971, Richard D. Irwin, Inc., p. 108.
7. Drucker, P.: Managing for results, New York, 1964, Harper & Row, Publishers, p. 5.
8. Drucker, P.: Management; tasks, responsibilities, practices, New York, 1974, Harper & Row, Publishers, pp. 430-431.
9. Skarupa, J.: Management by objectives; a systematic way to manage change, J. Nurs. Admin. **1**(2):52-56, 1971.
10. Brady, R.: MBO goes to work in the public sector, J. Nurs. Admin. **3**(4):44-52, 1973.
11. Bittel, L.: Management by exception, New York, 1964, McGraw-Hill Book Co., p. viii.
12. Flippo, E.: Management; a behavioral approach, Boston, 1970, Allyn & Bacon, Inc., p. vii.
13. Bennis, W.: Revisionist theory of leadership, Harvard Business Review **39**(1):26-36, 1961.
14. Davis, K.: Human relations at work, ed. 3, New York, 1967, McGraw-Hill Book Co., p. 19.
15. Levitt, T.: The managerial merry-go-round, Harvard Business Review **52**(4):125, 1974.
16. Barnard, C.: Functions of an executive, Cambridge, Mass., 1938, Harvard University Press, p. 21.
17. Torgersen, P.: A concept of organization, New York, 1969, American Book Co., pp. 37-38.
18. Sisk, H.: Principles of management, Cincinnati, 1969, South-Western Publishing Co., p. 10.
19. Adams, B.: The theory of social revolution, New York, 1913, Macmillan, Inc., pp. 207-208.
20. Gross, B. M.: The managing of organizations, vol. 2, New York, 1964, The Free Press, pp. 477-478.

CHAPTER 3
EXAMINATION OF NURSING CARE

The relationship between administration and nursing care is an intimate one, and one of mutual dependence. Excellence in one is nearly impossible without excellence in the other.

Administration of the nursing service consists of the activities, resources, and personnel in the correct amount, kind, and relationship necessary for the purpose of providing nursing care to a specific group of patients. This purpose is paramount; however, nursing care must be *rationally defined* and *deliberately accepted* if it is to generate competent and effective administrative behavior and strategy.

Brown[1] cautions us "not only to understand intellectually the nature of this greatly expanded role (nursing care), but to internalize its meaning in order to incorporate it into practice."

As with administration, the more one can internalize nursing (express it in different terms, see its component parts and how they relate to each other, and observe the points of contact or overlap with other health services), the closer one will come to possessing a coherent view of nursing. Both intellect and will are necessary to achieve the overall view. Intellect makes knowledge one's own, and will enables the nurse to carry out this knowledge.

Acceptance of a rational definition is vastly different from deliberate acceptance of nursing components and activities (nursing care). Time and conscious effort are required to fuse knowledge of the wording and the acceptance necessary to perform the work as described. It is probably safe to say that the great majority of nurses who engage in and faithfully discharge the myriad components and activities that comprise nursing do so without deliberation. This is not to deprecate all that is done in the name of nursing, for it is a phenomenal achievement, but to point out the great need for constant consideration that will bring nurses closer to the ultimate definition. Internal familiarity with the meaning of nursing makes deliberately accepted nursing care possible.

DEFINITIONS OF NURSING CARE

Nursing care is far from being defined completely, though it can be said that those who have struggled toward the essential, albeit partial, definition have done so rationally.

Ramey proposes that nursing practice is

a process which involves assessing the patient's state of being, developing short- and long-term health objectives, planning and implementing appropriate nursing measures to help the patient reach those objectives, and evaluating the effectiveness of these nursing measures using scientific principles as a theoretical basis. Such nursing measures include not just those aimed at curing pathological conditions, but also prevention, rehabilitation, and health teaching.*

Johnson[2] classifies the ingredients of nursing practice as care (independent of medical authority), delegated medical care, and health care. Stabilizing and maintaining the patient's condition are distinctly nursing functions. A triad of stability, constancy, and equilibrium characterizes conceptualization of the desired outcomes of nursing. Management of the physical and psychological environment accompanying

---
*Ramey, I.: Meeting today's challenges to nursing service and education, Nurs. Forum 8(2):183, 1969.

nursing interventions designed to protect and sustain the patient's defenses and adaptive mechanisms are the means of securing these goals.

Mauksch[3] address the interdependent-dependent-independent aspects of nursing to a greater degree than most authors. He defines nursing goals as care (shared by nursing with other services of the hospital), cure (the physician's province, with portions delegated to nursing), and coordination (those functions deriving from the "holding" position, or continuous presence, of nursing). He elaborates the care component by showing the interdependence in this function as paralleling in some ways the dependence in the cure component, and uses the feeding of patients to illustrate this interdependence.

For example, there are patients for whom the nurse's only responsibility is to observe and record the amount of food taken. Even this small contribution to the patient's nutritional needs is obviated in such locations as minimal care units, where it is assumed that patients can manage their dietary needs without recourse to nursing, once the initial direction for food has been given to the dietary department. This initial direction constitutes one of nursing's coordinating duties, that is, the relay of physician's orders to the dietary department. It is only when the patient's condition demands that the nurse prepare, assist, or feed the patient that the nursing component comes into play. Likewise, in dietary instructions to the patient the nurse must first coordinate (request the instruction) and then interpret, reinforce, and help the patient to assimilate the instruction—a participative but not primary nursing function. Completely independent nursing duties decrease when nursing is viewed within the total hospital context.

Brodt[4] sees the care-cure-coordination [view of nursing] in terms of six nondiscrete dimensions of nursing action directed toward:

1. the preservation of body defenses;
2. the prevention of complications;
3. the reestablishment of the patient with the outside world;
4. the detection of changes in the body's regulatory system;
5. the implementation of the physician's prescribed therapeutic and diagnostic activity; and
6. the provision of comfort.

As an example, she uses the synergistic drug model. Two drugs given in combination produce different effects than when they are given independently. Likewise, nursing interventions are altered either favorably or incompletely as a result of the interplay of the above six dimensions or any combination of them that would be involved in the nursing intervention.

Donovan[5] sees four divisions: nursing care and functions deriving from the medical plan, which comprise the largest part of nursing; the range of functions derived from or relinquished to collateral services, that is, fluctuating services such as efforts to provide therapeutic exercises in the absence of physical therapists or the duties once the province of nursing that are assumed increasingly by inhalation therapists; those functions accruing from the holding position, such as the collaboration in the dietary plan; and independent nursing care and functions in the total care-cure-comfort domain, such as personal hygienic care, psychological support, and instruction within a vast area of clinical conditions.

Levine[6] describes nursing in an innovative and effective way within the context of conservation. The categories of conservation apply to the energy and the structural, personal, and social integrity of the patient. She introduces the notion of trophicogenic, or nurse-induced, disease. This formalization of nursing failure to meet the needs of patients is important because it strengthens the use of formalized nursing theory in practice, so that failure to comply to standards is readily identifiable. This is related to the sage observation of Norris [pp. 18-21],[7] who suggests that nurses are practicing their own brands of nursing rather than engaging in comprehensive nursing care, because there is no specific model or theory to which they are directed by their employers.

As a result of curriculum-planning projects, Finch proposes "a descriptive model of professional nursing care which is based on the assumption that all nursing care is carried out through the nurse-patient relationship." The components of a nurse-patient relationship were identified as: "(1) a patient who is in a state of disequilibrium that can be resolved by nursing care; (2) a nurse who is prepared to assist in the resolution of this state of disruption; and (3) the termination of the relationship when equilibrium is restored."*

In addition to the above examples, there are definitions that attempt to break nursing down into physical, spiritual, mental, emotional, socioeconomic, and teaching compondents of care. With this view in mind, Sr. Olivia Gowan says:

> Nursing in its broadest sense may be defined as an art and a science which involves the whole patient —body, mind and spirit; promotes his spiritual, mental and physical health by teaching and by example; stresses health education and health preservation as well as ministration to the sick; involves the care of the patient's environment—social and spiritual as well as physical; and gives health service to the family and community as well as to the individual.†

In all of the above definitions, there is an overriding quandary: other health care personnel may view their services as similar if not identical to nursing functions. Donovan [p. 12][5] cites two nurse leaders who caution against extending nursing beyond its true scope, giving itself a wider function than that to which it is in fact entitled, and ignoring nursing's participative role in carrying out and evaluating the medical plan. There is a danger of artificiality in the efforts of nurses to define and describe nursing if collaborative efforts in the health care spectrum are not acknowledged. Evasion will not get us around the large part of nursing that derives directly from the medical plan.

Attention to definition is necessary if we are to make wise decisions about the expansion of nursing. Lynaugh and Bates[8] caution us to move carefully into this area. For example, there are nurses who must know how to do physical examinations (a skill not easily achieved) because of their extension into medical care. A clear view of nursing is necessary to answer the question of which nurses and how many need this skill.

It is possible that the fluctuating components of nursing will never be settled, because they are contingent on changes in medicine and collateral health services. Therefore, the perfect definition of nursing may never be reached.

DEFICIENCIES IN NURSING CARE

Any of the above definitions (or one's own definition) serves to provide a frame of reference with which nurses can compare their own or their institution's practice.

Psychological needs of patients. Hospital nursing consists mainly of physical or custodial care: the bathing and feeding of patients and the carrying out of physicians' orders. There is some emotional care, but too often it is limited to brief remarks of comfort, with little or no individualization or listening component. We have scarcely begun to utilize the vast and growing body of knowledge about psychological needs of people and their relationship to nursing care. We are woefully backward in availing ourselves of studies that demonstrate the relationship of personality to illness, the rate of recovery, and even longevity, and in bringing them to bear on our day-to-day practice.

For example, the psychic trauma of maternal separation on small children has been known for at least two decades, yet many pediatric departments still perpetuate the practice of stringently restricting

---

*Finch, J.: Systems analysis; a logical approach to professional nursing care, Nurs. Forum 8(2):183, 1969.

†From Gowan, Sr. M. Olivia: Proceedings of the workshop on administration of collegiate programs in nursing, Washington, D.C., 1944, Catholic University of America Press, p. 10.

visiting hours for parents. We have not used such resources as psychiatric nurses, social workers, and psychologists. Additionally, we are certainly among those who avoid meaningful contact with the dying, despite their needs as found in the research of Kubler-Ross.[9]

Spiritual needs of patients. The spiritual needs of the sick are not well met, though a category called spiritual illness is beginning to be found in the literature.[10,11] There is expanded training for hospital chaplains, and they are increasingly found on health care teams; yet the spiritual aspect of nursing remains minimal. While we have always tried to contact a clergyman of the patient's choice, what of those who have no religious affiliation? Do they not have spiritual needs? If nurse-patient relationships were deeper, would we be able to fill these needs? Besides human relations skills, what preparation do nurses require to meet these needs?

Discharge planning and referral. Discharge planning, of which referrals are an important part, is only beginning to receive the attention it has long needed. Although information has long been available, the first national forum on discharge planning[12] did not take place until 1973. Rossman,[13] in describing extensions of the justly famous Montefiore home health program to transport chronically ill patients to the hospital regularly for services, expresses disappointment at the limited extent to which this proved program has spread. Nurses must assume considerable responsibility for failure to encourage parent organizations to move in the direction of such an excellent program. Moreover, we should be encouraging physicians to use community resources for their patients.

An exciting thrust in the direction of strengthening discharge planning and referrals is found in Hartford, Conn. As a part of continuing cooperative planning, nursing service directors meet with both the directors of nursing of facilities to which their institutions transfer patients and representatives of the Visiting Nurse Association, in order to resolve difficulties and effect appropriate and smooth transfers among the institutions and services [O'Neil[14]].

Instructing patients in self-care. Teaching patients to care for themselves has been minimal and, for the most part, random and diffuse. Perhaps instructing the diabetic patient has been most widely practiced, and yet even this is not universally done.

• • •

Serious attention to definition of nursing should help us to assume responsibility for our collective failure to integrate long-known knowledge into practice. Assumption of responsibility should in turn speed the day when our practice is routinely comprehensive.

CHALLENGES TO NURSING PRACTICE

Strauss and associates[15] suggest new challenges in patient care. For example, because of the nature of the organizational setting, there may be differing and conflicting attitudes toward pain, as in the delivery room when the mother may wish to endure the pain and staff are accustomed to alleviating pain. Rather than administering pain killers or anesthetics, nurses can adapt their practice to helping the laboring patient by instructional and psychological support, to the satisfaction of both patient and nurse. Related to this example is patient expectation of conflict between obstetrical staffs and those mothers who are members of La Leche League and are dedicated to breast feeding [Knafe[16]]. These mothers should be assured that every effort will be made to assist them in their choice to breast feed, if they are able, by knowledgeable and specific support.

An exciting foray into preventive medicine, with implications for nursing, has been made by Methodist Hospital of Indiana, Indianapolis.[17] In the form of proscriptive medicine, it pinpoints risk factors for individuals, with a view toward projecting the degree of longevity each person being assessed may attain.

We cannot ignore or override such challenges, but must provide for them in our nursing care, in order to achieve a universal practice of comprehensive nursing care.

OBJECTIVES OF NURSING SERVICE

Compilation of objectives of nursing service reflects or is definition. Objectives describe what is to be achieved—the goal or purpose. The official pronouncements of the American Nurses' Association *Standards for Nursing Services 1973* and the National League for Nursing *Criteria for Evaluating a Hospital Department of Nursing Services 1965* both place the need for written statements of philosophy and objectives in first place.

Nurses often experience difficulty in writing objectives, for the same reasons they have difficulty in defining nursing. Ellis[18] cautions us that both generalization and particularization are necessary in theorizing about nursing; both are necessary and valuable in helping to isolate and practice nursing care.

Working from generalizations permits us to see our work in a larger framework, which in turn permits viewpoints not to be found in examination of day-to-day activities and routines. However, one must be aware of generalizations as a trap when deliberations stop at that point instead of being carried on to particularizations. There is considerable evidence that nurses have indeed stopped short of particularization and in fact have sought refuge behind generalization. Specificity and precision are not our fortes. Norris [p. 10][7] believes that nurses overgeneralize to avoid the rigors of dispelling ignorance by closer examination.

Providing optimum nursing care is a good objective for a nursing service, but it cannot be reached or even evaluated for potentiality until it is taken from general to specific terms. Only by such concretion can nurses know clearly what they are attempting to accomplish, or even what they *are* accomplishing.

Besides objectives relating directly to nursing care, there are those directed to the workers, and appropriately so because the goal itself and the means of achieving the goal are inseparable. This is the core of the message of administration. It is the purpose that sets the administrative process in motion, but that purpose should be clear as well as worthy.

Most nursing departments do have objectives of nursing care, composed by one person or even a group. However, they often remain in a drawer, from which they are drawn to show visitors or inspectors but less often used for staff deliberation and explanation or for appraisal or comparison with existing nursing practice. That the gap between the ideal and the real is wide is not so great a problem as the absence of knowledge of what is ideal and real in a given clinical setting. There is no easy way of getting nurses to think and deliberate about nursing care, but by hard, time-consuming, persistent, and patient effort nurses will come to know intimately what they are doing and, more importantly, what they could be doing.

There are sufficient helps, however, to make a real dent in the process of defining and examining nursing care. The literature is not sparse, and there are many more illustrations than those cited. There are institutions that have written down their collective view of nursing. We shall examine some of these efforts in Chapter 5, particularly within the context of the philosophy and objectives of nursing services, because they serve as a base for planning. The relationship between the definition, or at least the description, of nursing and objectives of the nursing service is very close—so close that they will be achieved simultaneously.

The nursing process

There are various devices that help illuminate the study of definition and objectives. One is the concept of nursing

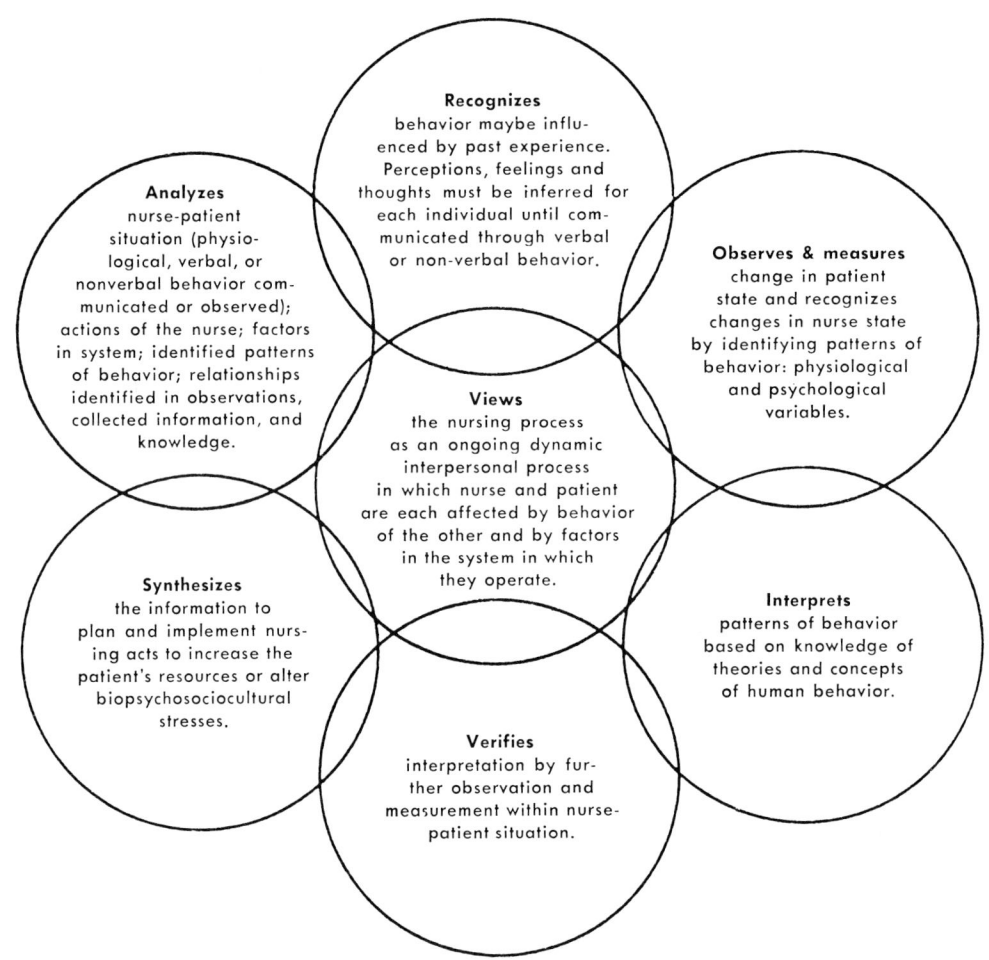

Fig. 1. Methodology for the study of the nursing process. (From Daubenmire, M., and King, I.: Nursing process models; a systems approach, Nurs. Outlook **21**(8):515, 1973.)

process. This view draws heavily on systems analysis. According to Daubenmire and King, there are

three general systems—personal, interpersonal and social—[with man] in the center. . . . Nursing process is viewed as the vehicle through which nursing is practiced. The nursing process is defined as a dynamic, ongoing interpersonal process in which the nurse and the patient are viewed as a system with each affecting the behavior of the other and both being affected by factors within the situation.*

The comprehensiveness of a systems approach and the nursing process within this framework is shown in Fig. 1. All possibilities are included for consideration, and the nurse is presented with a stated overview from which to choose intelligently and apply skills.

Carlson[19] describes the nursing process as "the sum of the activities jointly performed by the patient and the nurse." She sees this sum of activities as "a three-part problem-solving approach: (1) assessment (including nursing history and nursing diagnosis), (2) intervention (includes nursing orders and care plan), and (3) evaluation (includes nursing prognosis)." She favors a nursing order sheet as a permanent part of the patient's chart, with transcription to a nursing care plan as in the case of medical orders.

---

*Daubenmire, M., and King, I.: Nursing process models; a systems approach, Nurs. Outlook **21**(8): 512-513, 1973.

Mauksch and David[20] go so far as to say that the future of the profession itself is dependent on the use of the nursing process. They see it as a radical departure from present nursing care and the only means for nurses to achieve "accountability, service to client, scientific competence, peer review and control over conditions of practice."

But is nursing really a process? Ferkiss[21] describes structure as being process in slow motion. In this context, then, is the structure the comprehensive nursing care that has evolved from the process of administering that care? To entertain this question, we must think of structure as being capable of movement and change, as indeed is comprehensive nursing care.

Since process is a series of operations in the generation of something, there is an element of confusion in the use of this term. Nursing care itself is not the series of operations, but the result of them. The series of operations seems more nearly to approximate administration than it does nursing care itself. For example, checking an order for correctness and timeliness, preparing the exact dosage, checking the patient's identity and pulse, and recording the action comprise the process involved in administering digitalis. Likewise, acquiring the knowledge to hear and respond to the verbal and nonverbal cues of a patient about to undergo surgery, supplying specific information in response to these cues, taking required action, informing appropriate colleagues, and recording these activities comprise the process of nursing care known as patient reassurance.

All that contributes to the end is process. The end itself is nursing care, the purpose served by that process, or the production deriving from that series of operations.

Does this current preoccupation with process deflect us from the nursing care itself? Do the process promoters assume that comprehensive nursing care is so universally known and assimilated by practitioners that only the means of arranging it remain to be attended? Do these promoters assume that process, or the system of operations producing the nursing care, includes the nursing care itself—that the process is both method and content rather than essentially method?

Is it, rather, a case of needing to be so familiar with the nursing care itself that the method of giving it (the process) will be executed more satisfactorily; to be so familiar with the art of administration that one will go about achieving the objective (the specific nursing care) in the most expeditious way possible: with determination of purpose, planning, implementation (which includes organizing, staffing, and directing), evaluation (controlling), and recording of the nursing care (intervention, transaction, or service in meeting the particular needs of a particular patient)?

We must decide very carefully whether the nursing process includes the goal or is the means of achieving the goal. It in fact is not a question of either/or, but both. This may seem to belabor the point, but it is essential that we nurses see as precisely as we can what we do and the elements comprising it. It requires us to analyze and use language as carefully as we can.

Problem lists

Another device that provides a framework for nursing care is the following List of 21 Nursing Problems:

1. To maintain good hygiene and physical comfort
2. To promote optimal activity and exercise, as well as rest and sleep
3. To promote safety through prevention of accident, injury, or other trauma and through the prevention of spread of infection
4. To maintain good body mechanics and prevent and correct deformities
5. To facilitate the maintenance of a supply of oxygen to all body cells
6. To facilitate the maintenance of nutrition of all body cells
7. To facilitate the maintenance of elimination
8. To facilitate the maintenance of fluid and electrolyte balance
9. To recognize the physiological responses of the body to disease conditions—pathological, physiological, and compensatory
10. To facilitate the maintenance of regulatory mechanisms and functions

11. To facilitate the maintenance of sensory function
12. To identify and accept the positive and negative expressions, feelings, and reactions
13. To identify and accept the interrelatedness of emotions and organic illness
14. To facilitate the maintenance of effective verbal and nonverbal communication
15. To promote the development of productive interpersonal relationships
16. To facilitate progress toward achievement of personal and spiritual goals
17. To create and maintain a therapeutic environment
18. To facilitate awareness of self as an individual with varying physical, emotional, and developmental needs
19. To accept the optimum possible goals in the light of limitations, both physical and emotional
20. To use community resources as an aid in resolving problems arising from illness
21. To understand the role of social problems as influencing factors in the cause of illness*

Such a list provides nurses with ideas about nursing care so that they can broaden and deepen the care they give.

Acronyms

The acronym is another device to help nurses see the care they give in a deeper context and more comprehensively. One acronym used is *self-pacing: s,* socialization and special senses; *e,* elimination and exercise; *l,* liquids; *f,* foods; *p,* pain, personal hygiene, and posture; *a,* aeration; *c,* circulation; *i,* integument; *n,* neuromuscular control and coordination; *g,* general condition. Many suggestions and ideas are contained within each of these headings.[22]

Another acronym is the *SOAP* process, part of the problem-oriented medical record system in which nursing and medical care meld in treating and recording the problems of patients. Problems arise and are selected from a data base for each patient, consisting of chief complaint, patient profile, present illness, past history and systems review, laboratory and x-ray diagnostic review, and well-defined social history. Problems are then dealt with by this *SOAP* process: *s*ubjective, patient's complaint and information from others; *o*bjective, nurse's observations, pertinent data, physical examination, and laboratory tests; *a*ssessment, feelings and interpretation of *s* and *o* data; *p*lan, diagnostic, therapeutic, and eductation plan for nursing care, both immediate and future, and discharge planning [Wakefield and Yarnell[23]]. This acronym describes a method of looking at problems rather than constituent parts of nursing care, but does suggest some ingredients of nursing.

Additional factors

Besides the unequal and incomplete development of component parts of nursing, there is current concern about the expanded role of nursing and the technical-professional dilemma.

Expanded role of nursing. The expanded or extended aspect of contemporary nursing will make an impact on nursing as it is practiced now and in the future. It is currently of great concern to the profession that the American Medical Association looks to nurses for a substantial number of physicians' assistants. This proposal, made without consultation with the American Nurses' Association, assumes too much. Yet physicians have always had nurses available to do what was needed, such as take blood pressure readings and give intramuscular injections, intravenous infusions, and rectal examinations during labor. Other tasks such as cast and suture removal, taking of initial histories, and giving physical examinations seem to fall in line with this practice. There are collateral questions of whether nurses should subsidize the work of physicians (who enjoy the highest income of any group in the country) and whether the independent part of nursing will suffer as a result of this expansion or extension into the medical area. As always, the impact of this movement in the direction of nurses providing primary medical care, after some

---

*Reprinted with permission of Macmillan Publishing Co., Inc. From Abdellah, F., Beland, I., Martin, A., and Matheney, R.: Patient centered approaches to nursing, New York, © 1960, Macmillan, Inc., pp. 16-17.

special preparation, will be felt wherever nurses and nursing are found.

Recent events have strengthened the autonomy of nursing, at least in its essential conflict with medicine. The passage of a new nurse-practice act in Washington State, and in other states, seems to pave the way for some "diagnostic and drug-dispensing activities" for nurses in highly specialized areas such as intensive care units and emergency departments.[24] Isolated rural areas or inner cities are other locations where the effects of this new nurse-practice act will likely be felt.

Autonomy of nursing is also strengthened by the emergence of the nurse practitioner in private practice in different parts of the country. This nurse usually works from his or her own office, as the physician does. Nurse practitioners may eventually provide concrete data about what constitutes nursing, because they are separated from traditional relationships.

Technical-professional dilemma. The prodigious expansion of the technical component of medical care, with its consequent effect on nursing care, most persistently raises the question of professional versus technical nursing. Does it require a professional nurse to manage the intricate and complicated equipment found in coronary care and intensive care units, or can this care be provided by technicians or licensed practical nurses? Where care contingent on equipment is routinized, contained, and limited, though crucial in nature, can it be performed by a technician or licensed practical nurse? Routine in this use is not casual, but fixed by order and system. Will technicians or licensed practical nurses assume an important role in such settings, thereby releasing professional nurses for more specialized or overall responsibility?

This professional-technical dilemma, which seems to date from the American Nurses' Association Position Paper of 1965, persists largely because diploma and associate degree nurses are thought to be technicians, and baccalaureate degree nurses are considered professionals, even though they all take the same examinations. The claimed differentiation of objectives of the three programs seems more illusory than real to some. Also, complaints continue that the baccalaureate nurse has not been able to achieve a major impact on nursing, that the nurse with an associate degree requires a longer period of orientation to become proficient on the job, and that the diploma nurse lacks an intellectual base.

In 1973 the American Nurses' Association reopened the Position Paper in an effort to redress the alleged wrongs done by it. Among other points in this 1973 review, a task force will be established "to reconsider the contemporary relevancy of the terms 'professional' and 'technical' to distinguish basic preparation for nursing practice and to recognize all registered nurses as professionals."[25]

A related problem is the question of whether nursing is a profession. If "a body of knowledge, a code of ethics and a professional organization [Gross[26]]" are the marks of a profession, then nursing is one. It must be admitted, however, that the body of knowledge is heavily derivative, as is the case with teaching and social work. Also, nurse practitioners run the gamut from pure technician to the highest caliber of professional.

Gross[26] speaks of teaching or administration as tangential professions, in contrast to medicine, law, and engineering. The "professional teacher should be wedded both to teaching and to the subject he teaches. Similarly, an administrator must administer something." A case could be made for nursing as a tangential profession in the same way as are teaching and administration. For Etzioni,[27] nursing constitutes a semiprofession, as distinguished from the classical professions of medicine and law. These semiprofessions are characterized by less autonomy, shorter training (under 5 years), noninvolvement with questions of life and death or of privileged communication, and knowledge that is communicated rather than created. These semiprofessions are closer to the principle of administration than to the principle of knowledge.

One might question the assertion that involvement with life and death or with privileged communication is not part of nursing. It is less easy to question the administration principle. This seems to be one of nursing's main difficulties—a difficulty often addressed as we try to extricate ourselves from being all things to all people or available for anything that needs to be done.

One must admit that the professionalism of nursing is not yet definitely established and could be described as in a fragile state.

All these questions must be faced and answered by availing ourselves of all the logic and expertise possible. Nursing care must be strengthened along with administration, or it is only partial and self-defeating. The content (the nursing care) is as important as the method (the administration); they are mutually dependent. Without nursing care, nursing service administration would not exist.

REFERENCES

1. Brown, E. L.: Nursing reconsidered; a study of change. Part I. Philadelphia, 1970, J. B. Lippincott Co., p. 211.
2. Johnson, D.: The significance of nursing care, Am. J. Nurs. 61(11):63-66, 1961.
3. Mauksch, H.: The nurse; coordinator of patient care. In Skipper, J., and Leonard, R.: Social interaction and patient care, Philadelphia, 1965, J. B. Lippincott Co., pp. 251-265.
4. Brodt, D.: A synergistic theory of nursing, Am. J. Nurs. 69(8):1674-1676, 1969.
5. Donovan, H.: Toward a definition of nursing, Supervisor Nurse 1(5):12-15, 1970.
6. Levine, M.: The four conservation principles of nursing, Nurs. Forum 6(1):45-59, 1967.
7. Norris, C.: Delusions that trap nurses, Nurs. Outlook 21(1):10, 18-21, 1973.
8. Lynaugh, J., and Bates, B.: Physical diagnosis; a skill for all nurses? Am. J. Nurs. 74(1):58-59, 1974.
9. Kubler-Ross, E.: On death and dying, New York, 1970, Macmillan Inc.
10. Frankl, V.: The doctor and the soul, New York. 1955, Bantam Books, Inc.
11. Ford, P.: The healing trinity, New York, 1971, Harper & Row, Publishers.
12. News, National League for Nursing 22(2):1, 1974.
13. Rossman, I.: The Montefiore Hospital after-care program, Nurs. Outlook 22(5): 325-328, 1974.
14. O'Neil, C.: City-wide planning for nursing service, Nurs. Outlook 22(9):569, 1974.
15. Strauss, A., Fagerhaugh, S., and Glaser, B.: Pain; an organizational work—interactional perspective, Nurs. Outlook 22(9):562-563, 1974.
16. Knafe, K.: Conflicting perspectives on breast feeding, Am. J. Nurs. 74(10):1848-1851, 1974.
17. Will he live 10 more years? Idea Forum, Hospitals 48(21):30, 1974.
18. Ellis, R.: The practitioner as theorist, Am. J. Nurs. 69(7):1435, 1969.
19. Carlson, S.: A practical approach to the nursing process, Am. J. Nurs. 72(9):1591, 1972.
20. Mauksch, I., and David, M.: Prescription for survival, Am. J. Nurs. 72(12):2189-2193, 1972.
21. Ferkiss, V.: The future of technoligical civilization, New York, 1974, George Braziller, Inc., p. 216.
22. Geitgey, D.: Self-pacing—a guide to nursing care, Nurs. Outlook 17(8):48-49, 1969.
23. Wakefield, J., and Yarnell, S.: Implementing the problem-oriented medical record, Seattle, 1973, Seattle Medical Computer Services, pp. 13-14 (Weed, L. L., major contributor).
24. Where RN's can diagnose and prescribe, RN 36(8):31, 1973.
25. ANA issues statement on diploma graduates, Am. J. Nurs. 73(7):1137, 1973.
26. Gross, B. M.: The managing of organizations —the administrative struggle, New York, 1964, The Free Press, p. 823.
27. Etzioni, A.: The semi-professions and their organization, New York, 1969, The Free Press, pp. xii-xiii.

CHAPTER 4
HUMANIZING THE ENTERPRISE

Because administration is directed to achievement of purpose, it is heavily dependent on human resources. We have noted the alternate points of view of administration: the scientific method, with emphasis on structure and component parts; and the human relations method, with people dominant. These approaches are not mutually exclusive. However, because of the overriding emphasis on people, both in staffing the enterprise and on patients receiving the ministrations of this service, it is useful to think about the various means of maximizing personhood for personnel and patient alike.

PERSONHOOD

Personhood is comprised of essence (that with which one is endowed, or is innately) and existence (that which one becomes). It is more than physical existence. It means living fully—having life in which the needs of existence are met, but, more important, the higher needs of the person are met. It is life in which one's faculties are brought to fruition; where one lives more thoughtfully and deliberately; where the sensate, emotional, and intellectual components are brought into proper relationship and focus; where one makes choices and is in charge of his or her life, rather than being buffeted by others or by circumstances.

Personhood is an achievement that is worked for and acquired gradually. It is growth of the personality in the direction of maturity, or integration of the components of personality. The intellect must prevail, because the mind is man's unique and distinguishing feature.

Personhood, though individual, has a relational aspect. The quality of relations with others will be determined by the degree of personhood (maturity or personal integration) of those interacting in the relationship. This determinant obtains whether the relationship is intimate, formal, or distant. Interactions are not necessarily equal, because there is an infinite variety of personalities at various points on a continuum, and each individual maintains his or her own degree of personhood. However, one person may reflect another's stage of development. For example, demonstrated maturity, or personhood, may be imitated by the other person in the relationship (as with a parent and child). One is variously on the giving or receiving end of such conduct in relationships. Self-delusion is insidious and subtle; therefore, the varieties in degree and elements of personhood and the prevalence of neurotic behavior in our society must be kept in mind.

There is little uniformity in the acquisition of personhood, because endowments are wide-ranging and opportunities for their exploitation differ. Free will and choice determine exploitation of endowment. It is true that there are societal factors so overriding and personality weaknesses so compelling that free will and choice seem to become or are inoperative. These factors and weaknesses are brought into perspective when the meaning and pursuit of personhood dominate. In short, people are in charge of their own destinies, despite the real and powerful conditions that may prevail. History is replete with examples of people who have overcome towering obstacles and disadvantages to rise to great heights of being and achievement. Viktor Frankl, the Viennese psychiatrist, in his moving account of life in concentration camps in *Man's Search for Meaning,* tells of the ultimate freedom left to him: the decision not to grovel for a crumb of bread.

Personhood is an ideal as much as an accomplishment, and deterrents are numerous. It is both a cliche and a truism that we can put men on the moon but cannot solve our domestic problems. We are far better at establishing efficient methods than we are at securing or keeping cooperative, willing workers. Where people are involved, as in political and social enterprises, no matter how sound the theory or precise the mechanism, success hinges on the goodwill and maturity of those people. Conflict, tension, and frustration are at the heart of social disorganization. The more mature the persons involved in such disorganization, the better the chance of conversion to organization. Although adding to the complexity, conflict and tension can be used to help us make more appropriate choices. At best, we can hope for and try to minimize conflict, tension, and frustration by attempting to achieve personhood ourselves and assisting others, especially those for whom we have responsibility, to achieve it also.

CONTRIBUTIONS TO HUMANIZATION

Achievement of personhood is closely related to the process of humanization. The means are many and varied. The continuing effort to examine, understand, and put into action the growing body of knowledge directed to human relations and communication is important. This knowledge addresses itself to the heart of the matter, that is, the quality of the interactions of people, providing benefit and consequent effect on life, family, work, or community. The morale factor derives from this body of knowledge and is an indicator of the relational quality and change or growth in individuals and the enterprise. Closely related is the application of philosophical concepts of logic, ethics, esthetics, politics, and metaphysics, which keep deliberations within a larger framework for coherence and universality. These concepts also provide us with the tools to see more objectively, so that we are better able to distinguish reality from illusion. Additionally, viewing stress—a dominant feature of our society and health care institutions—in relationship to human relations, communication, and their derivatives, within this philosophical framework, contributes to humanizing the enterprise.

If we are to maintain satisfied, productive workers providing optimal nursing services, we must admit the depressing state of human relations as a first step in trying to improve them. This is a two-part effort, concerning interrelationships with patients also. Improved relationships with co-workers should result in improved relationships with patients, and vice versa. Strengthening of human relations should produce general rather than categorical improvement.

EFFECT OF GOALS OF THE ENTERPRISE

A prime consideration in developing and maintaining good interpersonal relations is whether the goals of the enterprise are worthy of commanding the loyalty of the workers.

Nursing is indeed a noble service to mankind, but we have noted the failure of nurses to exploit this nobility. The service of nursing must be spelled out, deliberated about, and communicated to all workers. The immediate goal of getting daily tasks accomplished will never be as energizing and satisfying as when duties are seen in terms of patient care and protection of the healthy in a meaningful way; where patient needs are realistically appraised, assigned priority, and met. The message is not that the work must get done, but that the needs of patients must be particularized in such a way that even routine activities can be shown as important in attaining the larger goal of high-quality nursing care. It is important that all workers give the goal their unstinting loyalty; how well this goal is communicated in all its detail and attendant importance will determine in large measure the workers' loyalty. For example, when time off for meetings is limited to management personnel, others may view this time off as a double standard, which produces cynicism that undermines loyalty.

DIGNITY AND WORTH OF THE INDIVIDUAL

Respect for the dignity and worth of each person is the base for good human relations. Such consideration is not compartmentalized: when patients are treated with consideration, colleagues are also. As an illustration, when the father of a young head nurse died, she was absent from work for 3 days by arrangement with the nursing office. Her close friend, another head nurse, also was absent for the same 3 days, and had duly notified the nursing office. On her return, she was reproached by the supervisor for taking the days off to support her friend in her bereavement when nursing coverage was so short. The incident occurred before the days of contracts or personnel policies that might provide a determined number of days a year for personal business. It took a long time for the supervisor to see this absence for what it was: a good friend giving support to her friend in need of such help, rather than abdication of responsibility to the hospital.

Sensitizing oneself to genuine respect for others is a lifelong pursuit, demanding that we acknowledge our violations of such respect for others when they occur so that our sensitization can be ongoing.

Openness and human relations

The pursuit of openness, an important ingredient of respect, is a lifelong exercise too. Essentially, it is recognition of one's own biases and, if they cannot be eliminated, prevention of their influencing reactions and decisions. Because nursing is essentially a middle-class occupation, nurses must guard against judging all persons by those standards. An illustration is shown in the embarrassment of a nurse who saw a diabetic patient's liquor license (in a state and at a time when a license was required to purchase liquor) as it accidentally fell from his wallet. Nothing was said by either the patient or nurse. Instead of embarrassed silence, could it not have been possible for the nurse to use the occasion to comfortably inquire whether the patient realized that alcohol must be counted as a carbohydrate and therefore alteration of diet or insulin dosage might be required? Such incidents abound in our experiences, not only where a therapeutic opportunity is lost, but where an opportunity to better know and appreciate a fellow human being is missed. There is a growing phenomenon in the health field —the founding of clinics in deprived areas —that attests to our collective failure to respect people's dignity and worth. They are forsaking the technical excellence of hospital outpatient departments for the empathic treatment they get in these grass roots health centers. If our attitudes drive people away from the care they need and want, surely we must try to understand the alienation and alter our attitudes positively.

There is a corollary in the work situation where consciously or unconsciously we devalue the work of persons lower in the hierarchy or jealously guard our title or status. Allied to such behavior is the sharp rebuke or thoughtless cruelty to a subordinate, which leaves a scar and reduces the relationship permanently. There was a time when nurses' aides were not allowed to listen to change of shift reports, and even today caps and name-position plates are worn protectively. There is ample evidence of role strain in nursing and nursing services. It is generated by the proliferation of levels and jobs in and out of the nursing service and by the wide variety in modes of preparation for nursing.

Human relations research in industry

Industrial research corroborates the importance of respect for the dignity and worth of the individual in human relations. In research for Western Electric Co., Inc.[1] "It was proved beyond the shadow of a doubt that a close relationship exists between the productivity of workers and their social and psychological relations with one another [p. 6]."[2] Where mutual respect and trust are found, good interpersonal relationships are present and the common enterprise is carried forward. This may account for the camaraderie and goodwill one sometimes encounters in units of an organization where the staff actually enjoy each other while they go about their serious business. An interesting sequel to the landmark research of Roethlisberger and Dickson is their account 25 years later of a counseling program set up at Western Electric to meet workers' needs identified in the original research.[3] The program covered keeping a job, friendship and belonging, felt injustices, authority, and job and individual development. That these men should have the opportunity to write a progress report of their research so many years later is a tribute to continuity.

In the aircraft industry in Southern California during World War II, Mayo and Lombard[4] found a sense of responsibility to and for the job where the work group was integrated or involved in a satisfying way with one another. Respect is an indispensable ingredient of the mutual caring in such integration. Gardner and Moore [p. 353][2] also found this integration where the supervisor deliberately established goals that the employees could support and helped them achieve these goals.

Human relations and society

The raising of societal consciousness and awareness attests to and states the importance of human relations. Surely this consciousness raising has its roots in the dignity and worth of the individual. Sensitivity training, or T groups, are widespread attempts to help people develop this very basic respect and to accept other human beings as they are, be they husband, patient, client, co-worker, or stranger. Such development of sensitivity enables us to sense the panic of the paralyzed and the quiet desperation of the distraught, to respond to the needs of older workers or patients, and to use friction to good purpose.

The dignity-and-worth concept is often found translated or broken down into components of need. For example, the Maslow[5] hierarchy of needs—physiological, safety, love, esteem, and self-actualization—seems to spell out the ingredients of respect for the dignity and worth of a person, allowing him to develop to his full potential as a human being, while keeping in mind all the resources at hand.

Patients' rights

The growth of patients' rights reflects the concept of the dignity and worth of the individual. Its emergence coincides with, if not stems from, the Civil Rights Movement in general. It is also part of the consumerism phenomenon, accompanied and supported by an increasingly knowledgeable and sophisticated citizenry.

Probably the first such statement on the subject of patient's rights was made in 1959 by the National League for Nursing. Entitled "What People Can Expect of Modern Nursing Service," it appeared in *In Pursuit of Quality* (National League for Nursing, 1964). This statement was prepared by a committee that included wide representation and was reviewed by hundreds of people in the field, including aides and orderlies. It became the base for *Your Nursing Services Today and Tomorrow*, Public Affairs Pamphlet No. 307, 1961. It deals with seven items, among which are adequacy of care, preparation and sensitivity of the worker, and obligation to provide instruction and continuity of care, appropriate records, and an appropriate environment.

In 1973 the American Hospital Association published its Patients' Bill of Rights. It consists of twelve points addressed to considerate care, full information about a diagnosis, adequate information to ensure an informed consent, refusal of care, privacy, confidentiality, admission, information about hospital relationships to other agencies, participation in research, continuity of care, full information about the patient's bill, and the rules and regulations governing patients.

At about the same time, a few hospitals individually prepared patients' bills of rights. One that received national attention was that of Beth Israel Hospital, Boston. Essentially, it included the same points as the AHA statement, with the additions of assistance in getting financial aid if necessary; opportunity to call or write staff members about possible unfair or improper treatment during hospitalization; and responsibilities of the patient to keep appointments, provide information necessary for personalized care, control visitors' behavior, and pay promptly.

Also in 1973, a more forthright and aggressive statement was put forth by H. Denenberg, Insurance Commissioner for Pennsylvania [in Quinn and Somers[6]]. It contains twelve points addressed to quality, continuity, and economy of care, personal dignity, full information, access to one's records, participation in decisions, refusal of care, grievance procedures, consumer advocacy, and information about the hospital, especially in regard to possible conflict of interest, and broad representation on boards of directors. It is apparent that this is a much stronger statement than that of the AHA and might even be construed as a rebuttal. Mr. Denenberg had a previous record of outspoken patient advocacy: his office prepared a *Shopper's Guide to Hospitals* in the Philadelphia area in 1971, which provides information about 101 hospitals relative to per diem charge, per diem cost, occupancy, average length of stay, total bed capacity, type, participation in preadmission testing program, and number of nonconforming beds by category according to Hill-Burton program figures.

Another strong and similar statement of patients' rights was offered in 1974 by Annas.[7] He omits the grievance procedure and hospital data items of Denenberg, but suggests that patient advocates be paid independently of hospital management to ensure patient-versus-hospital loyalty. By considering four cases and a range of questions about each, Annas and Healey[8] further expand this concept of patients' rights.

The Pediatric Bill of Rights[9] was introduced in 1974. Directed to the needs of minors, it ensures treatment for venereal disease and drug and alcohol abuse and provides birth control and abortion without parental consent. It follows the trend of the times in which parental rights over dependent children are in jeopardy and the fragility of the family is at an all-time high, as evidenced by the divorce rate. In arguments for this children's bill of rights, health professionals proffer that either they circumvent parental consent or the child will not seek treatment. The fallacy here is that it is not an either/or situation. Two other options to consider are enforcement of parental responsibility for the care of minor children and legal intervention in the event of parental delinquency. As a rule, parents do not refuse treatment for their children; they do try to curb promiscuous behavior when they have knowledge of it. By denying parental consent for treatment, this bill of rights may in fact protect the child's promiscuity. Logical scrutiny is useful in reviewing this children's bill of rights.

Popular magazines too are contributing to the patients' rights movement. One gives advice in dealing with physicians, hospitals, or both, such as being selective, changing physicians, and getting more than one opinion; demanding a reasonable amount of time and attention; getting full information; refusing treatment; participating in research; and determining costs.[10] It parallels similar advice on all aspects of living, from best use of one's car to funeral services.

The increase in number of malpractice suits further attests to the growing patients' rights movement. A federal malpractice commission composed of lawyers, insurers, consumers, and health professionals concluded that the growing number of malpractice suits was indeed caused by injury to patients. It recommended relicensure tied to continuing education for physicians, reexamination for specialists and stricter disciplinary procedures, inclusion of lay members on state licensing boards, improved treatment, and closer doctor-patient relationships. It also supported patients' bills of rights.

Little has been done to extend participatory democracy to specific patient populations, especially in long-term or chronic illness and nursing home situations. Patient councils in which patient representatives deliberate about issues affecting them and submit consequent recommendations to those in charge of the facility would bring the same advantages as participatory councils do elsewhere. They should be introduced and nurtured forthwith.

There is a growing number of patients' advocates, ombudsmen, and other representatives, who interview, intercede, and generally follow through on patient complaints, though Annas' caution that who pays the piper calls the tune may be a determinant of the effectiveness of such personnel in really representing the patient population. The growing hospital response to the patients' rights effort attests to and demonstrates their goodwill and concern for the humanizing of institutions. There have always been nurses who advocated patient participation in planning their own care, and the AHA statement reinforces such efforts at humanization. These are good beginnings and must be practiced faithfully, but they require the goodwill and effort of all engaged in the health care setting.

Nurses' rights

Fagin has isolated seven rights of nurses, as distinguishable from the rights and responsibilities heretofore enunciated, which addressed responsibilities far more than rights.

1. The right to find dignity in self-expression and self-enhancement through the use of our special abilities and educational background.
2. The right to recognition for our contribution through the provision of an environment for its practice, and proper, professional economic rewards.
3. The right to a work environment which will minimize physical and emotional stress and health risks.
4. The right to control what is professional practice within the limits of the law.
5. The right to set standards for excellence in nursing.
6. The right to participate in policy making affecting nursing.
7. The right to social and political action in behalf of nursing and health care.*

This list should receive the same serious attention as that given to the declared rights of others. It provides a fine base for deliberation wherever nurses are engaged in nursing.

PARTICIPATORY GOALS

Another aspect of the dignity-and-worth concept is a voice for people in the conduct of affairs in which they participate. The concept is violated where the participatory factor is denied, whether to worker or patient. It is at this point that the defender of respect for personal dignity and worth is put to the acid test: does he or doesn't he provide full and continuous opportunity for workers to make their opinions and thoughts known in an atmosphere free from fear? This voice for the worker is sometimes called participatory democracy. Though "participatory" is probably redundant because participation is inherent in democracy, it

---

*Fagin, C.: Nurses' rights, Am. J. Nurs. **75**(1):82-85, 1975.

does represent an attempt to correct the failure of democratic institutions and organizations in meeting this part of their obligation. Follett[11] speaks about the need for the voice of both the expert and the worker, whose experience melds with the information of the expert to produce cooperative experiences and activities flowing toward greater effectiveness. A similar point is found in Myers'[12] effort to involve the worker in planning and controlling, as well as doing the work, for both job enrichment and goal achievement. Both are variations on the participatory theme.

There are unlimited opportunities for such participation at early stages before final decisions are made involving, for example, work patterns, equipment, time utilization, and such, accompanied by consequent evaluation of such decisions. This kind of participation makes every employee a "manager," or demonstrates respect for the dignity and worth of the employee within the framework of human relations by allowing him not the privilege but the inherent right to a voice in affairs that concern him in the specific work situation. By combining consideration of every employee as manager with demonstrated respect for the person, one sees relationships that are mutually supportive though deriving from different sources, namely administrative and human relations theory. The combined consideration illustrates the interpenetrative nature of both administrative and human relations theory. Nor does the type of ownership of the enterprise, be it private or public, make any difference, because the employee is deserving of and indeed possessed of the right to such participatory involvement regardless of type or arrangement of ownership.

A long-standing practice has been the open-door policy, whereby the worker can approach a superior at any time about points of dissatisfaction or problems, and there *are* superiors who consider these contributions of the workers in the conduct of affairs. Yet, the greater number of workers are not heard, because rare is the employee who will take anything of a controversial nature to a superior on his own and by himself. For this reason, a staff organization is necessary to provide the worker with a formal, scheduled, and ongoing opportunity to discuss with peers his ideas about the conditions of work and the work situation and to make recommendations for improvement. Where the democratic principle is firmly upheld, individual groups at all levels hear minutes of other group meetings, so that they know what becomes of their own ideas and contributions.

This formal structure does not replace informal solicitation of workers' opinions. This kind of exchange generates ideas to enrich the superior's proposal or program in order to carry forward the goal of the enterprise. It broadens the base for and tempers decision making and provides a modified check-and-balances system. It also utilizes the potential contribution of the worker beyond routine work and enhances commitment to the job. This kind of two-directional communication flow demands that such ideas be reflected in subsequent decisions. Not all can be incorporated, but there is direct or indirect evidence that such ideas have been considered.

• • •

These two principles—respect for the dignity and worth of persons and their right to a voice in affairs affecting them —are bases for all kinds of actions and decisions within the enterprise, either permeating it with goodwill and generosity of spirit or, conversely, with bad or reluctant will and niggardliness of spirit. They underpin the human relations component of administration.

COMMUNICATION

Communication is the other pervasive and far-reaching determinant in human relations. It will vary directly as the respect principle varies, because communication is always transactional and mutually influencing. Communication has many constituent parts—speaking, listening, looking, writing, reading, silence, facial expression, touch, and body movement—all in multiple variations and degrees. (A survey at the 1974 ANA convention showed that nurses favor touching over verbal communication in importance in nursing practice.[13]) Basically, however, communication consists of three ingredients: inception, transmission, and reception of the observation, idea, or message, often accompanied by emotional messages.

Probably the most difficult part of communication, and the one most crucial in human relations, is the listening component. If one does not hear, he or she cannot respond, help, make decisions about, take actions, or be changed. Listening and hearing are synonymous here; they both imply thoughtful attention, perception, and appreciation. Not only must we give complete attention, but we must try to listen empathically, that is, try to hear what is said while simultaneously appreciating the person speaking, regardless of status or personal characteristics.

There are a few categories of people who especially need empathic listening, such as the inarticulate, the negative, and the repetitive. They require patience and acceptance. Moreover, the empathic listener may help by gentle probing so that the one groping to convey his ideas is assisted rather than stopped in the process. The negative are often stopped in the encounter because the listener closes his mind to the irritation. The negative point of view is seldom popular; yet one must guard against hasty rejection, so that inherently sound ideas are not also rejected. The repetitive are often rejected, without benefit of further consideration of their ideas. Listening and responding to these people are difficult because often we do know better than they, although not always nor perhaps as often as we think we do. In responding to people, the more we recognize our own biases the better we can listen and respond to the communication.

Listening, like all other facets of communication, can be learned, practiced, and evaluated. Skills can be developed and applied to a growing area of nursing care as well as to group and individual relationships. From social workers and psychiatrists, we are learning how to listen, evaluate, and respond to patients and to each other. The demanding, ungracious patient or co-worker may be telling us of his anxiety, fear, or frustration, and is never helped by deprivation and retaliatory response but may improve if we can determine the cause of the unpleasantness and respond effectively to it by increasing attention, solicited or not, and softening or deepening the response in a variety of ways.

The mirror technique is another method of listening, whereby the listener tries to reflect the concerns stated by the speaker so that the speaker can see himself and his statements more clearly and insightfully. Pertinent but open-ended and unstructured responses can facilitate speaker satisfaction. Great lengths of time are not necessary for satisfactory communication; insightful, receptive, open people can and do reach the heart of the matter and the other person in amazingly short time spans. The groping and troubled employee or patient can be helped almost immediately by one person, yet flounder indefinitely with another.

Carl Rogers,[14] though he and his colleagues are masters of techniques in nondirective and related schools of therapy, maintains that the intent of the person to help is more important than the use of any formula. He praises concerned persons turned hot-line counselors and emphasizes that this person-to-person contact is essentially a more important relationship than that between professionals and lay people. When and if one can be real and nonjudgmental, the relationships and communications will be richer, more productive, and more satisfying.

Communication with the dying

Barbus makes some important statements about communication in three articles. In an insightful piece on death and dying, she addresses the loneliness and isolation experienced by the dying when everyone abandons them out of ignorance, anxiety, or self-denial, often with mutually stated or unstated agreement. She cites the case of a psychiatrist[15] who was deserted not only by his family but by colleagues as well, on the assumption or evasive thinking that professionals can handle their own problems including such a monumental one as death. Indeed, thinking of death as a problem rather than a solemn experience for every man, and as a professional rather than as a man, may be a secondary abandonment of reality. Communication in this instance is withheld or evasive, based on false assumptions, and nonreality centered. Nor are these characteristics of communication confined to persons surrounding the dying; they occur in many kinds of relationships and situations. Such illustrations, however, give us concrete material to consider for the purpose of strengthening our own communication quotient and those of others as we engage in the managerial process. Barbus's work has culminated in a *Dying person's bill of rights.*[16]

Danger of stereotyping

Barbus[17] addresses the stereotyping potential of communication whereby a patient is catalogued precipitously and finally by labels. She cites the case of Mr. Allen, who was described, stigmatized, and classified as old and terminally ill, which in turn determined the attitudes and nursing care ministered to him. The labels froze the nursing care at a very unsatisfactory level—routinized, unthinking, and impersonal. Precipitous labeling is an enemy of communication, because it actually obviates or stops discourse and dialogue at an early stage. Barbus goes on to observe that lack of curiosity contributed to or indeed caused the freezing of this unfortunate situation. No questions were asked of the patient, despite his frequent efforts to communicate. All were construed as reinforcement of the established stereotype, until one nurse quite accidentally happened on the situation, communicated with the patient, and set personalized nursing care in motion. This illustration is not extraordinary. Collectively, we are missing such opportunities to personalize nursing care, as well as collegial and managerial relationships, because of blanket labeling and lack of communication, curiosity, or interest. Freezing communication at premature levels and positions blocks any possibility for growth, completion, or satisfaction.

Precision and clarity

Barbus and Carbol[18] note another aspect of communication, that is, the need for precision and clarity in describing what is meant and understood by complete bed rest. They conducted a study that turned up considerable variation in understanding of this concept. It raised such questions as whether feeding oneself or reaching for objects on the bedside table are permitted within this directive. The range of questions and responses illumined dramatically this commonplace item in nursing care and also kept deliberations and understanding moving in the appropriate direction. This same range of questions and responses elicited precision and clarity by their precision and clarity, but it required much organized communication to achieve the desired end.

Indirect communication

The work of Barbus illustrates another facet of communication, that is, communication by indirect and remote contact. It consists of communication between people, though no direct contact is involved. Remote contact can occur directly or indirectly. For example, Barbus' interest and discussion of death probably originated from her extensive work in a terminal unit of a large hospital where she and I were employed. Her article on the subject spoke to me directly about death. The indirect aspect of communication by remote contact occurs when others interested in the subject read the material and share the information by recalling similar or companion cases and incidents, though there is no personal common background with the author. This is both linear and lateral communication, varying in time and place, related to history but differing in that there is reciprocal though unspoken exchange by way of remote contact through the written medium.

Overcommunication

It should be noted that overcommunication also exists. We are inundated by repetitive and almost constant communication in our society, by way of the omnipresent transistor radio, television, and so forth. This overcommunication is found in the health care institutions as well. There is a tremendous proliferation of messages of all kinds and in various media. There is some justification for this proliferation, because the complexity and sophistication of modern organizations require it. The point, however, is that there could be reduction, consolidation, or integration of communications if we become aware of the danger and its destructiveness. Concerted effort could tighten, organize, and refine communications. Lack of appropriate administrative practice may indeed contribute to undue proliferation.

Easy consensus

Another hazard of communication is "groupthink," identified and described by Janis.[19] It is the danger of premature or easy arrival at consensus where the group making the decision is cohesive and cooperative. Wisest and best decisions may thus be prevented. He illustrates with cases from high government places. The degree of harmony and intelligence pervading the group promotes this phenomenon. It may get encouragement from concepts of group dynamics and various sensitivity group programs where cooperation is a goal; however, the influence is potentially destructive to the purpose of arriving at sound decisions. Special effort is needed to bring all alternatives, including unpleasant ones, into view, even with overemphasis to offset this phenomenon. This is a case of where the negative, groping, and repetitive persons of whom we spoke can be assets to group deliberation. It also points out the obligation to dissent and the need to encourage such dissent, in order to help prevent the bad effects of this phenomenon. Harris[20] speaks to this point when he says opponents and divergent ideas should help us grow and develop ourselves and our ideas; seeking truth is more important than vanquishing our opposition. Earlier he had noted how argumentation threatens the interpersonal relationship in Americans, whereas with Europeans arguments do not alter the friendly relationship.[21] Reston[22] sees the need for honest discussion about the extraordinary things happening to and around us and their relationship to values and purposes. Searching, rather than neat deliberations and probing of the fashionable, is necessary.

From her experience with a large number of nurses, O'Brien formalized opinions that more or less concur with and elucidate those just elaborated:

Honesty
Directness, with tact
Listening, with follow-through (that is, action, refusal, or a more careful examination of the situation should be communicated)
Giving the reasons for policies
Establishing an open-door policy and giving support when needed
Balance between congratulations given and constructive criticism offered
Respect for the individuality of the person*

Communication and confused thought

Gill[23] finds that nurses almost universally complain of problems in communication. They are seldom able to elaborate or spell out exactly what these problems are. He

---

*From O'Brien, M.: Communications and relationships in nursing, St. Louis, 1974, The C. V. Mosby Co., p. 105.

speculates very shrewdly that this inability may well mean that they do not know the exact nature of the problem. It may not in fact be communication, but something else such as emotional state, tangled work relationships, or imprecision in analysis. He claims that communication in management is not two-way, but three-way, because it involves lateral and cyclical activity. Such activity increases the complexity and margin for error and requires greater care, while providing wider and deeper input.

This common complaint of nurses about communication may be related to inarticulateness, deprivation experienced, lack of precision in both nursing and management of nursing, or other factors that affect them directly and indirectly. Whatever the cause, there are knowledge and resources with which nurses may reduce and overcome the problem.

MORALE

Morale is the indicator of level of goodwill, cooperation, or esprit de corps of a group. It is demonstrated by the location of the staff on a continuum between commitment and alienation. It is the effect of the sum total of interpersonal relationships and communications between each member and among the total staff.

Personal and organizational aspects

Total staff means all employees distributed in their respective positions in the organization. This means staff members as individuals and staff members as position holders making decisions in the organization. All staff members react to these decisions from the vantage point of their position, either favorably, unfavorably, or indifferently. These reactions to decisions and policies help to form the morale factor by their effect on all personnel. In short, there are two kinds of reactions and responses operative: to individuals as persons and to individuals as part of the decision-making management. Morale is influenced by both co-workers and policies and decisions of the organization. It is illusive and pervasive, because the reactions and responses evoked may be conscious or unconscious. It is subtle, because the reactions and responses may be directed toward secondary or tangential aspects of persons or conditions as well as primary targets. It is direct, because it is related to the attention given to explaining reasons, pointing out various points of view, the quality and amount of briefing, and engaging of personnel in the concerns of the enterprise.

Equanimity and detachment, or objectivity, of personnel play a part in the morale quotient. Some people know the difference between what can and cannot be changed. They also know how to go about changing what is changeable and accepting without undue regret what cannot be changed. One can ameliorate a situation or must endure it, for many reasons good and bad.

Roy[24] speaks of morale as hope for whatever is anticipated, for example, victory or success. The sufferings and difficulties encountered as one pursues a goal contribute to morale also. If nursing is understood in terms of benefits to people and society, not only is worker tolerance increased but there is correspondingly higher morale. Care must be taken, however, not to overburden workers; victory or success is not justified by overburdening, except in a crisis situation. This view of morale is complementary to any other, not a replacement.

A study done in England, directed by Revans[25] and reported as *Standards for Morale,* showed that the quality of communication in an institution is related to staff stability and reduced length of patient days. Approachability of authority figures and clarity of communications constituted the two emphases of the study. Action-learning played a significant part; learning was accompanied by application to insure its having occurred. This concept is akin to the integration concept of E. L. Brown: knowledge or information must be internalized by the learner-performer before it becomes readily operative.

As noted, we are indebted to industry for much theory and knowledge of morale.

From industry we also learn something of the measurement of morale. Absenteeism, employee turnover, and grievance rates are three measures of the morale of an organization; and the morale quotient varies directly with the turnover, absenteeism, and grievance rates. Turnover rates are high in institutional nursing services. Salaries may be a contributing factor to turnover, but they are not always the first concern. Poor utilization of personnel, poorly defined work situations, and poor communication, personal relationships, and supervisory techniques also are found to be reasons for turnover. Such conditions are crucial factors in the status of morale in any given institution.

Hagen and Wolff[26] point out and their findings confirm the close relationship of morale to the quality of leadership. They found high morale related to supervisory personnel with considerable concern for patients, their families, and visitors; greater expectancy of higher standards; and the giving of less direct care except when the purpose was to help subordinates. Supervisory personnel were critical of themselves for any breaks in composure in dealing with personnel; were more concerned for the health and welfare of staff; solicited suggestions from and gave credit to subordinates; gave explanations for changes or inability to comply with requests; and provided more incidental teaching and showed greater appreciation of such teaching.

It sometimes happens that one or a few key people in an otherwise rigid and arbitrary organization can provide those for whom they are responsible with a sense of belonging and participation and the reality of decision making by conscious effort and skillful, judicious intervention. This accounts for the islands of harmony and goodwill one finds in certain units of an organization. Contrariwise, it has happened that a few key people of a rigid and arbitrary bent have succeeded in suppressing the goodwill of a substantial number of employees in an otherwise open organization. One cannot overestimate the sphere of influence of each person, especially those in leadership positions at various levels. Leaders' performance and attitudes can be an open and growth-producing or a subtle and inhibiting influence on staff.

Change and its management

How change is handled will affect staff morale. It is a fairly universal maxim that the more those who must change are involved in the planning for the change, the greater their acceptance will be. The input of those affected will do much to determine not only the quality of the change and its implementation but their response as well. Nothing inhibits response quite so fast as arbitrary, unilateral, sudden decisions. Even inertia should be overcome with persuasion, if at all possible. Times when direct immediate orders are required are rare. Good communication skills and use of logic help. Reinforcement of status that is threatened by the proposed change is also important. A current problem is getting nurses to relinquish appropriate duties to others. The latent anxiety caused by such relinquishment can be reduced by reinforcing and expanding the nursing component energetically. Effecting change is another application of participatory democracy.

Change stems from positive as well as negative forces. We tend to think of it as being problem-based. However, the problems arise from the successes of the enterprise as well as from difficulties encountered. Change is concerned with corrective actions, but also with developmental actions. It can be seen as closely related to growth, or maturation, of people and enterprises.

Although change has many positive aspects, one must always ask whether a proposed change is in fact necessary. The aphorism credited to the Duc de la Rochefoucauld, "Plus ça change, plus c'est la meme chose" (The more things change, the more they stay the same.), deserves deliberation. Changes have a way of eventually reverting to the original situations. There are numerous illustrations of this. Recent joint position appointments for management of service and education in the university setting is a return to joint positions, the separation of which began in the 1950s. The current emphasis on assessment, planning, implementation, and evaluation of nursing care is an approximate restatement of the goal-setting and problem approaches to nursing care found in classical team nursing two decades ago. Continuous comprehensive nursing care is necessary and is implied in both cases.

With our current penchant for and adulation of change (there are instances that almost make it look like obsession), questioning should be encouraged. It may provide some restraint, because it will require at least review of reasons for making a change. This is good, and perhaps deeper probing will show alternate routes, variations of the status quo, or that maintenance of the status quo is best. Questioning may also illumine areas of collateral disequilibrium or dysfunction. It may show the change as addressing symptoms of a problem rather than the essential problem. A current example found within the ANA is the regrouping of nursing service administrators into a Council of Nursing Service Facilitators, presumably to strengthen their position. In fact, use of such a nondescript word for administrator may well weaken their position.

Etzioni's[27] commentary on change emphasizes the need for the right kind of change. He points out quite factually the limited effect education, re-education, or compensatory education has had on such major social problems as drunk driving, drug abuse, and disadvantaged populations. He suggests that our high expectations of education to solve our problems are illusory, whereas efforts such as treating the problems by such interventions as breath analysis for drivers suspected of being inebriated, use of methadone and antabuse, and so on, are more effective. The phenomenal decline in the highway death rate in 1974, attributed to reduced speed limits to conserve gasoline after years of unsuccessful educational efforts, supports his view.

Norris[28] corroborates Etzioni's point in her insightful and forthright review of nurses' delusions. For example, she amasses a quantity of telling material to show the fallacy of the belief of nurses that knowledge will prevent disease. She does not say how to get out of the world of fantasy, though she would be one nurse who could begin to get us out of Plato's cave of illusion and into the light of reality.

A brake on the "change" mentality is necessary, because change is no panacea. Detailed attention and care are required to bring the concept back to reality. Qualification is always necessary. We do need change, but the base for it must be solid so that it will contribute to achievement of goals rather than to floating problems.

Etzioni's idea of making changes closer to the problem rather than to the person (as for example through education) has a parallel in the case of the individual. Rather than assume that everyone is perfectable in a uniform way and completely susceptible to the good influences of administration, comprehensive nursing care, and so forth, perhaps we should try to work around or integrate people's neurotic behavior, which can be strength as well as weakness. For example, consider the rigid behavior of a central supply room supervisor who, while insisting on everything being done correctly so that her operation would be the excellent one it was, scolded and stormed when material was returned from the floors improperly rinsed or incomplete. Though her rigidity and anger greatly disturbed the messengers, usually aides who probably were not directly responsible for the condition of the goods, the fact remained that she ran a very tight operation in a very crucial area.

RESOLUTION OF CONFLICT

When one has done and continues to do all in one's power to affect the climate of an organization and its relationships positively, there is still residual conflict. It cannot be wished away or ignored, but must be treated in as open, fair, and healthy a way as possible. Listening to both sides of a story, attempting to put the facts in as objective a light as possible, sharpening them by careful questioning, weighing them for seriousness, and avoiding irritation and anger as much as possible can all help in reducing conflict.

Follett's "authority of the situation" is a valuable means of treating conflict of change (or giving orders). It consists of depersonalizing the issue—getting it externalized and visualized as thoroughly as possible—with the expectation that the solution will emerge from the very logic of the situation rather than the positions held by the participants [in Metcalf and Urwick[29]].

The following illustration, with minor variations, is a common one to which this principle is applied. A head nurse found the 8 AM medications poured and set up by the night nurse on a unit, though this nursing service had a rule that "the one who poured must pass." On questioning, the night nurse said she had done it to help the day nurses, who were faced with a heavy schedule of preoperative patients, among other duties. The supervisor reminded her of the rule and its reason—safety—and asked her not to do it. Some mornings later the same situation was found with the same persons involved. One must, in this situation, become firmer with the offending nurse, remind her again of the reason for the ruling and the need for all to subscribe to the rules for the sake of order, and perhaps ask that the medication procedure be reviewed by the appropriate committee or person. But what of the terrible stifling of this night nurse's spirit of goodwill and generosity? If the head nurse had pressed for review of the medication procedure, in light of the generosity of the night nurse, perhaps a system might have been devised that would provide safety and yet encourage such generosity. After all, many nurses were not taught that the one who pours must pass; and we have come to accept the unit dosage system that may provide for medication to be prepared by the pharmacist but passed by the nurse. We have tended to think of safety, or similar issues, alone and ignore the accompanying reservoirs of goodwill. Both should be feasible.

Another illustration concerns patients' visitors. A terminally ill man continued to go down to the lobby to see his children, who, because of age, were not allowed in the patient units; to do without pain medication so that he could go into the hall in a wheelchair to see his family, to avoid the "two to a patient at a time" rule; and connived with his roommate to have two of his relatives be the roommate's "visitors" when he had none. If this harsh arbitrary treatment of patients and their visitors were viewed within the framework of the therapeutic as well as the deleterious effect of visitors (their "inconvenience" to staff in caring for patients), more humane policies could exist in our institutions. It is an illustration of our biases prevailing over a rational total review of a patient's visitors. It is heartening to note the appearance of "visitors" on nursing interview forms, making them a matter of nurse-patient decision rather than arbitrary house rule.

Logic and argumentation are not highly prized or developed skills in our society. The decline of the art of debate and rhetoric, the encouragement of verbal participation for its own sake instead of its merit, the unstructured format of deliberations to encourage verbal participation, and the "bandwagon" mentality sometimes prevailing in regard to fashion in ideas all militate against logic and sound argumentation. These influences, while working against deliberate, precise reasoning, can be identified, treated, and reduced. However, the emotional appeal sometimes found in argument must be protected, because it is capable of stemming from sound logic as much as is the dispassionate argument. One's response should be to the argument in whatever climate it is carried and not to the climate itself or to the personality of the one arguing.

Logic in resolution of conflict

The return of a formal structure to discourse would reduce destructive actions and maximize achievement in defined and refined ideas and decisions. The platonic dialectic provides such a structure enabling the participants to deliberate with greater concentration and lucidity on the subject at hand. It always permits of fallibility on everyone's part, and it always requires evidence. Essentially, the platonic method of discourse consists of words or names that are defined. Definitions are followed by examples, in pursuit of and on the way to knowledge and understanding.[30] Such procedure tends to prevent premature or immature freezing of the issue being deliberated.

For example, remember the above illustration relating to visitors. Nurses have tenaciously held the position that visitors interfere with their ministrations to patients and prevent the patient from getting needed rest. Others in the hospital think similarly, and the relaxing of visiting hours, where it has occurred, has been greeted with much reluctance. Patients have many responses to visitors: enjoyment, moral support, fatigue, perhaps annoyance at or exhaustion from having to be a host or hostess while ill, appreciation for assistance such as with walking or eating, a quiet presence, or a contact with the outside world. Is it possible to bring order and satisfaction out of such a welter of diverse reactions and responses? Definition of the term visitor would yield categories, such as family, primary or extended; loved one; surrogate relative; friend or neighbor, fellow parishioner, or business associate—all with a wide range of claims on and obligations to the patient. Examination and examples of the composite of the patient's visitors could yield a therapeutic plan for visiting. Such discrimination might then remove the obstacles to care giving of which nurses so frequently speak. The scheduling of nursing care could be made around these considered visits or worked into the individualized visiting plan or pattern with the patient. Consultation with visitors who are part of this plan could bring about alterations helpful to the staff and yet convenient for the visitors' schedules too.

When the patient is a child, the obligation to facilitate rather than discourage the presence of a parent or other significant person is great if we are really serious about giving individualized care that respects the needs of the patient. It requires that ignorance of patient needs be dispelled, consequent attitudes changed, enlightened decisions made, and actions altered accordingly. There is abundant knowledge about parent-child separation to justify such intensive inquiry and action.

Follett wants reliance on careful, complete, and orderly examination of the issue, using all the pertinent evidence that can be gathered and from which will come the wisest decision. Yet the decision may change, because new evidence and fallibility of the persons involved will always be operative.

No less a nursing leader than Stewart[31] cautioned us over 50 years ago that knowledge of logic would enable us to identify and expose fallacies, straighten out misrepresentation and misstatement, and gain greater public support. Though we have nurse-sociologists, nurse-anthropologists, and so forth, we still have no nurse-philosophers. Part of the deficiency stems from the notion that philosophy and its components are considered to be acquisitions, as social grace or lofty nebulous themes, rather than concrete bodies of knowledge. This error pervades our culture, too, of which we are a part, making incorporation of philosophical concepts in management doubly hard.

CONSIDERATION OF STRESS

Another gross threat to the humaneness of the hospital is stress. Because health restoration of patients is the essential nature of the hospital's purpose, there will always be patient and personnel stress in varying amounts. We have been slow to acknowledge and come to terms with stress and anxiety. It is significant that in England Revans, whose work we have noted, calls the hospital a cradle of anxiety. Yet at St. Christopher's Hospice near London, patients, their families, and the staff face the reality of death compassionately, beautifully, and with reduced tension, in contrast to our anxiety-generating subterfuge.

Acknowledgement is the requisite to correction or reduction of stress and anxiety. Physicians' offices are generously sprinkled with nurses who left hospital work because of its strains (often named is the aloneness and responsibility of the evening and night shifts). Stress derives from or is associated with conflict, tension, and frustration. In their extensive hospital studies, Georgopoulos and Mann[32] found levels of tension and pressure directly related to the quality of existing coordination, and the quality of care directly related to tension and pressure levels.

Nurses are noting such stress and its effect on thinking, claiming that the busy medical-surgical ward militates against the thought and action necessary for giving comprehensive nursing care [in Cleland[33]]. Johnson and Campbell[34] point out the need to state frankly the condition prevailing in the unit day by day, so that adjustments can be made in assignments and procedures accordingly, thus eliminating anxiety, frustration, and guilt feelings present during nonadmitted, nonaccommodated pressure times.

The advent of critical and coronary care units has contributed to illuminating the problem of stress by both concentration of critically ill patients and the complicated lifesaving devices that nurses must understand and operate. Stress here is constant; there are no respites as are found in regular units. Reres[35] proposes the use of a mental health consultant, whose skills would help the staff in their care of these special patients and in coping with their own anxiety and stress. As nurses understand and upgrade their nursing care, nurse-patient interactions should become smoother and more satisfying, further reducing stress. The question of compensation for work in high-stress areas has not been met, if in fact it has even been raised. It probably awaits more sophisticated wage and salary administration in hospitals.

We should not take for granted the anxieties of patients in our care. Recognition is the starting point here, too, because if we do not consider this aspect of the patient we are treating and nursing him as something less than a feeling, thinking, ailing human being.

Bettelheim[36] points out the dichotomy of the "good" patient—the uncomplaining, cooperative, passive, accepting one—and the "bad" patient—the complaining, crying and demanding, who reacts in ways the staff finds troublesome and irksome. This dichotomy, he says, represents a reversal of good and bad mental health responses. Passivity, cooperation, and such, while pleasing to the staff, represent poor mental health, whereas complaining and demanding represent good mental health in the face of the anxiety-ridden position in which the patient finds himself, isolated and virtually imprisoned in an unknown and seemingly hostile environment of treatments, medications, surgery, and so forth. He describes an instance of individualized nursing care at its most independent where the nurse, overriding protocol and the decision of the resident, telephones the patient's physician at night at the patient's insistent request, to the satisfaction of both patient and physician. There are innumerable instances where such nursing intervention would place the nurse in trouble with the physician as well as the resident and those in charge of protocol, procedures, and policies. The occurrence illustrates how much nursing intervention is controlled and limited by other authorities, adding to the stress of the patient's situation. Would an insightful supervisor have supported the nurse and patient or the resident and hospital policy? One thing is clear: patients sometimes need heroic tenacity and psychic strength to remain a part of the decision making in their own health care. Nursing requires comparable tenacity and strength in meeting patient needs.

Occasionally a patient can verbalize his terror and anxiety by reporting that the clanging elevator nearby, rather than awakening and annoying him, reassures him that he is still alive. Another will tell of her fear of drowning in the tubes and bottles of fluids to which she is connected. However, the vast majority of patients keep their fears and panic to themselves or display them in other ways. We speak of patients entrusting themselves to us, but where in all the decisions they make do they have less choice or less knowledge about the alternatives, if any, than when under our care? We can do no less than conscientiously and diligently try to allay such anxiety by identifying and exploring it with both the patient and the staff.

ETHICAL CONSIDERATIONS IN HUMANIZATION

Logic is not the only philosophic tenet to safeguard humane behavior. Ethics has traditionally pervaded health care; unfortunately, it has been eclipsed for some decades, perhaps by the scientific-technological revolution and perhaps by the relativistic tenor of the times. A resurgence is overdue, because ethical problems are proliferating rapidly. Current ones in the health field, such as abortion, euthanasia, organ transplants, and genetic engineering, have strong ethical ramifications, and application of ethical inquiry is mandatory. Accountability to patients should have demanded ethical inquiry by nurses in the widely publicized cases of the Tuskeegee syphilis study and recent sterilizations without understood consent.

An account of current problems under consideration by multidisciplines at the National Center for Bio-Ethics, Hastings-on-Hudson, N.Y., corroborates the urgent need to reinstate the study of ethics [in Rilton[37]]. It discusses such subjects as abortion because of the sex of the child; forcible shock therapy; buying blood from countries where the people are impoverished; decision revolving around finding an extra Y chromosome, generally thought to indicate proneness to violence; the need for good kidneys for transplant while people who die accidentally are buried with transplantable kidneys; and the relationship of psychosurgery to criminality. Our society is flooded with such considerations and practices that cry out for ethical consideration.

Frankel reviews the enormity of biomedical consequences:

> Rightly or wrongly, people in the past could make decisions about the introduction of technologies without thinking about the consequences. In the case of biomedicine that fine freedom is gone. Its various techniques may be widely adopted, and the consideration of consequences may be minimal but the process will involve a conscious and deliberate refusal to think. Biomedicine has eliminated the insouciance with which most people have embraced technological progress. It forces consideration not simply of techniques and instrumentalities but of ends and purposes.*

It can be said that these are problems of doctors, and perhaps in the final analysis they are. However, nurses and others who demand participation on the health team also must share responsibility for distressing and painful decisions. Moreover, because such decisions require the input of other professionals, such as lawyers, philosophers, and scientists, they certainly deserve the input of nurses, who after all are second in seniority on the health team. Also, as we grow in professionalism we must move from the concrete to the general and speculative. The study of ethics will provide material for reflection and speculation.

ICN and ANA ethical codes

A review of the Code for Nurses of the International Council of Nurses (1973) and the Code for Nurses of the American

---
*From Frankel, C.: The specter of eugenics, Commentary **57**(3):27, 1973.

Nurses' Association (1968) shows two features that address themselves to current ethical problems. These deal with protecting the patient against inept or improper care and working with health colleagues and the citizenry in meeting health (and social ICN) needs. These features seem to authorize or justify the nurse's engagement in wide-ranging ethical problems of health care.

Although both codes speak of the dignity of man, there are two noteworthy omissions in the ANA code: respect for life (which appears in the ICN code) and rights of man. Conservation of life was present in the ANA code immediately prior to the 1968 revision; perhaps its deletion was a result of the pro-abortion movement at the time.

There are ethical considerations for nurse managers beyond those deriving from biomedicine. They could be said to derive from the concept of justice, because they deal essentially with the economic rights of workers. The trade union movement is replete with examples of unethical behavior on the part of the employer, not only in the economic sphere but in hindering the right to organize. The Economic and Welfare program of the American Nurses' Association is likewise full of such examples. There are many and subtle ways to defraud the laborer of wages and keep him defrauded. But the ethical violation of justice is not confined to employers; it is incumbent on employees to provide a fair day's work for a fair day's wage if they are to behave ethically. A fair day's work and wage here are literal, but must be flexible, because they represent related personnel policies.

Timely resurgence of the study of ethics and its application to problems in health care will require concerted effort at revitalization to equal the enormity of the problems. We convene conferences for research and other far-reaching subjects; why not for ethics? Perhaps ethics should be on the agenda of physician-nurse meettings, or joint practice meetings as they are currently called. The National Endowment for the Humanities encourages and supports teachers and physicians in the quest for greater humaneness. Perhaps nurses should and could tap into such resources and interests.

ESTHETICS

One could make a case for the importance of the remaining branches of philosophy for nurses, for they too generate the humaneness we all seek.

The esthetics of the environment of some new or renovated hospitals, incorporating muted colors, subdued lighting and sound, scenic vistas, plantings, art exhibits, and such, attest to the importance of esthetics to architects and secondarily to the administrators where such amenities exist. Esthetics are not confined to new construction or renovation; they occur elsewhere in hospitals of all vintages. If esthetics played a larger part in our lives, we would provide and expand them. Esthetics is a point of view and value system more than it is possession and arrangement of selected materials, though it influences such selection. An esthetic sense is ongoing, because when one appreciates the assault of our environment on our and our patients' senses and sensibilities, it becomes a continuous task to devise ways (both internal and external adjustments) to reorder the environment, in order to reduce or eliminate the assault.

POLITICS

Politics, which is the correct ordering and arranging of the institution, is extremely influential in one's humaneness. The better the order and coherence of the management in which one is involved, the more humane one is. Cast in this light, the whole point of this book, devoted as it is to means of improving the operation of nursing service administration, can be viewed as contributing to a higher level of humanity for everyone engaged in the enterprise. Subscribing to the notion that "politics is dirty" denies the good that is possible where political arrangements are cohesive and well organized. Perhaps it is tying the good and beautiful to the mundane task of ordering means to ends in the health care setting that liberates the person to become humane. In addition, use of the term nonsystem to describe the state of health care denies that it is, in part, a political entity. The system, however incomplete or ineffective, exists; examining, renovating, innovating, and tying the political entity to the whole is a healthier, more realistic view of the health care system.

METAPHYSICS

Consideration of metaphysics, with its concern for being, becoming, existence, universe, and interrelationships, should not only soften us for greater appreciation of man and the universe but also help us check our own brutish impulses and recognize and try to ameliorate these impulses in others. Moreover, such metaphysical considerations contribute directly to the realities of life and death, helping us to deal with them knowledgeably and compassionately rather than evade them both personally and professionally. Death should have more meaning for us than that the patient died, and birth should connote more than a clean, safe delivery.

MORAL ATTRIBUTES

It is currently unfashionable to speak of moral attributes such as kindness, compassion, and patience, but many cherish and seek to develop these traits in themselves. If one can verbalize them, so much the better, because they can bring a humanizing effect to all our relationships despite the derision or embarrassment they may evoke. Such attributes are not to be confused with gushiness or sentimentality. They are, rather, related to empathy and rapport, which bring a personal dimension to often impersonal and shallow relationships.

• • •

Like people everywhere, hospital personnel and patients are seeking participatory democracy: the right to have a voice in affairs in which they find themselves, without fear of reprisal and with dignity and justice. It is indeed their right. It is possible where administration impregnated with humanizing influences, sound human relations, and communication principles prevails. Morale plummets or soars in proportion to how personnel are treated by superiors and co-workers. The climate that prevails determines in large part not only the policies and practices of, but the interrelationships with and within, the organization. An excellent summary admonition is to brief workers and co-workers continuously; in so doing you are maximizing opportunities for knowledge and exchange of ideas about the work at hand or the goals to be achieved and directly involving personnel in achieving them. A philosophical framework enhances the exploitation of such opportunities.

REFERENCES

1. Roethlisberger, F. J., and Dickson, W. J.: Management and the worker, Cambridge, 1939, Harvard University Press.
2. Gardner, B., and Moore, D.: Human relations in industry, Chicago, 1950, Richard D. Irwin, Inc., pp. 6 and 353.
3. Dickson, W. J., and Roethlisberger, F. J.: Counseling in an organization, Boston, 1966, Harvard Business School, Division of Research.
4. Mayo, E., and Lombard, G.: Teamwork and labor tunover in the aircraft industry of Southern California, Business Research Studies, no. 32, Boston, 1944, Harvard Business School, Division of Research.
5. Maslow, A.: Motivation and personality, New York, 1954, Harper & Row, Publishers, pp. 88-106.
6. Quinn, N., and Somers, A.: The patient's bill of rights, Nurs. Outlook **22**(4):242, 1974.
7. Annas, G.: The patient rights advocate; can nurses effectively fill the role? Supervisor Nurse **5**(7):20-25, 1974.
8. Annas, G., and Healey, J.: The patient rights advocate, J. Nurs. Admin, **4**(3):25-31, 1974.
9. Children's bill of rights gives a voice to minors, News and Reports, Nurs. Outlook **22**(6):353, 1974.
10. Knox, G., and Rothman, L.: What are your rights as a patient? Better Homes and Gardens, April 1974, pp. 6-11.

11. Follett, M.: Creative experience, New York, 1951, Peter Smith, p. 213.
12. Myers, M. S.: Every employee a manager, New York, 1970, McGraw-Hill, Inc., p. 69.
13. Nurses rate touch over words for communication, Nurs. Outlook **22**(9):545, 1974.
14. Rogers, C.: From a speech given in Portland, Ore., March 24, 1972.
15. Barbus, A.: A nurse looks at the death of a psychiatrist, Psychiatric Opinion **7**(2):16-25, 1970.
16. Barbus, A.: A dying person's bill of rights, Am. J. Nurs. **75**(1):99, 1975.
17. Barbus, A.: The hospitalized Mr. Allen; the non-person, The Michigan Nurse, part I, July 1970, pp. 9 and 22; part II, October 1970, pp. 6-7.
18. Barbus, A., and Carbol, K.: Experiences in problem-solving for the baccalaureate student in nursing, J. Nurs. Educ. **2**(3):11-20, 1963.
19. Janis, I.: Victims of groupthink, New York, 1973, Houghton Mifflin Co.
20. Harris, S.: Enemies should help us grow, Vancouver, Wash., The Columbian, March 28, 1974.
21. Harris, S.: Thoughts, Vancouver, Wash., The Columbian, March 12, 1974.
22. Reston, J.: Honest discussion needed in nation today, Portland, Ore., The Oregonian, August 23, 1973.
23. Gill, W.: Key concepts in management for nursing, Supervisor Nurse **3**(3):75, 1972.
24. Roy, R.: The administrative process, Baltimore, 1958, The Johns Hopkins University Press, p. 154.
25. Revans, R.: Psychosocial factors in hospitals and nursing staffing; research on nurse staffing in hospitals, publication no. (NIH)73-434, Washington, D.C., 1972, Department of Health, Education, and Welfare, pp. 137-150.
26. Hagen, E., and Wolff, L.: Nursing leadership behavior, New York, 1961, Columbia University Press, pp. 142-145.
27. Etzioni, A.: Human beings are not very easy to change after all, Saturday Review, June 3, 1972, pp. 45-47.
28. Norris, C.: Delusions that trap nurses, Nurs. Outlook **21**(1):19-20, 1973.
29. Metcalf, H., and Urwick, L., editors: Dynamic administration. In The collected papers of M. P. Follett, New York, 1940, Harper & Row, Publishers, pp. 58-59.
30. Seventh epistle. In Plato: The epistles, Indianapolis, 1962, The Bobbs-Merrill Co., Inc., p. 238 (translated by Morrow, G.).
31. Stewart, I.: Popular fallacies about nursing education, Mod. Hosp. **27:**1, 1921.
32. Georgopoulos, B., and Mann, F.: The community general hospital, New York, 1962, Macmillan, Inc., p. 399.
33. Cleland, V.: Effects of stress on thinking, Am. J. Nurs. **67**(1):108-111, 1967.
34. Johnson, B., and Campbell, E.: It's time to be realistic about the work load, Am. J. Nurs. **66**(6):1282-1284, 1966.
35. Reres, M.: Coping with stress in the ICU and CCU, Supervisor Nurse **3**(1):29-33, 1972.
36. Bettelheim, B.: To nurse and to nurture, Nurs. Forum **1**(3):72, 1962.
37. Rilton, B.: Doctors' ethics in upheaval; tough questions from the brave new world of medicine, Family Weekly, September 9, 1973, pp. 4-10.

PART II

FRAMEWORK FOR STUDY OF NURSING SERVICE ADMINISTRATION

Outlines or diagrams are often the base for study or consideration of a project or process, serving to insure consideration of the various components individually so that they may better be seen in relationship to each other and to the whole. This method has application to administrative theory. Deliberate and clear thought on components of the process is encouraged by working through a compartmentalized breakdown of the process. Though the process is dynamic, that is, subject to change induced by the interaction of diverse persons in diverse times and places, it can still be viewed best through its component parts, despite the static nature inherent in viewing parts of a process.

Tead[1] states that administration is "a variety of component elements which together in action produce the result of getting done a defined task with which a group of people is charged. . . . It is the inclusive process of integrating human efforts so that a desired result is obtained." For Urwick[2] administration consists of forecasting, planning, organization, coordination, command, and control, all undergirded by investigation. Appropriateness undergirds organization and coordination, while order does the same for command and control.

Henri Fayol, the French industrialist, is thought to be the father of modern administration. Finer uses his schema: *posdcorb,* an acronym for *p*lanning, *o*rganizing, *s*taffing, *d*irecting, *co*ordinating, *r*eporting, and *b*udgeting. Within this schema we shall correlate the elements and activities of the nursing service necessary to provision of the best possible nursing care—its purpose. We shall double the *c* in the acronym and consider *c*ontrolling specifically, as many management theorists do.

Finer adds an *a,* for *a*ttuning, or sensitizing oneself to the ethos of the purpose. In nursing this is especially important. Nursing has a long history of service to mankind and has made a generous contribution to one of society's greatest needs. Indeed, two of nursing's biggest problems, those of diffuse definition and identity coupled with inability to restrict its efforts to a defined purpose, may be a result of this generosity. It is little wonder that the American Medical Association looks to nursing for medical assistants, and its lamentable unilateral statement about recruiting such assistants speaks eloquently to the unstinting willingness of nurses to do what is needed, when it is needed, in meeting health needs of people. It should be noted that nurses have been the forebears of the newer professions, including dietetics and social work. This broad historic and continuing commitment to care of the sick and to health promotion does indeed provide an ethos for attunement. It is possible that the reticence to exploit this ethos is one of the deterrents not only to sound nursing service administration but to the dilemmas of identity, definition, and preparation.

Evaluation

Evaluation is a part of administrative study, though not included in the schema. It deserves and will get special attention because, though very difficult at best, evaluation is crucial in order to determine whether the purpose is being achieved substantially, in part, or not at all. It is an essential part of control (see Chapter 10).

Development of personnel

One view of nursing service administration is that of optimal nursing care (the purpose) given by happy productive workers (the means of achievement). This view has the advantage of singling out the persons giving the care, who are certainly the most important resource. When personnel are supported by material, services, good policies, and healthy attitudes, job satisfaction is maximized and high-quality, expeditious nursing care is provided.

Finer imposes the notion of economy. It is economy in the widest sense—not only monetary, but of effort and material. It requires that the overworked, understaffed record of nursing be scrutinized most precisely so that not only corrective action can be taken, but perhaps more important the system can be revised and realigned so that waste of money, resources, and personnel can be eliminated and their adequacy can be provided. A carry-over from the long-standing procedural economy of nursing arts is useful in considering administration.

Human relations and communication

Human relations and communication pervade the administrative process and were considered under the wider view of humanizing the enterprise (see Chapter 4). Though they are thought about individually because they color and permeate all aspects of the enterprise, they do join with other humanizing influences to treat the whole man, in an attempt to render him a more complete person, whether he be worker or patient. Moreover, human relations is embedded in wider philosophical concerns that favor and encourage a holistic view of man.

Systems analysis

Some concepts of systems analysis will be included. Its mathematical precision can present a more stringent view of administration, because systems analysis insists on thorough evaluation at all points in the process and requires a discipline conducive to a clearly defined, enunciated, and articulated understanding of administration.

• • •

In the following chapters we will consider these aspects of administration as well as the individual components of *posdcorb*.

REFERENCES

1. Tead, O.: Administration; its purpose and performance, New York, 1959, Harper & Row, Publishers, p. 2.
2. Urwick, L.: The elements of administration, New York, 1942, Harper & Row, Publishers, p. 13.

CHAPTER 5
PLANNING

All management theory respects the need for planning a carefully detailed program of action to achieve a given objective that has been assessed in a deliberate analytic way. Planning is difficult, because this kind of thinking can be more demanding than action. However, the sense of accomplishment is great, especially when evaluation accompanies it so that the plan can be maintained or revised to maximize its effectiveness. It is a first and vital step in administration; without it there can be no carrying forward of the rational definition or deliberate acceptance of purpose.

There are societal factors operating against planning that affect planning for nursing service and care. With the tremendous complexity of everything (medical care, foreign aid, welfare service, education, and so forth), it becomes increasingly difficult to see component parts and their relationships, let alone the many philosophies surrounding these complicated enterprises. This same complexity gives rise to the feeling of helplessness and frustration in dealing with these complex enterprises.

This complexity is accompanied by a decline in philosophical and analytical thought. The predominant pragmatic view that "if it works it's all right" may be correct sometimes, but it negates the need for a wider ranging examination of all facets of a solution, in depth as well as breadth. Harris[1] notes the disdain of our culture for analyzing and theorizing. He points out the need to think before acting —or plan—if we are ever to come to grips with such societal problems as overcrowded jails, run-down homes, broken families, understaffed hospitals, and exhausted financial resources. His solution is to think diligently, not to commit more money. Because there is a current tendency to regard federal funding as an indispensable ingredient of achieving an objective, it should be noted that much is possible within existing budgets. Improvement may be achieved by internal rearrangement, effort, or insight, as well as financial resources. There can be parallel sets of plans. One would be put into effect if possible added resources become available; the other would be utilized if these resources do not materialize. This is an application of flexibility in planning.

Harris's plea also has relevance for nursing considerations. For example, legislation to provide contraceptives to minors without parental consent may indeed cut down on illegitimate births and physicians will be able to treat minors for venereal disease, but it also may give children a whip with which to beat their parents, reduce parental authority and family stability, increase promiscuity, or reduce human sexuality to animal level, among other undesirable results. Likewise, restricted visiting hours in pediatric wards (or elsewhere) may allow nurses to get their work done and safeguard rest and sleep for patients, but it also may produce anxiety in any of its many guises, psychic damage if the anxiety is severe enough, and reduce nurses' effectiveness in carrying out the medical regime by depriving them of parental help. It may also damage the emotional tone of the unit by forcing parent-child separation and fostering staff insensitivity.

Adequate time allotment for serious and

systematic planning is necessary. Though there may be flashes of insight and some easily available information, there is need to deliberate about the aim in such a way that the contributions of as many as possible are included in order to determine the best plan. It also helps in execution of the plan. A mix of a sense of urgency that motivates the group and a sense of calm to ensure the development of a thorough, effective plan is desirable.

Ours is an age of instant satisfaction, pleasure, and solution. There is little of the instant quality to planning. Though expeditious and exciting as that instant quality seems, the error margin is greater than when time is taken to review all aspects, including the unpopular or negative ones, so that the best solution, action, or plan can be selected. The frustration level is reduced by the same total review. Tangential thinking can be returned to the mainstream. Too, there is the sobering realization that one must accept or allow for error in planning, so that it can be faced frankly and remedied more realistically when it does occur.

BENEFITS OF PLANNING

Decisions must be made, and the more thoughtfully and deliberately they are made, the more satisfactory the outcomes should be. When plans are made in advance of emergencies, the emergencies can be minimized or eliminated, with consequent improved function. Good plans that anticipate emergencies allow the worker to function more calmly and deftly when an actual emergency arises. For example, when orange juice can be produced quickly 24 hours a day and where equipment that might be useful in treating an incoming patient in a diabetic coma is assembled (intravenous fluid set, glucose, catheter set, insulin, and so forth), care for that patient is begun faster. Likewise, civil defense plans and the hospital's part in them ensure greater effectiveness if and when disaster falls. In something so complex as civil defense, where many units of the community must be synchronized, one sees the absolute need for planning even minute details. Good plans assure economy of time, space, and materials and the highest use of personnel. In short, a well-articulated plan that can be seen and studied can be executed more effectively than one vaguely proposed.

DECISION MAKING IN PLANNING

Many decisions are made as a plan develops; however, one application of the consultative process that pervades good administration is that decisions be made as close to the point of application as possible. While any plan will work better when those concerned with the project are consulted and involved in the deliberations, planning is essentially the responsibility of those in authority, involving the group or individual who must utilize its implementation. The more input before finalization, the better.

Along with consideration in decision making, one must realize that there are times when decisions are inappropriate at a given time. Even in careful, deliberate planning there may be areas of the plan or timing of elements that do not yield to decision. The indeterminate parts, as well as factors relating to them, should be isolated and possible decisions should be projected. By keeping these in mind, time and events may then suggest the proper decision. Decisions deferred until more data are available or the right time has arrived are usually more comfortable and fruitful, though deadlines must be respected.

PHILOSOPHIES IN PLANNING

Philosophies exert considerable influence on planning. If the institution is devoted to research, there must be staff in sufficient numbers and with sufficient expertise to support the research goal. Public hospitals have different obligations, and hence philosophies, than private (proprietary or nonprofit) hospitals. These latter, often thought of or in fact named community hospitals because they serve a specific population, are entering a new stage in the hospital-community relationship. They are seeing their roles as more participative, and personnel from these hospitals are found much more frequently where social conditions of the community are being considered, especially the health care component. As we will note later, they occasionally provide specific, minimal-cost, community health services as community service projects. These community involvements constitute a definite philosophical change for these hospitals and demand changing plans. The hospital operated by a religious group may have a different philosophy than the specialty hospital (for example, the rehabilitation or long-term illness facility). Indeed, there probably is an overlap of philosophies, which enriches any particular one.

This overlapping may require special attention to make certain that conflicting philosophies do not exist in or are forced on an institution. A case in point is the occasional move to require Catholic hospitals to permit abortion, sterilization, and such operations because they (like most hospitals) receive federal funds for one reason or another and therefore are obligated to provide all legal surgical procedures to patients. Clearly stated philosophies are necessary so that disputes of this kind are settled appropriately and satisfactorily for all concerned.

City of Hope Medical Center

The philosophy of the Nursing Department of City of Hope Medical Center is essentially one of adherence to the Thirteen Articles of Faith and the Torchbearer's Creed of this institution. These statements are extremely impressive because they encompass not only the usual aspects of a medical center but also a view of the patient and society that is both realistic and altruistic. This view embraces the whole man as man and his human needs and resources.

THIRTEEN ARTICLES OF FAITH*
WE BELIEVE
ARTICLE I

Since the span of human life is short, compared to the long procession of time, and

Since disease constantly threatens and often succeeds in abbreviating life before the course is run,

It is incumbent upon us to rescue those who are physically ship-wrecked and help them round out their full span of years.

ARTICLE II

Since major diseases are difficult to diagnose and costly to cure, and

Since people who suffer from major diseases require specialized attention,

It is our duty to offer such people the best physical, medical and surgical care known to science.

ARTICLE III

Since the patient's recovery often depends on his confidence in the care he receives, and

Since specialized diagnosis and treatment of major illnesses can best be carried out in a properly staffed, well-equipped medical center,

It is our duty to create a center where work is performed by fulltime doctors, technicians and nurses, unhampered by outside interests, and augmented by the knowledge and experience of specialists in private practice who are able and willing to give their services.

ARTICLE IV

Since the conquest of major diseases must be carried on not only in the clinic, the hospital, the conference room, but more especially in the laboratory, and

Since a medical center which has well-equipped and specialized hospitals, clinics and laboratories is the logical place for medical education,

It is our duty to develop to the utmost degree facilities for basic and clinical research, as well as for medical education.

ARTICLE V

Since the fight against major diseases requires maximum physical and mental strength, and

Since the cost of financing the cure of a major disease is often beyond the reach of the patient,

---

*City of Hope, Los Angeles. Reprinted by permission.

It is our duty to give the patient all necessary care and treatment on a free basis in order to set his mind at rest and enable him to obtain a more certain and speedier recovery.

ARTICLE VI

Since the high spirit of the patient is most vital in the fight against disease, and

Since in this modern age the feeling of being a recipient of charity lowers the morale of the patient, and

Since we feel there is no profit in saving the body if in the process we destroy the soul,

It is our duty to maintain the dignity of the patient by avoiding all implication of charity in our service.

ARTICLE VII

Since the home is the foundation of our civilization and our happiness, and

Since to save the life of a loved one stricken by catastrophic disease, the family is willing to dispose of the home, the means of livelihood, and even go into debt, and

Since these factors pauperize the family, destroy the home, and adversely affect the recovery of the sick one,

It is our duty to assume the responsibility of the patient's care, thereby helping to maintain the dignity of the family and the security of the home.

ARTICLE VIII

Since the patient who suffers from a major disease will recover more rapidly under gentle, kind and considerate care, and

Since such care can be given only by those who have a personal rather than an impersonal attitude,

It is our duty to bring into our service only such people as are motivated by a deep humanitarian impulse.

ARTICLE IX

Since we do not always succeed in our fight to save life, and

Since it sometimes becomes necessary to prepare a patient for departure from this world,

It is our duty to create for such departure an atmosphere of kindness, love and compassion.

ARTICLE X

Since the restoration of health and the saving of life should be the concern of all mankind, and

Since such unique service requires the wholehearted voluntary contributions and voluntary efforts of a great many people,

It is fitting that the work of the City of Hope should be carried on by a People's Movement.

ARTICLE XI

Since every human being has the right to life, health and happiness, regardless of race, creed or nationality, and

Since the sick should not be denied healing because of race, creed or nationality, and

Since the worker or student should not be discriminated against because of race, creed or nationality,

It is our duty to adhere to a broad nonsectarian policy in all our services, thereby strengthening the American principle of democracy.

ARTICLE XII

Since "man does not live by bread alone," and has a hunger and a need for spiritual nourishment, and

Since the City of Hope has created values which form a more enriched spiritual diet, and

Since helping others offers rich sustenance for the spirit,

It is true that wholehearted participation in the City of Hope movement will give people enriched spiritual nourishment.

ARTICLE XIII

Since materialism is rampant in our society, and

Since the antidote for such materialism is a return to spiritual, moral and ethical values, and

Since the City of Hope is fostering such values,

It is incumbent upon us to bring to the attention of the people of our nation our philosophies, our aims and our objectives.

TORCHBEARER'S CREED*

We bear witness to individual worth and human dignity. Our stress on the sacredness of man, formed in God's image, repudiates the cynicism that "life is cheap." If our concept is fully accepted, could there be wars to snuff out lives, dictatorship to enslave people, crimes of violence and greed?

We bear witness to the necessity for enhancing the personality of the human being. This is an age of conformity and everyone

---

*City of Hope, Los Angeles. Reprinted by permission.

is being forced into a common mold. We reject the mass man and insist on bringing out the richness of genius, of dissent, of differences. The American heritage takes pride in the principle of e pluribus unum—unity in diversity. In this fashion we bring out the finest potential in every person. Self-realization and self-fulfillment will assure the maximum contribution to our culture and society.

We bear witness that democracy, properly organized and intelligently directed, can develop a large reservoir of leadership. Democracy is becoming a faceless thing, a mere matter of counting noses, which encourages the "one leader cult." Organizations like the City of Hope must resist this trend, making it possible for people to be somebodies in a world of nobodies.

We bear witness to the responsibility of each of us to be our "brother's keeper." This means more than the social obligation of rescuing those plunged from the bright sunshine of health into the despairing darkness of disease. It involves a framework of social justice, emphasizing our larger social responsibility and man's humanity to man.

We bear witness that life can be lived to the full only by giving more fully of ourselves. Many people are lonely because they build walls around themselves, rather than bridges to others. We affirm that to "love thy neighbor as thyself" is as important for the one who gives love as the one who receives it.

We bear witness that the resources of mankind must be mobilized for constructive and not destructive purposes. "Atoms for Life" has been the theme of the City of Hope for many years and this symbolizes our conviction that the wealth and talents of men should be directed to the advancement of the sum total of human welfare.

We bear witness that spiritual values and humanitarian impulses must guide our everyday lives. Today people have lost their moorings and drift aimlessly, living empty lives. Men and women will accept a creed that gives life a purpose and each day a meaning.

Illinois State Psychiatric Institute

The philosophy for the Illinois State Psychiatric Institute spells out nine concepts in terms of function, problems, and stereotypes. This philosophy is a veritable minicourse in psychiatric nursing, intentionally constructed as such to provide guidance for administration, teaching, and supervision of nursing in that institution while still retaining the overview or broad-base philosophy from which the practice derives. Its concreteness goes a long way toward helping staff operate within this philosophic framework, closing the gap between what should be and what is the state of nursing care in a particular setting.

1. Man is an integrated biological, emotional, and intellectual organism. Life experiences which affect one aspect of man affect man in totality.
2. Man cannot live alone. What he is endowed with at birth is developed by his contacts with others. Man becomes much of what he is through interpersonal experiences. The kind of living experiences he has makes the difference between health and illness.
3. Man cannot be understood apart from his culture.
4. The human being has worth.
5. Behavior is goal-directed and purposeful.
6. Anxiety is a dynamic force, common to all people, which serves to inhibit or motivate receptivity and function.
7. People interact in terms of mutual needs.
8. A person's needs must be met at his level of development before he can move to a more mature level.
9. Behavior changes within short periods of time. Sufficient stress can cause marked behavioral changes within short periods of time.*

Concept 6, which deals with anxiety, has wide applicability. The following shows the development of this concept in the total philosophic construct:

Concept: Anxiety is a dynamic force, common to all people, which serves to inhibit or motivate receptivity and function.
   A. Function: Because the concept is so, nurses:
      1. Recognize and understand the various manifestations of anxiety.
      2. Evaluate the level of anxiety present to determine whether it is useful or inhibiting.
      3. Are aware of the patient's capacity to tolerate various living experiences; use interpersonal and technical skills to reduce anxiety when it overwhelms the patient or interferes with his functioning.
      4. Anticipate and participate in preparation of patients for new experiences as a way of

---

*From Norris, C., and associates: Administration for creative nursing, Nurs. Forum **1**(3):106-117, 1962.

preventing unnecessary anxiety. (The nurse can help patients meet new experiences in healthier ways when she has been adequately informed of admissions, research projects, administrative changes, treatment changes, etc.)
   5. Observe patient behavior and share information with allied disciplines to collaboratively plan means of reducing patient anxiety.
   6. Attempt to examine their own anxiety and how this contributes to patient and staff anxiety.
B. Problems: Interference with the development of creative roles occurs because nurses:
   1. May manifest anxiety which is reflected in patient groups.
   2. Are under pressure to make changes which are not based on identification of realities of the situation.
   3. Are expected to make changes which are not based on staff understanding and readiness to accept.
   4. Are often not able to deal with new situations properly, due to being given information too late to plan adequate communication.
   5. Are often anxious and concerned over overstepping their role, or are unclear where roles do overlap.
C. Stereotypes: Stereotypes in relation to this concept:
   1. The nurse operates at the "do level" rather than the skill level.
   2. The nurse operates interpersonally only on an intuitive basis.*

One can see the profundity of these concepts that, by their skillful elaboration, are translated to statements more easily applicable to mental health, as well as other branches of nursing.

OBJECTIVES IN PLANNING

Whether explicit, as goal determination is incorporated in management by objectives, or implicit, as the rationally defined purpose of administration for which achievement plans are made, goal or objective is the sine qua non of planning. Also, this goal or objective must be so familiar to planners that they can view it from many points in order to plot the design for the orderly disposition of the array of persons and material involved.

---
*From Norris, C., and associates: Administration for creative nursing, Nurs. Forum 1(3):106-117, 1962.

By so doing, the purpose, subsequent planning, and execution can be achieved in the most deliberate and economical way possible. It is essential that the goal or objective, including breakdown of its parts, be stated in writing. This leads to refinement, clarity, and precision as the plan develops and as personnel are continuously involved in this formulation of goal or objective.

So far we have used goal, purpose, and objective interchangeably; they are essentially the same. Aim could be added too. Something toward which effort is directed, an object or end to be attained, and purposeful directing of effort all share meaning in these terms. For greater precision and in practice, however, there are usages that, if not crystallizing the issues, at least provide common terminology. For the most part hospitals and nursing services use the term objectives, which flow from a philosophy or occasionally a purpose. If there is a purpose, it is a broad and overall statement from which the philosophy and objectives derive.

It is interesting and heartening to find a description of nursing care that places the primary emphasis on physical care, such as the objectives for the nursing service of the City of Hope Medical Center, below.* It is so often taken for granted or assumed to be satisfactory, whereas other components such as psychological and patient teaching that are known to be unsatisfactory are consequently featured. The frankness of the statement is valuable in thinking about priorities in nursing care:

   1. To give the highest possible quality of nursing care in terms of total patient needs. This will involve physical needs which must always have priority in nursing service, followed by spiritual, psychological, social, rehabilitative, and educational needs as they are defined by nursing service personnel and diagnosed in order of priority.
   2. To assist the physician in the medical care of the patient, and to carry out such therapy as he prescribes.
   3. To promote programs of nursing education; to provide facilities for the development of all categories of nursing service personnel.

---
*City of Hope, Los Angeles. Reprinted by permission.

4. To promote and encourage nursing research studies in order that the quality of performance may be improved and maximum utilization of personnel obtained.

5. To assess the quality of the nursing service and continuously build facilities and prepare personnel to improve on this quality.

6. To promote participation in the allied health organizations and supportive community activities.

These objectives remind one of a similar statement by Blake,[2] a veteran practitioner: "I needed much more experience before I could be free to see the individuality of the child, before I could relate to the child more than to the equipment and routine procedures. It was not that I was oblivious to the child's need for emotional support; it was because I could not give it until I had mastered the skills necessary to provide the physically protective nursing care required."

• • •

From the philosophy and objectives of the hospital and nursing service will come departmental and unit statements. Their variation will be essentially directed to clinical specialities or settings: the constant, sophisticated vigilance of the coronary or intensive care units, the patience and persistence of long-term care, the swiftness and precision of emergency procedures, the familial emphasis of the obstetrical units, and so on, will characterize such statements and will be variations on the primary and comprehensive theme of the nursing service.

Harper Hospital (a division of United Hospitals of Detroit)

The following current (1975) philosophy and objectives of Harper Hospital reflect the contemporary concern for professional accountability, consultative management, and commitment to the team approach.

PHILOSOPHY OF NURSING FOR THE NURSING DEPARTMENTS*

The nursing departments of the Harper Division of the United Hospitals of Detroit believe that nursing is a process of identifying and meeting the physical, socio-emotional, and spiritual needs of the patient. This requires collaboration with the physician, as well as other health professionals and departments of the hospital.

The patient care environment of Harper Hospital is characterized by complex, ever-changing internal and external situations, which require immediate decision making and plans for action. Therefore, the organizational structure must permit adaptiveness to a situation at a given point in time under a particular set of circumstances. Furthermore, we believe the control of patient care and personnel performance can take place best at the operational level (nursing unit). We believe that patient care in this kind of setting can be best organized around a team approach. Due to the increased complexities of patient care, we also believe that, whenever possible, patients should be grouped according to the level of care required, or a specialty service.

Competent staff available for all positions in adequate numbers are essential to provide quality care. Therefore, salaries and fringe benefits must be reviewed at regular intervals and adjusted accordingly to keep positions competitive with those of the community. We believe that all employees of the Nursing Department must be afforded a comprehensive orientation program, as well as continuing staff development programs. In addition, we expect each professional to assume responsibility for their own professional growth and development. Whenever possible, promotions without discrimination with regard to sex or race will take place from within.

The nursing departments of the Harper Division believe that patient care and nursing education are supplementary and complementary. Therefore, the nursing departments will conduct educational programs when appropriate and/or participate and support educational endeavors of the health professions whenever possible.

The nursing departments also believe that, as a major medical-surgical component of the Detroit Medical Center, we have the responsibility and obligation to continually seek ways to improve the delivery of patient care. Thus, the staff is encouraged to be involved in research endeavors related to patient care and support those of other professionals.

*Courtesy Harper Hospital, a division of United Hospitals of Detroit.

Lastly, the nursing departments believe that, for any organization to remain viable, there must be periodic evaluation of all levels of the organization, and provisions for necessary changes as needed, in order to maintain its effectiveness.

The objectives for the nursing departments of Harper Hospital are as follows.*

1. Develop an organizational structure that will:
   a. Permit the nursing staff to meet the physical, socio-emotional, and spiritual needs of the patient.
   b. Permit adaptiveness to a given situation at a given point in time.
   c. Permit decision making at the level the action takes place.
   d. Exact accountability for the job at each level of the organization.
   e. Foster a team approach to patient care.
   f. Allow for grouping of patients by level of care and/or specialty service.
2. Develop a competent staff in adequate numbers:
   a. Maintain an active recruitment program.
   b. Maintain an active Staff Development Program.
   c. Recognize superior performance by promotion whenever possible.
   d. Collaborate with Administration and Personnel to keep positions competitive with community practice with regard to salaries and fringe benefits.
3. Develop and/or support educational programs:
   a. Maintains educational programs as needed to meet community or educational needs.
   b. Supports and/or participates in educational programs in the medical center and community.
4. Seeks ways to improve patient care:
   a. Encourages and supports research endeavors of the staff.
   b. Participates in research programs conducted by the university and/or other health professionals.
5. Strives to increase organizational effectiveness:
   a. Periodic evaluation of all departments.
   b. Makes necessary revisions/changes as indicated.

CLARITY AND INTEGRITY OF PURPOSE

Clarity of purpose is the requisite for planning. It must always be seen in relation to the work to be accomplished, but must go hand in hand with reality. If this relationship does not exist, reality may be bypassed. This has happened often where the preoccupation of the planners has excluded their own real world as they assembled lofty phrases often gleaned from the literature. Goals and plans should represent real possibilities and be attainable, while reaching up to high standards as well. Sometimes reality is truly stark where sheer numbers to be cared for obviate the individualized care or semblance to the comprehensive care stated in the objectives. In circumstances where stated goals seem out of reach, even minute amounts of time spent with or for patients, within the framework of the goals, will be valuable.

Schlotfeldt[3] reminds us of the discrepancy between what we claim to do, as demonstrated in philosophic statements, and what we do in actual practice. Cantor[4] points out this discrepancy and recommends the application of reality to objectives and the essential understanding of those charged with the implementation of the objectives. She says in another way what Peterson[5] said in 1963: nursing objectives must be specific, practical, and attainable if they are to have any real meaning or application in actual nursing practice. Whether it is closing a gap between the ideal and the real or making stated objectives consonant with nursing practice, we can never achieve order and coherence in practice until progress is made in reconciling objectives to practice. It remains essentially a problem of raising the quality of nursing care until it equals that nursing care we know is possible and which we enunciate in objectives. Objectives, like nursing care plans, assignments, or any other administrative ingredient or device must be vitalized by appropriate nursing performance if they are to be realized. These objectives will remain sterile unless an all-out attempt is made to have them operative in the particular setting.

Gross's concept of "teletics" is helpful here [p. 469].[6] He regards purpose and purposefulness as being the ingredients of teletics. By considering purpose and purposefulness together, we might hasten the

---
*Courtesy Harper Hospital, a division of United Hospitals of Detroit.

day when the gap is closed between the ideal and the real. By directing attention of all to purposefulness and by intent, resolute, and ongoing attention to the purpose (ideal care), we may succeed in doing what we say should be done. We must close this gap if we are to achieve the unity necessary to carry forward nursing's goals. Without clarity there is danger that the diffuse or imprecise view of the purpose will carry over into planning and subsequently into execution of the plan. For example, in planning for the staffing of a hospital, floor, or unit, the exact duties of each worker must be known so that the staffing plan and consequent budget will reflect these exact duties. If nurses are doing 30% nonnursing duties, the staffing plan is not precise, nor is the budget. The plan may provide for equitable compensation, fair distribution of desirable hours, generous fringe benefits, and so forth, but be deficient because the planners did not take into consideration optimal utilization of personnel. Such a plan does not go far enough to cover the whole job.

This necessary precision in goal clarification demonstrates the need for sound collateral investigation (such as consideration of staffing and budgeting together) in order to arrive at a refined goal. Plans deriving from the refined, examined goal have a greater chance of successful achievement.

GOALS OF WORKERS AND ORGANIZATION

The closer one can mesh the goals of the organization and the goals of the workers, the better. The goals of workers are unlimited. The overriding goal is probably financial compensation, for a variety of reasons—a house, vacation, education of children, sole or partial support of a family, and so forth. Added to these are interest in the hospital or health field, need to feel useful outside of or escape from the home, a strong service orientation, and companionship, among other reasons. A worker's goals may or may not coincide with those of the hospital; yet through open and frank discussion, seemingly incompatible goals can be brought at least closer, if not together. Working for money is not bad, nor does it rule out altruistic goals on the secondary level. Indifference of the worker to the goal of the nursing service may be due to lack of understanding or knowledge of what the goal of the nursing service is. We have been notoriously poor at communicating to workers the goals of the nursing service. Morever, if we do not understand the goals ourselves, we cannot communicate them adequately.

Arendt and associates'[7] observation about the effect of teacher attitudes on students has application here. They cite the need for teachers of humanities to believe that what they are teaching is important, not just beautiful or interesting. Likewise, it behooves managers of nursing service to convey the importance of the goal to which nursing is devoted, so that the workers can appreciate it to a higher and growing degree.

Since people, especially the young, talk much these days about values in our society, perhaps it would be helpful if we try to assimilate into the goals of the enterprise some general and various values held by workers. It is not a matter of low compatibility so much as low communication; when values are explored, analyzed, and conceptualized, compatibility of workers' and institutional values is highly probable. It is the amorphousness of values rather than the values themselves that may prevent their absorption.

For example, the considerable value placed on environmentalism in our culture has potential correlation to the goal of optimal nursing care. This particular commonly held value can be elaborated to show its contribution to quality nursing care by control of the internal environment of the patient in terms of quiet, nonobtrusive, rest-producing measures of nursing care, or of achieving simplicity and order amid complex, conglomerate materials. As the mutuality of environmentalism and nursing care is explored, the applications become more apparent. Talking nicely to plants to encourage them to grow, a perhaps whimsical aspect of environmentalism, has many corollaries in the patient setting. It is the conceptualization of the value and the goal that brings congruence.

In addition, the goals of the organization must be not only clear, but relevant and command the loyalty of the workers. If competent and compassionate nursing care is the goal, then areas where critical care is given must be staffed appropriately by adequately prepared personnel. If for reasons of budget deficit or short supply staff is removed from or not available for critical care areas, workers see the goal eroded, and they become cynical and incapable of loyalty to the goal. Compromise is possible here too. There may be other valid ways to compensate for these cuts in personnel so that the integrity of the workers' loyalty to the goal is maintained. However, all elements of the compromise must be known to staff to assure continuing loyalty. If the noble purpose of nursing could be communicated and faith in the splendid outcomes demonstrated difficulties and hardships could be more easily borne, though they must receive appropriate attention.

FORECASTING

Forecasting is important to planning. It describes the ultimate condition or projections that provide general incentive and direction to planning. It also provides time for planning, which crises and immediacy prevent. For example, the rising public clamor about hospital care, measurable by a systematic survey of popular magazines in the last two decades, provides forecasting material that can give general incentive and direction to planning for the overall upgrading of nursing care or the selection of key areas to be upgraded. Similarly, documentation of the nurse shortage is an illustration of forecasting that has given rise to planning for optimal utilization of nurses. There is clinical forecasting, too, as medicine is refined and new procedures come into existence. Open heart surgery, renal dialysis, and coronary care units all illustrate the forecasting component of planning and staffing.

INTERNAL MOVEMENT OF PLANS

Movement from the general to the specific is an aid in planning, because it allows goals to become guidelines, which in turn become policies. Guidelines and policies have commonalities. Gross supports the need for generalization in working through plans [p. 17].[6] He says that it expands the view, thus removing one from regular, routine activities; illumines or points out alternatives, often imaginative, thus making selection easier; keeps the person selecting more judiciously from copious materials; and points out the comforting universality of problems. A planning committee representative of all levels of nursing and time for selected individual formulation of tentative plans or for projected outside contacts provided to a nursing assessment committee seem to partake of both generalization and specification. Policies (generalization) can then be developed into procedures (specification). Standards are operative at all stages, which help the plan to be developed in an orderly way; provide ultimate specificity so that loopholes, vagueness, and error may be reduced or eliminated; and help in the execution, control, and evaluation of the plan. The philosophy of the Illinois State Psychiatric Institute (pp. 54-55) demonstrates development from the general to the particular.

An interesting and helpful distinction in planning consists of repeat-use and single-use plans [in Haiman[8]]. Repeat-use plans are those that have been formulated and are repetitive, for example, staffing or audit procedures. The plan will be implemented successively each time the procedures are repeated. These plans are closely related to guidelines, policies, and procedures. Single-use plans are those which are completed when they are implemented. Projects to gauge time utilization of the professional nurse, to plan for the implementation of the audit procedure, for staff orientation and instruction, or to draw up an annual budget are examples of single-use plans. Planning the audit procedure, to be used over and over again, and one-time preparation of personnel to do the audit, show a combination of the two.

LONG- AND SHORT-RANGE GOALS

In planning for the nursing service one must look at the quality of the nursing care being given, deliberate about what kinds of improvements are indicated and possible, and then lay out the long- and short-range goals. For example, the long-range goal of improved nursing care given over a 3½-year period could be broken down into short-range goals, such as 6-month increments devoted to an assessment program, selection and priority setting, increase in discharge plans and referrals, upgrading of the psychological and emotional component of care, improved physical care, incorporation of rehabilitation techniques, and evaluation of progress in the achievement of these short-range goals.

In the 6-month nursing care assessment phase of planning, the nursing staff would read, examine, and collect data individually, then discuss and review findings with each other and with outsiders, in order to learn what is ideal. To reach a realistic appraisal of the institution's current nursing care, interviews and opinion polls with the nursing and medical staff, other services, patients, former patients, families and friends, and community can be used. This realistic appraisal becomes the baseline that provides direction to successive steps. It describes the nursing service in a given institution at a given time. Goals for improvement that are possible within a given institution's strengths and limitations will be found between this baseline of what current nursing practice is and what the ideal should be.

The time allocation and survey of the above sources of information in the appraisal phase constitute guidelines, or a first step, for carrying forward the plan for the goal of general upgrading of nursing care.

The short-range goal of assessment of existing nursing care in the light of what is ideal and capable of being achieved in the particular institution can be converted to a management by objectives format, because much is quantifiable, all levels are involved, and a time schedule can be provided. It can be a three-part objective: learning what is ideal, learning what is extant in the institution, and comparing the extant with the ideal.

As Palmer[9] points out, dialogues and memos, which are in effect contracts covering what exactly will be accomplished in a given time period, can be set up from the director of nursing to each associate, assistant, and supervisor, for the broad breakdown of review of ideal nursing by nature, definition, and component parts. Sources are essentially the literature, field visits, and interviews with experts. Dialogues and memos can be carried out between the associates, assistants, supervisors, and head nurses for more specific parts of this general review. An alternative would be having associates and assistants provide the library work for the supervisors, who would then confer with the head nurses and write down what they would be responsible for in reviewing ideal possibilities. This would allow natural opportunity for the clinical supplement to the common core of the nursing care.

The next step would involve much data collection as each component part of nursing is examined in the institution. Division of the assessment by categories for which there are dialogues and memos in the same arrangement as step one is a possibility. Considerable specificity is possible and called for here.

For example, in the physical component of care such items will need to be checked as the numbers of bed and partial baths; the components of partial baths; the facilities and utilization of bath and toilet areas, including surfaces for the patient's equipment; the number per day and nature of patients receiving backrubs and foot and toenail care; the numbers of patients positioned for maximum respiratory and/or circulatory facility; the number of patients to be fed completely, partially, or minimally, as well as observation of food and fluid intake by all patients; the kind and degree of exercise engaged in by or administered to patients; the appropriate amount of light and air; and proximity and security of call light, water, and so forth. A survey of untoward accidents and incidents, the number and nature of pressure sores, and hypostatic pneumonia or emboli for their possible physical component is of concern in assessing this aspect of nursing care. This is not an exhaustive listing of findings that can be counted.

Because provision for nursing care outside the hospital is one of the overriding weaknesses in nursing service in general, it might be given first priority as a short-range goal in the long-range plan. Moreover, it has the advantage of being quite visible when compared with appraising the physical aspect of care. On any day in any institution the number of patients for whom there are discharge plans can be determined, and it will be pitifully small! The next step is to determine by category how many patients require discharge plans. This is followed by a listing of services available inside and outside the hospital and then bringing together in specific terms the patients' discharge needs with the resources available.

In determining patients' discharge needs, checklists might be helpful in order to routinize appraisal. These provide standards to be used in carrying the plan forward. It should be noted that routine here means bringing order and clarity to the appraisal, so that items are not missed or left to chance. For the patient with congestive heart failure, a checklist could be prepared regarding diet, exercise, work, medication, weight and edema, living arrangements, life style, and so forth. This list could be modified for the patient who has coronary artery disease.

Checklists make it possible to appraise the needs for individual patients after discharge. Special diet is an important long-range need of the patient with cardiac disease. The plan should outline the steps to be taken well before discharge, in order to acquaint patients and their families with low-cholesterol, low-sodium diets and allow opportunity for a followup appointment with the dietitian for questions. One can see that a plan for dietary care of patients at home provides much more than the cursory visit of the dietitian to present a printed plan on the day of or prior to discharge. In fact, the beginning of the instruction can occur immediately following the crucial period of the hospitalization rather than at the end, ensuring time and opportunity to assess whether the instruction has been absorbed by the patient and family. The dietetic department will provide the outline and instruction. However, dietetic services are dependent on nurses for timing and scheduling so that the instruction can be carefully and thoroughly assimilated by the patient and family. Nurses also provide reinforcement for dietary instruction. There is a coordination factor, too, because the question of whether the dietitian or the nurse tells the patient about alcoholic restrictions arises when one works interdepartmentally on patient instruction. There are many such gray areas for which provision must be made.

Another facet of discharge plans for the patient with cardiac disease is help in utilizing the services of the state or local unit of the American Heart Association. One must know if these services are available in a given geographical area. For example, nurses should be aware of the kinds of literature that are available for public use and the number of times a year, dates, and content of public lectures that are offered. The services of the Visiting Nurse Association, the availability of home health aides, and volunteer services to the elderly are examples of other community resources that must be known about.

One must not assume that services are

not available because an area is small, remote, or rural; the enterprising nursing staff can find and list persons in the community who might take on volunteer or professional services for people in their homes. For example, the patient with terminal cancer who wishes to spend some time at home before death can be aided to do so if a family member is taught how to give injections and a nurse is found in the community to give the occasional intravenous infusion or whatever the patient might need during this time.

In planning for helping patients after discharge, one must also consider how to best utilize not only the resources of the hospital and community but of the nursing department itself. For example, must all nurses become proficient at appraising needs, giving instructions, and making contacts within and without the hospital, or should nurses be selected for various parts of the job? In answering these questions, staffs will have to assess the effectiveness of discharge plans where a public health nurse is part of the staff, including how effective she has been; whether her effectiveness depends on the appraisal skills of all nurses; and whether appraisal skills of the staff are developed by her, visits to homes and agencies, or other means. The absence of a public health nurse should not be a deterrent to planning a workable, effective patient discharge plan: the in-service department can contribute to establishing a plan of this kind; and nurses with special attributes, interests, or skills can be used in special ways, such as filling the role of internal clinical consultants. Medical staff and nurses should be supportive of discharge planning. The appraisal and analysis of all factors that can be brought to bear on setting up plans for improving the discharge planning for patients, or any other plan, must be thorough.

Besides the large-scale appraisal and upgrading of nursing in general, there are many long- and short-range goals for nursing services that need attention. Palmer[9] provides some fine examples, such as reduction in medication error by a specific percentage in a specific time, tightening the time for admission procedure after arrival of the patient on a unit, reduction in the number of back injuries suffered by nursing personnel by a specific percentage, study of feasibility of conversion to taped change of shift reports, conversion to cyclical staffing or team nursing, and decentralized budgeting to unit level.

EVALUATION

Evaluation of the plan must be incorporated in the formative stages, or it will be ineffective. Checks on progress achievement are best made at regular intervals during formulation and implementation of the plan.

The first step is the involvement of those responsible for carrying out and evaluating the plan in the initial stages, so that all aspects are considered. These people are familiar with the steps, having helped formulate, find, and determine them, and so are able to assess the success or failure of the plan. Moreover, they will have to be aware of the traps, so that they can avoid them, prevent others from falling into them, and evaluate the effect of the traps on the execution of the plan. For example, there is sure to be the complaint that provision for discharge planning would be too time consuming for the existing staff. The response to this complaint cannot be reprimand, but a concrete demonstration of the time involved to do it, step by step, showing how it can be fitted in or, if necessary, how something else can be left undone or postponed in order to do it. The plan can be shown to be streamlined. Alternative methods of expeditiously carrying out the plan can be delineated. The concrete demonstration can be accompanied by discussion, at various times and in various places, of how we always find time to do what we think necessary (for example, carrying out physicians' orders). There must be frank admission that there will indeed be times when a service will have to be deferred in favor of a more crucial one; recognition that there are patient needs just as vital to their welfare as what we now find time to do; asking if we are not avoiding the less familiar in favor of the familiar, rather than giving equal time to all of a patient's needs that can be met by the nurse; and wondering if these new means of helping patients will not become second nature to us.

Evaluation will be easier and more effective if it is thought about in the beginning of the plan. For example, the increase in the number of discharge plans for patients can be counted and compared with numbers in the time span prior to implementation. They can also be viewed and reviewed for their thoroughness and effectiveness. Followup with patients at home after discharge is necessary too, because only in this way can the plan's effectiveness be tested. This involves telephone calls, letters, and home visits for firsthand evaluation. Contact with the patient after discharge is almost nonexistent at present. Agencies that have been used will also need to be contacted for the same reasons. Followup will have to become a regular part of the nurses' work if they are to know whether their plans for discharge helped, and if not, why not, so that the plan can be reviewed, revised, continued, or terminated.

Another managerial device, developed by the U.S. Navy and others, that also contains the specificity and continuous evaluation of plans as they are implemented, is the Program Evaluation and Review Technique (PERT). It is a visual and mathematical schema known as a network which demonstrates the steps and/or parts of the plan, with accompanying articulations and timetables for purposes of monitoring, evaluating, and revising, if necessary, as the plan becomes actualized. Hence control of the implementation is continuous and built into the plan. Alternatives or exchanges can be initiated while the implementation is underway. It is yet another way of keeping close track of the operation by specific and precise formulation.

COMPREHENSIVENESS OF PLANNING

Comprehensiveness permeates the planning process when the difficulties of change are seen as determining the purpose and values, the use of staff and development of managers, communication, resistance or acceptance of change, conflict, or cooperation, and control [in Bennis and associates[10]]. It is an important part of the enterprise, providing the cornerstone from which other parts of administration emanate.

EXAMPLE OF HOSPITAL PLANNING

A beautifully sophisticated and detailed structure for hospital planning is provided by Webber and Dula.[11] Their work is based on a long-range planning committee for the hospital in which the current buffeting by regulatory agencies, consumers, and such is overcome by skillful, searching, open, and systematized planning. It parallels to some degree the planning for comprehensive nursing care described earlier (see pp. 60-62).

This committee work begins with the external analysis instead of the customary internal examination. Environmental scanning is part of this first stage in which all sectors—administrators, physicians, lay board members, and perhaps community members—engage in data collection to provide a base. The next stage consists of internal analysis, or the collection of data necessary to see the hospital's responses to data from external analysis, such as unmet needs of various communities for services, utilization, and cost containment. Issue analysis comprises the third phase, in which specific issues are examined, such as overbedding, decline in obstetrical care, and consolidation. After deliberation of these stages comes alternative analysis.

Only after the committee has worked through to alternative proposals followed as widely as possible by the hospital constituents is the hospital management in the appropriate position to decide among the alternatives and move on to goal setting within the framework of a long-range plan.

The committee work continues, relying on its educational support in overcoming resistance to change as the long-range plan is put into operation. Comprehensiveness pervades such planning work so that relationships are visible, the parts are articulated, and the hospital moves clearer and more realistic goals forward. These goals progress not unilaterally but interlaterally, in conjunction with the diverse forces affecting them. Systematic consideration of all elements enables the hospital to control its destiny.

• • •

Planning requires forecasting, generalization, analysis, detail, and specificity. It precedes action and should systematize and provide the base for action. Action is the implementation, or execution, of the plan.

Planning can be summed up by Urwick's characteristics of a good plan:

1. That it be based on a clearly defined objective.
2. That it be simple.
3. That it provides for a proper analysis and classification of actions, i.e., that it establishes standards.
4. That it is flexible.
5. That it is balanced.
6. That it uses available resources to the utmost before creating new authorities and new resources—really a special application of the principle of simplicity.*

---

*From Urwick, L.: The elements of administration, New York, 1942, Harper & Row Publishers, p. 34.

REFERENCES

1. Harris, S.: America should plan ahead, Vancouver, Wash., The Columbian, October 13, 1973.
2. Blake, F.: In quest of hope and autonomy, Nurs. Forum **1**(1):10, 1961-62.
3. Schlotfeldt, R.: Planning for progress, Nurs. Outlook **21**(12):766-769, 1973.
4. Cantor, M.: Philosophy, purpose and objectives; why do we have them? J. Nurs. Admin. [Refresher] **3**(4):21-25, 1973.
5. Peterson, G.: Specific, practical and attainable objectives, Nurs. Outlook, **11**:341-343, 1963.
6. Gross, B. M.: The managing of organizations, vol. 1, New York, 1964, The Free Press, pp. 17 and 469.
7. Arendt, H., and associates: Values in contemporary society, New York, 1974, Rockefeller Foundation, p. 21.
8. Haiman, T.: Supervisory management for hospitals and related health facilities, St. Louis, 1965, Catholic Hospital Association, p. 84.
9. Palmer, J.: Management by objectives, J. Nurs. Admin. **3**(5):59, 1973.
10. Bennis, W., Bennis, K., and Chin, R.: The planning of change, ed. 2, New York, 1969, Holt, Rinehart and Winston, Inc., p. 65.
11. Webber, J., and Dula, M.: Effective planning committees for hospitals, Harvard Business Review **52**(3):133-142, 1974.

CHAPTER 6
ORGANIZING

The terms administration and organization are often used to describe the nursing service. This common practice suggests that administering and organizing are a pair of activities used together to achieve a purpose. In a general sense, when someone or a group makes arrangements, contacts people, sets up schedules, and so forth, they are frequently referred to as organizing a project. However, they are doing more, because the term organize in this context may embrace other administrative aspects, such as staffing, planning, directing, controlling, and so on. Though organization often is used loosely as a synonym for administration or management, it is actually a clear-cut and important component of administration or management. Likewise, juxtaposition of terms as above presents an imprecise picture that works against the exact use of the concepts of administration and organization. They are indeed related; the relationship, however, is not one of equality, but one of inclusion. Organization is a vital part of administration. Similarly, organizing does not embrace other elements of administration, but works in partnership with them to achieve purpose. They are all cooperating elements of administration, directed toward achievement of objectives.

To further discourage this common tendency to equate organization and administration, or impregnate the term organize with other functions of administration, the use of the term enterprise (an activity that is systematic and purposeful) is useful; though they mean essentially the same thing, enterprise is free of the generic denotation of organization.

CHARACTERISTICS

An organizational structure is dynamic: it is people in their infinite variety occupying positions and interacting in prescribed ways to achieve a purpose (for example, nursing care). The arrangement may be altered as new methods are tried or old ones modified; new persons, procedures, or services are added or others eliminated or regrouped; or by expansion of plant or bed capacity, or both, in the complex hospital enterprise. Attention should be paid to economy of resources an essential criterion of administration. The organizational structure needs frequent appraisal to ensure the continuing appropriateness of positions and their articulations as an enterprise moves through changes. Insuring the growth to be engendered by change requires thoroughgoing review of the structure for viability. However, overhauling it is a major operation and should not be taken lightly.

Drucker[1] cautions against reorganizing too frequently and without sufficient reason. He says that reorganization is justified when basic changes are introduced, such as those enumerated above, or as objectives shift.

There is a corresponding hazard in making required changes on a piecemeal basis, without reevaluating the total organizational structure so that the principles of precision and economy are respected. This hazard is especially applicable to nursing, because of the newness of the use and application of administrative theory and our penchant for doing instead of thinking.

Other things being equal, the greater the attention given to establishing and maintaining a viable organizational structure, derived from deliberation and understood by all, the better will be the performance of the workers and the quality of the nursing care given. The visualization of the organizational structure—the organization chart—has not attained the widest possible use in nursing services. It is there for inspectors to see, but whether it is used for the ongoing direction and evaluation of the nursing enterprise is problematic. The organization chart helps to dispel the confusion deriving from the complexity of today's enterprises by allowing workers to see how their parts fit into the total work of the department and of the whole institution in meeting the known objectives and purpose. A sound organizational structure prevents overlapping, because it demarks areas of responsibility, thus illuminating the gray areas causing the overlapping and the possible consequent friction. It shows workers *to* whom they are specifically responsible and *for* whom they are responsible. The organizational structure provides stability and balance for workers, thus making their efforts more purposeful and consequently satisfying.

An organizational structure is a pivotal device in administration. It not only supplies the articulating apparatus for planning to achieve the purpose of the enterprise, but it also provides the skeleton on which to staff the function. The numbers and kinds of personnel are directly related to the organizational structure, because it represents the purpose of the enterprise. Management personnel direct, coordinate, and control the nursing care provided to patients, within the framework of the organizational structure from which these activities emanate.

Gill[2] suggests that nurses make their present operation work satisfactorily before replacing it with a better one. This is sound advice, because it insists that weaknesses and deficiencies be identified so that they can be corrected. Such identification and correction provide a much stronger base for change than seeking to impose change on confusion and inefficiency. An example is the move from team to primary nursing. The worth of primary nursing should be seen in relationship to appropriately functioning team nursing, not some remnant of it.

ACCOUNTABILITY

The organizational structure delineates responsibility, that is, to whom and for whom one is responsible, and also for what one is responsible, as visualized in the job descriptions. Responsibility has an intimate relationship to accountability, which suggests more carefully circumscribed, communicated, and controlled responsibility. If staff is liable for their responsibility, they will demand that it be clear cut and precise. Proof of the requirement for accountability is the tremendous need for and increase in malpractice insurance for nurses.

Passos[3] provides a masterful treatment of accountability in likening it to the price we must pay for our increasing autonomy. If we are not "handmaidens" but partners on the health care scene, then we must answer for our performance, increasingly more exactly and concretely. She cites interest evoked by a formal Position on Nursing Practice of the Michigan Nurses' Association, in which accountability dominated the other three components of the Position, namely, goal sharing with other professionals, clinical judgment, and responsibility for one's own educational growth. She points out that if true accountability is to be achieved, liability in nursing must be accompanied by willingness to subject our practice to monitoring and peer review. Whether peership is hierarchical or horizontal within the institutional nursing structure and whether the personnel evaluation system in use is geared to this precise organizational formation are important questions in the relationship of accountability to the formal organizational structure.

Passos raises another salient question, so far unanswered but at least partially clarified by the organizational structure, concerning to whom the nurse is accountable: the patient, the enterprise, or the profession? Because there is accountability to all three, perhaps the more cogent question becomes one of priorities. Accountability to the patient and the enterprise would include accountability to the physician, unless it is assumed that the physician and the enterprise are the same. Though the institution grants physicians the privilege of treating patients there, and by doing so it might be construed that they too are answerable to the institution for their practice, actuality shows otherwise. Nurses' accountability to the patients in an institution is not complete at this time; they must exercise it either through the physician who has ultimate responsibility for the patient or through the organizational structure of the enterprise. In actual practice, when nurses see something incorrect being done to or for a patient, they must inform the physician, who may be doing the incorrect thing, and/or report the occurrence to superiors through the chain of command in nursing to the hospital administrator and hence to the appropriate persons in the hospital medical structure who should see that the correction is made. This route may be unwieldy but necessary for appropriate responsibility. It should be noted that the urgency of the observed incorrect action may require reducing the number of steps and going directly to a higher authority immediately.

The coronary care unit is a location where nurses' accountability is tried, because their practice may conflict with that of a physician. Accountability in this crucial area must be supported by sufficient protocols to enable them to carry out obligations to patients appropriately. If there are no specific protocols, then at least there must be immediate and ready access to physicians as specialized as these nurses in meeting the critical needs of these patients. It is the obligation of superiors in the hierarchical order to ensure such necessary protocols and access. For illumination of problems in this area, the *RN* journal nationwide survey is valuable.[4]

Passos refers to the need for continuing improvement in the documentation of nursing care. This also is essential in discharging accountability beyond nursing care, because it is necessary that documentation accompany a report to superiors of the incorrect action of a physician. This is a highly sensitive area, and there is usually reluctance to commit such actions to writing. However, accountability can be discharged in no other way than by documentation, which either rules out hearsay, imprecision, and error or isolates them.

There is an aspect of accountability worth noting here. While accountability is most frequently thought of as going to a superior, it should also be thought of as extending down to the workers for whose performance one is responsible. This is an important safeguard for human relationships, because it generates trust and a sincerity of intention conducive to goodwill.

DELEGATION OF RESPONSIBILITY

A concept related to accountability and inherent in the organizational structure is delegation of a particular or general assignment to carry forward the nursing goals for a particular patient. Such delegation transfers responsibility for assignments to subordinates who are authorized or thereby empowered to carry out the assignments and are then held accountable for satisfactory compliance in doing so. Such assignments are not arbitrary, but are within the framework of the objectives of the enterprise and are mutually explored at the outset so that they are clear and understood. Goodwill and commitment to the goals of the enterprise are presumed.

Delegation, responsibility, and accountability are clearly interwoven. They form a triad that operates at every level and laterally at some levels, for example, at the unit level. One delegates; another assumes responsibility and accounts to the delegator for the conduct of the assignment or the nursing affairs in operation. Relative to delegation, authority, and responsibility, one has the right to assistance with a problem and its ultimate solution from the superior or whoever delegated the authority.

It cannot be assumed that the nursing affairs of a unit or area will always be satisfactory. Realistically, there can be, frequently are, and perhaps should be dissatisfactory aspects that become problems to be examined, analyzed, evaluated, and remedied. Frequently heard is the complaint that someone was delegated responsibility without the authority to achieve the particular goal. Often the person to whom the responsibility was delegated receives interference from other sources and even from the delegator, is not provided the material or personal resources to carry out the responsibility, is refused cooperation by subordinates, and so forth. In each case, the impediment to carrying out the delegated responsibility must be identified and removed, or dual responsibility must be assumed by the superior and the subordinate. For example, commonly one is given the responsibility for the satisfactory care of a given number of patients with a given number of personnel. If it is seen that the personnel are performing efficiently and according to the standards already set for the institution, but are unable consistently to complete the work within a given time period, the situation must be assessed and all possibilities reviewed in an attempt to identify ways in which the responsibility can be met. There may be unwieldy procedures or equipment, less experienced personnel, unusual or seasonal increase in patients' nursing needs, clashing personalities, and so on. If it is found that nursing personnel are doing many nonnursing duties, figures should be kept to show how often and what these duties are, so that the superior can take the problem to his or her supervisor and colleagues. The person who is responsible for the work must do all that is possible to rectify the problems or discrepancies, but has a perfect right to the assistance and guidance of the superior. Moreover, the superior has an obligation to see that the responsibility delegated is indeed being carried out satisfactorily. Accountability is an ongoing activity for both the one delegating and the one assuming the responsibility.

Perhaps it is the periodic checking on the ongoing achievement of the delegated responsibility that causes nurses to complain of being given responsibility without authority, because it can be construed or even be the case that this is interference of the delegator or superior rather than legitimate observation of the delegated responsibility in process. Understanding the clear-cut delegation and its consequent instructions may help reduce this interference. If it is in fact over-solicitude on the part of the delegator, or oversensitivity on the part of the one assuming responsibility for the delegated assignment, the differences or frustrations should be worked out together or a third party should be brought in.

DECISION MAKING

The organizational structure assists the decision-making process, because it provides appropriate groupings for deliberations that obviate randomness and enhances consultative management. The director of nursing has access to key people to assist in the decision-making process, namely associates, assistants, and department heads. Likewise, each department head has supervisors, head nurses, or both, depending on the size of the enterprise; and the head nurse has staff nurses for the same purpose. The final decision of the particular administrator is potentially better, either because of the input of these persons or because it has been tested by subjection to scrutiny. The decision, moreover, is enriched by this wider dissemination and consequent support from these people, who either formally or informally constitute executive committees. This is not to say that there is not input or testing of ideas elsewhere than in the organizational structure; however, the formal organization does provide the decision maker with ready access to appropriately related and responsible colleagues. Decision making by incorporating subordinates enlists cooperation, which increases the partnership aspect of supervision and reduces its authoritarian potential, thus generating goodwill and increased work production.

LINE-STAFF CONCEPT

The line-staff concept is one of the oldest organizational principles. It provides for two kinds of responsibility in the organization.

The line part of the concept, the older of the two, consists of the responsibility for carrying forward the goals of the nursing department through a chain of command, that is, the hierarchical order consisting of the director of nursing, associates, assistants, supervisors (often assistant directors in large institutions), head nurses, team leaders where they function as heads of groups of workers charged with the care for a certain number of patients, and charge nurses on any shift when they are relieving the head nurse. Each of these persons is answerable for a specific part of the total responsibility: the head nurse for a unit; the supervisor for a number of units, a floor, or a department; and the director of nursing for associates and assistants. Scalar process is another term for chain of command, or the arrangement of persons through whom responsibility passes.

All of these line relationships require the operation of the delegation-responsibility-accountability triad. This chain of command is mandatory, because it manages the very serious business of carrying out satisfactory nursing care for a designated number of patients, counted by the hundreds. There remains, too, the fact that orders can be given and obedience required. It is hoped that there are standards of practice operative that reduce the number of orders and required obedience, as well as that relationships are sufficiently cordial and mutually respectful and communications open and nonvindictive so that orders will be minimized. The power of ultimate decision, however, is inherent in the delegation-responsibility-accountability triad. This power can be used wisely or poorly, even maliciously. Though safeguards, such as periodic evaluation, grievance procedures, and so forth, have been introduced into organizations, people still suffer from the indiscriminate use of power. This wielding of power can be couched in altruistic terms or camouflaged in acceptable ways. The capable head nurse who is never promoted because she occasionally displays temper, without a much wider analysis and review of strengths and weaknesses by more than one person, illustrates this possibility.

It is incumbent on all persons in the organization, at any level, to have a conscientious regard for the uses and abuses of power, so that the reputation and integrity of persons who have been delegated responsibility, assumed it, and are accountable for specific work are not jeopardized. It is a moral aspect of the line position that must be honored by the person holding the position as well as by those above and below.

Because such terms as command and hierarchy have unfavorable connotations in our time, there are occasional efforts to soften or camouflage them. The use of the word coordinator, and more recently facilitator, for director is an attempt at such softening. However, the use of the word coordinator weakens the position and leaves the authority-responsibility role in confusion for people who understand and operate correctly in their relationships with the director, called coordinator. Conversely, there is a growing practice of strengthening the position of directors of nursing by calling them vice presidents or assistant administrators in charge of nursing and making them accountable directly to the hospital administrator and equal to other vice presidents or assistant administrators.

The autocracy sometimes exercised by directors has also fostered efforts to soften the title. It is not the title but the people occupying the position who must be softened, so that they will use consultative management principles in making decisions and so reduce the potential arbitrariness of solitary decision making. This is not to say that solitarily made decisions are opposed to those made after consultation; but consultation, besides building in a safeguard, increases the likelihood of staff cooperation in their execution of such decisions. Occasionally, persons charged with the responsibility may have to make independent decisions in the interest of previously examined and objective nursing care improvement. When persuasion cannot overcome inertia, orders are necessary: the terse change of shift report will be expanded to a comprehensive one; the critically ill will be visited together by charge persons at change of shift time; there will be periodic unit nursing care conferences; discharge plans will be ascertained on all patients well in advance of discharge.

Thus we see that there is no escape from the delegation-responsibility-accountability triad in organizational structure. The director of nursing is accountable for the conduct of the nursing service to the hospital administrator, either directly or through an assistant hospital administrator, usually one designated as in charge of patient care, though the latter injects an unnecessary level between the administrator and the director of the major service of the hospital. The administrator of the hospital is not free of such constraints, but is answerable to a board of directors, private owners, or a governmental body. This authority-responsibility factor inherent in the line concept of organizational structure pervades administration, in order that progress toward achievement of purpose can be measured and controlled.

Staff positions in the line-staff concept of organization are not vested with the delegation-responsibility-accountability triad except internally where a department, such as personnel or in-service education, requires two or more workers. These are positions of a specialized nature that depend on persuasion exclusively. These persons do not give orders. They both independently and collaboratively collect and analyze information and present their findings and opinions to the director or other appropriate person, but they are dependent on the line personnel to accept and utilize or reject their proposals.

It may seem that the distinction between line and staff position, that is, the use of persuasion and orders in line and persuasion alone in staff, is becoming more an academic question than an actual one, because all areas of nursing service are becoming more and more complex and dependent on the work of staff personnel. For example, an assistant director or supervisor cannot reject the contribution of the in-service education director in meeting an obligation to the staff for provision of educational opportunities, although necessary adaption or alteration might be contributed. Greater reciprocity and cooperative effort does blur line-staff distinctions; however, good order is served by understanding and using the concept.

A good example of how failure to think about the distinction between line and staff personnel produces considerable confusion and frustration is the current varied use of the clinical specialist. Some of these specialists have replaced the supervisor. They have become supervisors who have a very strong clinical background; that is, they are line officers in the organization. Some have become an enriching adjunct to the supervisor and use their strong clinical background to assist staff in upgrading their clinical care or in giving expert clinical care to patients for purposes of direct service, example, or research. Where the job description has been clearly drawn and the relationships have been seen appropriately and clearly, there has been less frustration and confusion. It is where the clinical specialist has been assigned without a clear-cut role that confusion, conflict, and frustration arise. Because this position is new, it is occasionally thought that clinical specialists should experiment and develop their own job descriptions after analysis of the duties involved. The final decision will be enhanced if the integrity of both administration and clinical practice is seen, understood clearly, and respected.

The dichotomy involved in the placement of the clinical specialist in the nursing service organization is discussed at length by Parkis,[5] who sees a clear need for management skills for clinical specialists so they will be able to achieve a higher level of nursing care through nursing personnel. Indeed, the argument for clinical specialists as supervisors also shows the value of line positions. Upgrading nursing care as expeditiously as possible will go faster when these specialists are supervisors in fact, if not in name, assuming they have the appropriate administrative abilities and preparation. As line people they have direct accountability for the performance of workers, which enhances their persuasive power in helping personnel improve the quality of the care. However, if clinical specialists are placed in a staff position and if the head nurse or supervisor cannot be persuaded of their value, other personnel too will reject or give only token acceptance to their ideas. The clinical specialists are then impeded from being effective, and the high cost of their service cannot result in improved nursing care for patients. Consequently, because of their various functions, the problem of placement of clinical specialists in the nursing service organization is yet to be solved. Understanding the line-staff concept puts the problem inherent in the utilization of the growing number of these specialists in manageable perspective.

The potential value of the staff position can be seen in another innovation that affects the organization of the nursing department, that is, use of a ward manager, who is coequal in the nursing unit with the head nurse and is accountable either to the nursing office or to hospital administration. Ward managers are charged with management of the unit, in order to release the head nurse for purely nursing responsibility. They assume responsibility for the maintenance and procurement of equipment and supplies; the good order of the physical plant; the relationship with collateral departments such as housekeeping, dietary, admissions, and pharmacy; and the preparation of time schedules. Formerly, the well-utilized ward clerk did many of these duties, especially where standards had been established, such as for equipment and supplies. However, the ward clerk was and remains accountable to the head nurse.

There is potential conflict at the head nurse–unit manager point of contact, for they are essentially coequal and report either to the same or to equal superiors; however, safeguards can be provided, such as clear-cut job descriptions, well-oriented personnel, and placement of persons with considerable flexibility in these positions.

The ward clerk and unit manager involvement in staffing has generated a corollary in the nursing office: the use of a lay person to direct and coordinate total staffing, working from prearranged patterns and directions.

SPAN OF CONTROL OR SUPERVISION

Span of control is an essential concern in an organization, because it is the decision about how many and what levels of personnel are needed to achieve the purpose of the organization. It is related to the numbers of persons one can supervise satisfactorily.

Size of the institution is one main determinant. In a moderate-size hospital of 200 to 500 beds, there might be supervisors for each of the usual clinical areas (such as medical, surgical, obstetrics, and pediatrics) and for special services (such as operating and emergency rooms and coronary or intensive care units), in addition to an assistant director of nursing. The titles assistant director of clinical nursing and supervisor (of clinical nursing) are usually interchangeable and determined by the size of the institution. Rather than have all head nurses in the organization report directly to the director of nursing, these assistant directors of nursing or supervisors report directly to the director of nursing for the units within their area of specific responsibility. The introduction of levels reduces the numbers of persons accounting to the head person; hence, there is span of control or supervision. It is intended to insure that persons in responsible positions are not overloaded by excessive numbers of persons reporting to them. It protects the integrity of a given position. At the unit level, all personnel—staff nurses, practical nurses, aides, orderlies, and secretary or ward clerk—usually report or are accountable to the head nurse. Where team nursing is used, the leader usually accounts to the head nurse for the work of personnel assigned to the team, and another level is thereby introduced.

Other factors that determine the span of supervision in a particular institution include degree of centralization or homogeneity of units, for example, the number of clinical specialties strong enough to be considered units (such as neurosurgery or urology). The degree of experience and excellence of the personnel likewise helps in determination of supervision. A stable, qualified staff or service may require less supervision than a volatile one with new personnel who have less experience or are using new techniques. The personality and experience of the supervisor enters into this determination. There are some who enjoy a wide span of supervision, whereas others prefer to manage an average number of units. Physical plant plays a part, in that one can supervise adjacent units easier than those spread throughout the hospital. The amount of support provided by staffing, in-service education, well-formulated policies and procedures, and so forth, will influence the span of supervision.

The purpose, then, of the span of supervision is to insure appropriate numbers of persons for whom one is accountable, so that the assignment is manageable.

Care must be taken that areas of responsibilities are seen firsthand regularly, in order that accountability be safeguarded. In other words, administrators must keep in personal touch with the work of personnel for whom they are responsible, as well as with the patients who are the recipients of that work. This applies at all levels. Reports will never replace direct observation. Moreover, supervisors remain reality centered when they see at the bedside-care level the problems and frustrations as well as successes and joys derived from giving nursing care in our complex time.

UNITY OF COMMAND

When all line personnel are personally observing the work situation, as they should, there is danger of overlapping supervision. Personnel work better when they are accountable to one supervisor. Corrections of or questions about care observed while the administrator circulates and evaluates should be directed to the person in charge of the unit where the finding was made or with the supervisor of the area if it is the director or an assistant who made the observation. That person can then respond, explain, and discuss the matter with the worker who administered the care.

Intervention with the worker, rather than reporting to the superior, is permissible when the issue might be critical, but such issues are not so common as we often think. Sometimes, too, the relationship of the supervisor to the unit personnel and head nurses is very close, and all are well known to each other and respected. In this case, the practice might be relaxed, but should still be remembered.

This procedure of indirect intervention may seem too time consuming; however, the results are well worth it in terms of satisfied workers, both those who were spared multiple corrections and those whose authority might be bypassed by direct intervention. Irreparable harm has been done to staff morale by overlapping supervision.

One situation in nursing where overlapping supervision is so far unavoidable involves the evening and night assistant directors of nursing or supervisors and the head nurse. We hold the head nurse accountable for staff around the clock, but unit personnel on evening and night shifts are responsible also to the evening and night supervisors. This possible conflict shows up most clearly when the head nurse is held accountable by a physician for something that went wrong. It is the head nurse who must collect details, see that the report is written, or do whatever investigation is called for. This may include consultation with the evening or night supervisor as well as evening and night unit staff. Knowing that this potential conflict exists can help eliminate it. It is impossible to state categorically that the head nurse or the evening or night supervisor has the ultimate responsibility for the work of the charge nurse, because occasionally both do.

A similar potential conflict point is that between head nurse and in-service instructor when nurses' aides or assistants are working on the units while still under the aegis of the in-service department. Likewise, the head nurse can be confronted with this kind of conflict when a physician's orders depart from the policies of the institution. In all cases, the possibility of conflict in dual or overlapping supervision can be reduced by recognition of its potential and by goodwill and clearly understood standards of performance. Unfortunately, jurisdictional jealousy can and often does underlie the conflict. Jurisdictional abuse remains a problem. Recognition, with all possible safeguards in operation, can reduce this potential for conflict where overlapping supervision does exist.

Because head nurses are frequently at the apex of such conflicts, it behooves the director of nursing, assistants, and supervisors to do everything they can to support the head nurses involved in multiple contacts. The head nurse should be made a full member of management, with the same well-acknowledged rights and obligations as other managers enjoy. We have failed almost universally to make this important position a fully integrated part of management; we have been far more verbose than effective in dealing with the real problems of the head nurse's position.

Roethlisberger[6] masterfully describes the comparable problem in industry, in which the foreman is victimized by similar separation from other management personnel and from the workers in his jurisdiction, by virtue of being only tenuously part of management.

SPECIALIZATION

There has always been the grouping by clinical specialty and of the critically ill, in beds or rooms close to the desk in former days and now in special units with ever-narrowing special care, such as coronary or intensive care units. There is no question of the importance to the goal of health restoration or maintenance of specific categories of patients by the use of specialized personnel and material in meeting nursing needs and medical needs. What one knows intimately can be done best. The continuous rise of specialty groups, despite efforts of the national organizations to maintain them in the general stream, gives evidence of the ongoing refinement and importance of special services and the consequent special needs of their practitioners. The difference between the postgraduate course of a former time and its companion in special preparation today is one of degree, not of kind. Proximity and access to a high-quality clinical area is still the sine qua non of institutions wishing to prepare specialized workers, whether these institutions are universities, regional medical programs, or whatever. Homogeneity is the root of specialization. Activities and practices are alike in nature and kind. They result in improved practice.

Decentralization often accompanies specialization, because of the intricacies of procedure and material involved. Because general administrative personnel know less about specialties, such as coronary care, personnel in these units tend to answer directly to the director of nursing. Supervision is self-contained, and decentralization occurs. Relationships in the operating room provide a meaningful and familiar example of such specialization and decentralization.

Geographic distribution of services also plays a part in the amount of specialization found in an organization and in the consequent work groupings. For example, pediatrics and the self-care unit might seem a strange combination of departments responsible to a supervisor if one did not know that they were adjacent units.

Specialization is a factor in organization. The organization may, for example, provide one or more supervisors for each division, on a clinical and numerical (patient) distribution. It should be noted that this arrangement tends to reduce specialization and increase the generalist component. Moreover, because of the great numbers of medical and surgical beds in our hospitals, personnel are often considered general anyway, at least in relation to obstetrics and pediatrics but less so to neurosurgery or urology. Specialization and generalization are both recognized. It has always been so and increases in direct ratio to the complexity of medical care.

General and special services, while having many differences, have a much larger common core, that is, the great body of common nursing care given, irrespective of special needs, though hopefully always respecting individualization of that care. Concentration on a common core of nursing from which specialties then extend would reduce the frustration that accompanies shifts to other specialties. Frequently a specialty is thought to be completely new, whereas it was in fact built on a common core, even if not fully recognized as such. For example, the need for exercise as an essential need of physically restricted patients is met by range of motion exercises in rehabilitation care, by isometric, limb, and respiratory exercises in postsurgical care, and in considerable physical activity in some types of neuropsychiatric care. Remembering that provision of such exercise is an essential aspect of nursing care renders the care more comprehensive and manageable, and the personnel providing the care are less thwarted and ineffective.

The advent of the nurse-epidemiologist in response to the need for increased attention to infection control brings another area of specialization to the hospital nursing scene. Because nursing is the largest service, it may seem logical that the epidemiologist be a nurse, though the clinical laboratories are ultimately accountable for epidemiology. Organizationally, this nurse-epidemiologist should correctly be answerable to the director of the clinical laboratories rather than the director of nursing. However, it may be more appropriate to have this epidemiological responsibility carried by clinical laboratory personnel, because it is clearly related to and affects other areas of the institution, such as food management, and to retain the respiratory therapy function, which has always been a nursing function.

There is a similar situation deriving from specialization in the case of responsibility for the central supply service. This has traditionally been a nursing responsibility. With the great increase and expansion of supply departments, two changes are emerging: the use of nonnurse personnel in charge of these departments, replacing nurses; and the separation of them from the nursing department and their alignment to purchasing and storing. In either case, there remains a need for strong nursing association, either directly or indirectly, because of great utilization of these supplies and services by nursing departments.

Gill[2] proposes another type of specialist for the nursing department: the functional specialist, whose job it would be to examine the enterprise for effectiveness and efficiency and work with and through the staff to identify problems and deficiencies and to plan and implement their improvement or replacement. This person would replace the outside consultant, frequently used in attempts to improve the operation of the enterprise. This position in some ways is analogous to the research and development staff in industry or operations analysts found in an increasing number of hospitals.

Careful analysis is necessary in our complex organizations to make certain that existing or new specialties are reduced to their essence, so that they will be placed within the appropriate jurisdictional division. Reviewing what might have been instead of what is should help us make more appropriate organizational decisions. There is no reason to believe that there will not continue to be specialization and its attendant problems.

STAFF COMMUNICATION

An organizational structure, besides showing the hierarchical relationships and communication of workers in accountability for parts of the total goal of comprehensive nursing care for patients given by qualified, satisfied personnel, must provide for lateral communication among the levels and classifications of workers. There must be formal provision for meetings on a monthly, quarterly, or annual basis, so that staff will have an opportunity to meet regularly to discuss their work and working conditions. Such meetings should be presided over and carried out by members of the group rather than superiors, although minutes of the meetings should be made available to superiors and other levels of personnel. It could be that the lower echelons might prefer to have a superior present at least initially, but superiors should attend only as requested.

Monthly meetings by clinical, categorical, or entire nursing staff to discuss means of improving nursing care, problems, and policies and of which minutes are kept constitute a standard for evaluation by the Joint Commission on Accreditation of Hospitals.[7] This standard implies that recommendations may be made; otherwise, the deliberations would be fruitless. If this standard is being met, one wonders why there is a concerted effort to introduce professional performance committees as part of contractual arrangements by state nurses' associations. The standard seems to fortify this effort of the state associations to secure input for staff in decisions about the quality of the nursing care of a given institution. There is little doubt that an organization must provide opportunities for staff to deliberate formally if it is to become and remain viable. Such provision gives stimulation and balm to the human spirit that cannot be found in any other way. Such formal deliberative opportunities parallel the line chain of command in importance.

Committees

Committees are essentially a coordinating device in that they assemble a group of people to do a job, either on a continuing or particular basis. They are an integral part of the organizational structure, because they provide a mechanism for decision making and deliberations necessary for carrying forward the goals of the enterprise. Standing committees deal with policy, procedures, and research.

The executive committee (sometimes called a cabinet) usually consists of associate and assistant directors of nursing and supervisors. Such a committee is indispensable to the director of nursing in conducting the nursing service. There is an emerging practice of rotating the positions of associate and assistant director with the clinical assistant directors, in the interest of keeping these high-level managers in touch with the total operation, so there will be cohesiveness and executive development of staff. This committee is a real testing ground for the consultative management skill of the director of nursing.

In addition to standing committees, such as procedure, in-service, and research, ad hoc committees are formed to do a specific job, for example, to develop ways and means to implement or strengthen discharge planning. The compact and comprehensive guide developed at Rancho Los Amigos Hospital [in David and associates[8]] can be used as an aid to this committee. Instilling the will to perform remains a formidable problem, but it is possible that the specificity of such a guide could be carried over so effectively by the committee that the staff would be motivated sufficiently to choose to implement such a plan.

There must be provision for nursing representation on hospital organization committees. The value of both nursing input and of participatory practice has long been denied nurse managers.

ORGANIZATIONAL SCHEMAS
Traditional

The traditional schema is most common (Fig. 2). Its structure resembles a pyramid, with the director of nursing at the apex, and an associate director on a line leading to the assistant directors and supervisors of clinical areas or departments and those

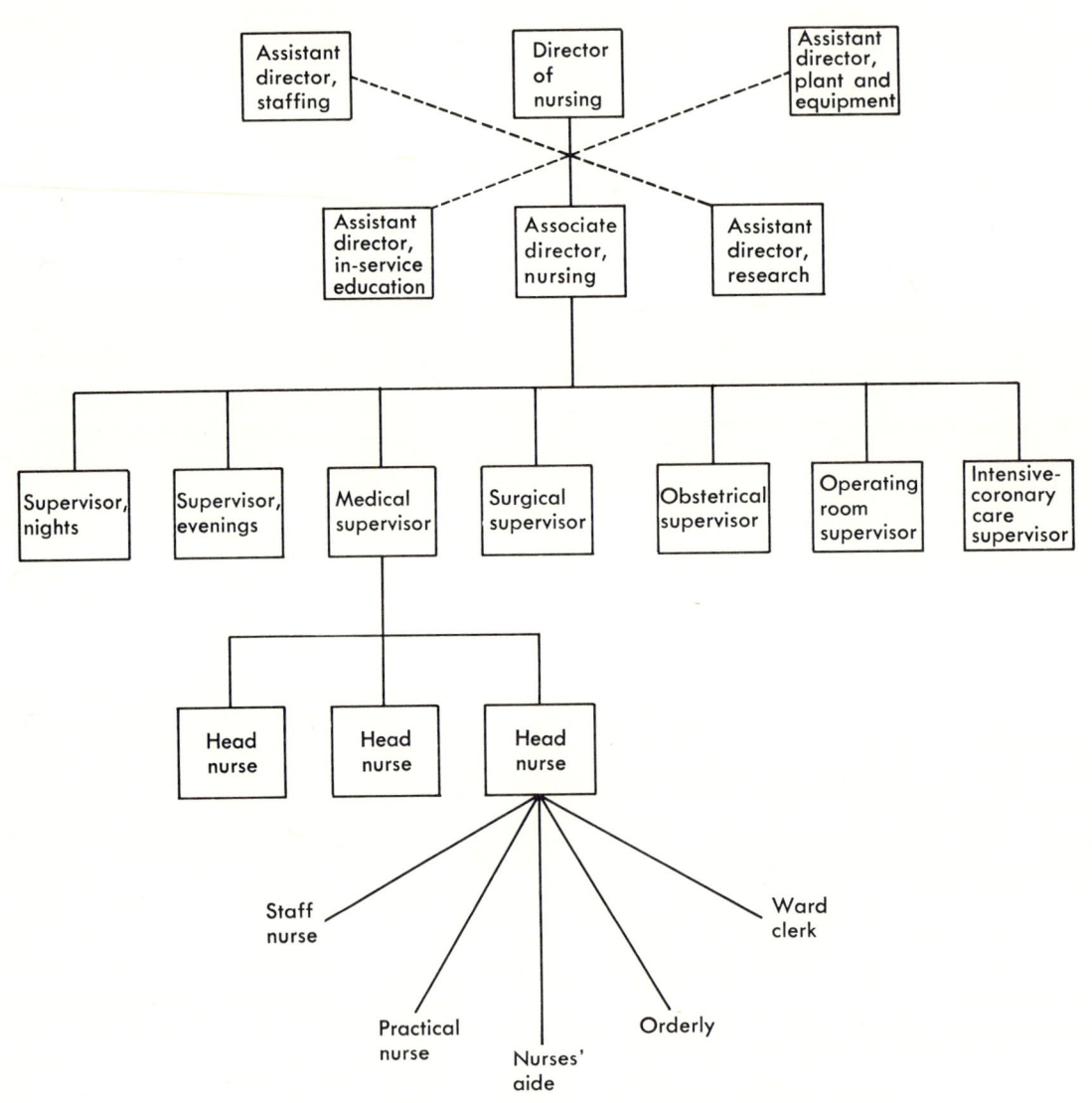

Fig. 2. Traditional organizational schema (pyramidal structure).

responsible for evening and night shifts. From each assistant director or supervisor, lines lead to head nurses at the unit level. All unit staff fan out from the head nurse, unless channelled through an assistant head nurse in the line. All lines denote delegation, responsibility, and accountability for carrying forward the goals of the organization in particular areas of jurisdiction. Dotted lines from the director of nursing denote staff positions such as assistant directors in charge of staffing (sometimes lay persons); in-service education; environmental factors such as physical plant, equipment, and supplies; research; and so forth.

Wedge. The traditional schema is sometimes represented as pie-shaped, with wedges of delegation, responsibility, and accountability assumed by assistant directors or supervisors (Fig. 3). This schema has the advantage of showing specific areas of responsibility more graphically. It is less graphic on the line-staff concept, because the line concept is visualized by the circular extension of responsibility of the evening and night supervisors around the clinical areas, and the staff concept by the absence of this extension around the four staff positions of assistant directors in staffing, in-service education, research, and plant and equipment.

Systems structure

Jehring[9] describes a systems model of organization that depends on the goal di-

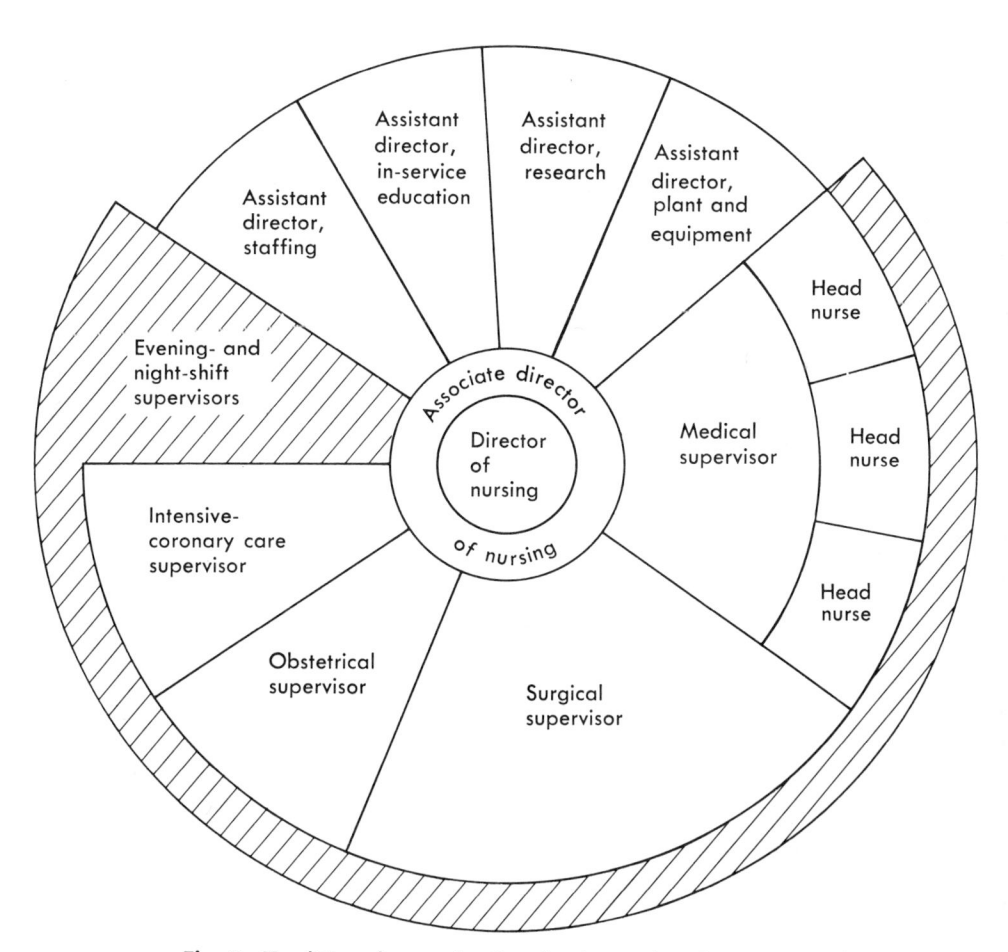

Fig. 3. Traditional organizational schema (wedge structure).

rectedness of personnel to supply the structure, along with the motivation for goal achievement. Because this schema seems nebulous, it might serve better as an adjunct to than a replacement for the traditional structure, because goal-related motivation is much needed in the traditional as well as any other organizational structure. However, there is the possibility that Jehring will eventually bring the clarity and precision of the traditional to his goals-system structure by developing and providing detail to it.

Kast and Rosenzweig[10] show the base for and impact of traditional–human relations administrative theory on their formulation of a systems structure. Their organization consists of five subsystems: goals and values, technology, psychosocial, structural, and managerial, within the encircling environmental superstructure. With the exception of technology, the subsystems partake of significant elements from traditional–human relations theory rearranged to advance the relational nature of systems theory.

Decentralized schema

There is a move toward flatter organizations in which there are fewer levels of control, as compared with the traditional schema. The early work of Worthy (in Gardner and Moore[11]) on decentralization demonstrated its merit in increasing morale by giving managers more freedom to achieve independently, as opposed to the greater structuralization of the traditional arrangement. It emphasized results rather than the details of process. This work was the forerunner and model for subsequent decentralization.

Similarly, Finer[12] notes the effect of decentralization on the morale quotient in his observation that the trust inherent in delegated responsibility is usually met with increased energy and sense of well-being, bringing the self and the goals of the enterprise into closer alignment.

Current nursing decentralization (Fig. 4) usually consists of dividing the nursing service between two assistant directors rather than three to five supervisors, for example, giving responsibility for surgical units, operating rooms, and obstetrical units to one assistant director and medical, pediatric, and intensive, coronary, or minimal care units to another. Though flatter, there is a greater span of control for each of these assistant directors. This decentralization attempts to provide the greater responsibility and freedom for decision making found in its antecedents. There is sometimes a concurrent move to strengthen the 24-hour responsibility of nurse managers, in the interest of increasing their autonomy.

Decentralization is an important concept for the nursing enterprise, because it will help reduce the traditional authoritarian stance. However, decentralization will have to be accompanied by clear-cut standards for nursing care and operation to insure enough homogeneity to carry forward the goals of such a crucial and complex enterprise.

Pigors and Myers[13] speak about recentralization, or the move back to some point on a decentralization-centralization continuum, as a result of speedy computerized information that is sweeping business enterprises, though nursing departments are not yet in the vanguard in using computerized information. As staffing is computerized, it will require more, rather than less, centralization. The movement is in the direction of greater computer service. Pigors and Myers reiterate the "magic formula," that is, the decision on decentralization or recentralization (or anything else of a structural nature) to be made by a representative management group.

Clinically directed schema

The concerted effort to upgrade nursing clinically has produced a change in the organizational structure, mainly in terminology. A current problem that is far from settled is where to place the clinical specialist, as noted in the work of Parkis.[5] Clinical coordinator is a new title for the

Organizing 79

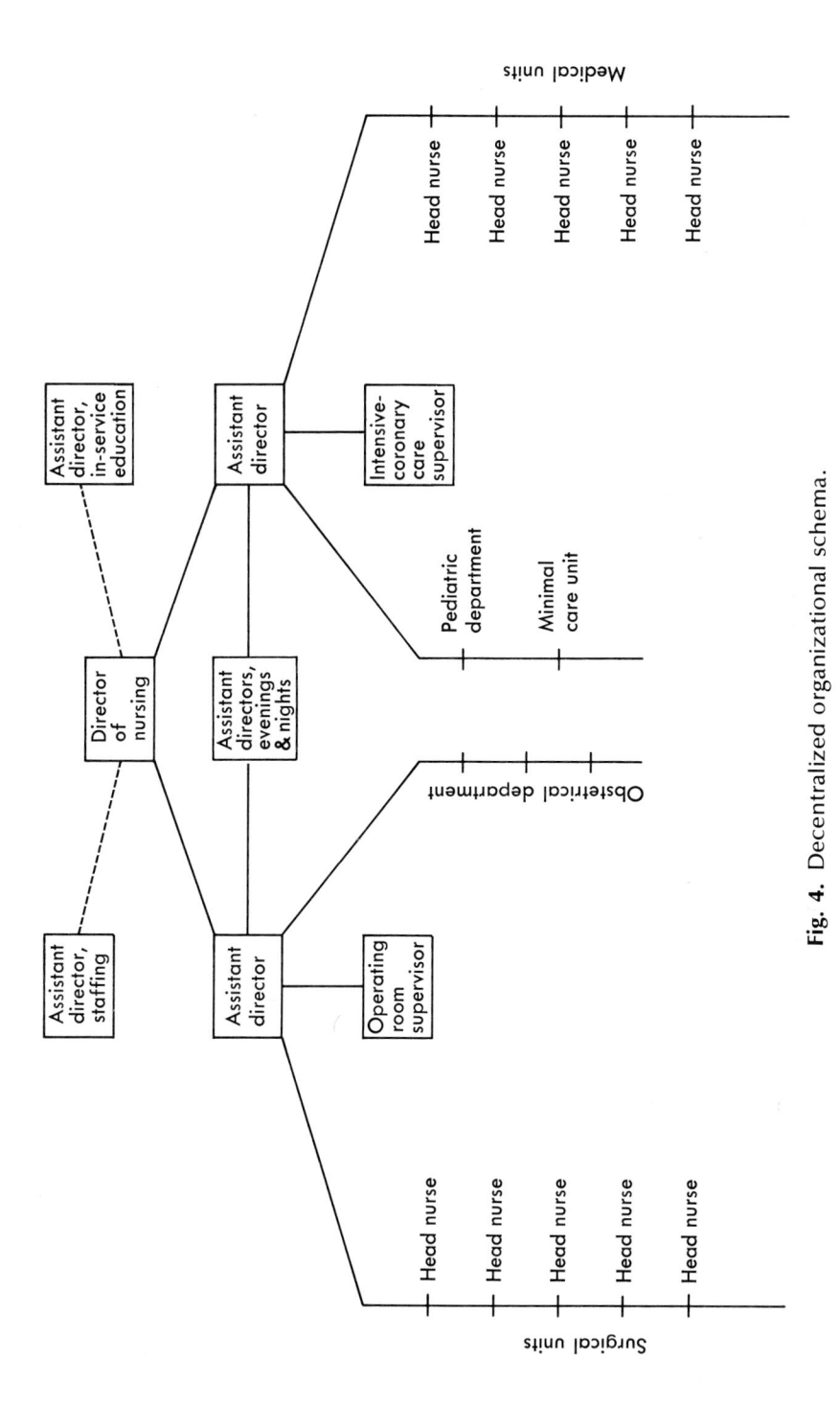

Fig. 4. Decentralized organizational schema.

supervisor. Clinical has sometimes been added to the supervisor's title, though Donovan[14] claims it to be redundant because clinical expertise is assumed where the supervisor functions appropriately. The supervisor does indeed coordinate, but is much more involved in carrying forward the goals of the nursing department within the delegation-responsibility-accountability triad. Head nurses are sometimes called nurse clinicians, and staff nurses have different clinical names sometimes too. In the current rash of name changing, we must be sure that the new names are logically and administratively sound.

One such clinically oriented reorganization is reported by Ayers, Bishop, and Moss.[15] Concern for more recognition for staff nurses, to encourage them to remain in staff nursing, resulted in a salary schedule respectful of lateral, or horizontal, progression within the staff nurse classification. Nursing care then was provided by practitioners ranging from the beginning nurse to the clinical specialist. As unit-service coordinators (ward managers) assumed the nonnursing and coordinating functions of head nurses, they shifted to a stronger clinical role. The supervisor's role also shifted in the clinical direction. Administrative nurses have been reduced by 63% in this shift of emphasis and practice toward clinical nursing.

The unit manager system that has been added to nursing units is also an effort to strengthen the clinical component of nursing by removing nonnursing responsibilities from the head nurse, as demonstrated above. The addition of this position directly affects the organizational structure of the nursing department. If responsibility for these workers rests with nursing, there must be a departmental superior, usually an assistant director in charge of unit managers. The alternative location, and one more logically sound, is to have these workers responsible to someone outside nursing, such as the general administrator of the hospital. If the responsibility for these workers remains within the nursing department, the principle of conservation of professional time, though respected at the unit level, is violated at the upper level.

Alterations in the clinical direction of the organizational structure, while consisting mainly of addition of unit managers and name changes intended to strengthen the clinical component, are found in both centralized (pyramidal) and decentralized (flat) organizational structures.

EVALUATION

Because the organization structure by its skeletal nature is so fundamental to administration, it provides a base for review, analysis, and evaluation. Where the parts are appropriately determined and articulated, institutional goals are more likely being carried forward, assuming of course that the goals are appropriate and well known. In the Checklist of Organizational Effectiveness (pp. 81-82), it will be noted that, for the most part, headings fall within the context of the organizational structure. The list suggests as well as provides items against which to check one's practice.

Prouty[16] uses the organizational structure as an evaluation device to the extent that reviewing and reformulating the existing organization are essentially evaluating too. Her organization chart departs substantially from what is conventionally contained in such a chart. The chain of command and span of control elements are missing; the head nurse remains outside management; and the evening and night supervisors seem to have less sphere of influence than do assistant directors and other supervisors. Directing and staffing are not given special consideration, but planning and evaluation (part of control) are. The question is begged as to why these two functions of management are given prominence. One can only regret that such excellent deliberations and thought resulted in an organization chart so oblivious to and incompatible with management theory.

CHECKLIST OF ORGANIZATIONAL EFFECTIVENESS*

1. Overall Planning

    Written Statements of
       Company Objectives _____
    Company Policies _____
       Sales _____
       Finance _____
       Production _____
       Personnel _____
       Other _____

2. Patterns of Leadership

    Primarily
       Authoritative _____
       Participative _____
       Appropriate _____

3. Organization Structure

    Departmentation
       Function _____
       Product _____
       Customer _____
       Geography _____
       Process _____
       Sequence _____

    Span of Management
       One over One _____
       Two or Three _____
       Three to Seven _____
       Eight or More _____

    Overall Impression
       Proper Balance _____
       Proper Emphasis _____

4. Authority Relationships

    Factors Limiting Effectiveness of Authority
       Overlapping Authority _____
       Superior Authority _____
       Provisions for Subordinate Acceptance _____

    Line-and-Staff Relationships
       Use of "Assistant-to" _____
       Limits of Line Authority _____
       Limits of Staff Authority _____
       Task Force Organization _____

5. Delegation

    Parity of Authority and Responsibility _____
    Absoluteness of Accountability _____
    Unity of Command _____
    Personality Factors _____

6. Decentralization

    Definition of Decentralized Unit _____
    Scope, Type, and Frequency of Decisions _____
    Availability of Controls _____
    Statement of Goals for Unit _____
    Degree of Decentralization
       Optimum _____
       Too Little _____
       Too Much _____

*From Sisk, H. L.: Principles of management, Cincinnati, 1969, South-Western Publishing Co., p. 381. Reproduced by special permission.

Continued.

CHECKLIST OF ORGANIZATIONAL EFFECTIVENESS—cont'd

7. Use of Committees

Committees	Ad Hoc	_____
	Advisory	_____
	Management	_____
	Composition	_____
	Benefits	_____
Board of Directors	Outside Members	_____
	Inside Members	_____
	Contribution	_____

8. Provisions for Control

Definition of Standards	_____
Units of Measurement	_____
Reporting of Exceptions	_____
Timeliness of Controls	_____
Strategic Placement of Controls	_____
Control Information for Line Managers	_____

The review by Prouty and our examination of that work are examples of the kind of evaluation we must bring to the organizational structure, which provides the platform on which personnel carry forward the individual contributions that result in goal achievement for the enterprise. Of such review and evaluation do refinement and clarity, as well as precision in achieving goals, consist.

Organizational arrangements as represented by organization charts are dynamic rather than static, as Prouty's work demonstrates. They must be scrutinized from time to time to make certain that they are in tune with the actual work situation, are brought into alignment with the actual work situation, or the actual work situation is brought into alignment with the formalized arrangement. Obsolescence of the organizational arrangement is a real threat unless surveillance and study are maintained.

In maintaining currency for the formal arrangement, Ferkiss's[17] observation about structure as process in slow motion illumines the need to keep relationships and functions in order, because the organizational structure is the firming up of the process of the assignments and articulations necessary to carry the goals of the enterprise forward.

REFERENCES

1. Drucker, P.: Management; tasks, responsibilities and practices, New York, 1974, Harper & Row, Publishers, p. 549.
2. Gill, W.: The concept of a strong centralized staff, Supervisor Nurse 3(2):15-16, 1972.
3. Passos, J.: Accountability; myth or mandate? J. Nurs. Admin. 3(2):17-22, 1973.
4. Robinson, A.: Professional conflict in the ICU/CCU, RN 35(5):40-45, 1972.
5. Parkis, E.: The management role of the clinical specialist. Part II. Supervisor Nurse 5(10):24-35, 1974.
6. Roethlisberger, F.: The foreman; master and victim of double talk, Harvard Business Review 43(5):23-50, 1965.
7. Annotated excerpts from JCAH nursing service standards, nursing service workshop, ed. 2, Chicago, 1974, Joint Commission on Accreditation of Hospitals, p. ST/15.
8. David, J., Hanser, J., and Madden, B.: Guidelines for discharge planning, Downey, Calif., 1968, Attending Staff Association of Rancho Los Amigos Hospital, Inc.
9. Jehring, J.: Motivational problems in the modern hospital, J. Nurs. Admin. 2(6):36-37, 1972.
10. Kast, F., and Rosenzweig, J.: Organization and management; a systems approach, ed. 2, New York, 1974, McGraw-Hill Book Co., p. 112.
11. Gardner, B., and Moore, D.: Human relations in industry, Chicago, 1950, Richard D. Irwin, Inc., pp. 346-348.
12. Finer, H.: Administration and the nursing services, New York, 1952, Macmillan, Inc., p. 231.
13. Pigors, P., and Myers, C.: Personnel administration, ed. 7, New York, 1973, McGraw-Hill Book Co., pp. 42-43.

14. Donovan, H.: What is supervision? Nurs. Outlook **5:**373, 1957.
15. Ayers, R., Bishop, R., and Moss, F.: An experiment in nursing service reorganization, Am. J. Nurs. **69**(4):783-786, 1969.
16. Prouty, M.: Making an organizational chart, J. Nurs. Admin. **4**(1):32-35, 1974.
17. Ferkiss, V.: The future of technological civilization, New York, 1974, George Braziller, Inc., p. 216.

CHAPTER 7
STAFFING

Staffing is the largest and a most crucial aspect of administration, because the quality of the workers and their performance will determine the degree of achievement of the goal of the nursing department. A good case can be made for staffing as the central point around which other functions cluster: the purpose of the enterprise, as well as the planning and organizing for its optimal achievement, would come to naught unless persons undertook to do it. Rational definition and deliberate acceptance of purpose are dependent on people. The staffing function is the means of keeping qualified persons in nursing service, with all that this implies in today's complex society.

Fig. 5 shows the staffing process in a systems context, with its support subsystems in relationship to each other and the whole and in turn in relation to the patient. The input is the sum of selected, qualified personnel giving to, receiving from, and interacting with patients in the ministration of nursing care. The output is the state of the patient as a result of the above activities, that is, improved, maintained, or unavoidably receding health. The subsystems that interact and interrelate with personnel and each other are the supports: classification of workers, recruitment, criteria for selection and placement, optimal utilization of personnel, staffing patterns, organizational behavior, communication, and personnel evaluation. Also of concern in staffing are in-service education; personnel policies and contracts; equipment; and legal aspects. These staff-related areas will be discussed in particular and to nursing service administration in general in Part III, Adjuncts to staffing.

Classification and procurement of personnel
VALUE OF STUDIES

A Report of the National Advisory Commission on Health Manpower, compiled by a distinguished panel of 68 persons (of whom only one was a nurse), notes the outstanding weaknesses in health manpower as they relate to the health needs of the nation and suggests possible courses of action to remedy these weaknesses. It states the national need for reactivation of nonpracticing nurses (of whom there are 500,000 to 600,000, half of whom maintain licensure) rather than increase in the output of new nurses. Accordingly, it is recommended that "nursing should be made a more attractive profession by such measures as appropriate utilization of nursing skills, increased levels of professional responsibilities, improved salaries, more flexible hours for married women, and better retirement provisions [p. 23]."[1] It is interesting to note that these very recommendations corroborate studies on nurse dissatisfaction done in the 1950s.

The findings of a job satisfaction survey done in the early 1970s are not much different. Benton and White[2] assessed satisfaction according to Maslow's hierarchy of needs (see p. 30), leaving out physical needs and moving from safety and security, social needs, and esteem to self-actualization. There is an essential equivalency between the earlier studies and the recent one: the ratings followed the same order, and salary and personnel policies were not found to be of high priority in any of the studies. Nurses in administrative positions were included in the later study. Considerable differences were found between ad-

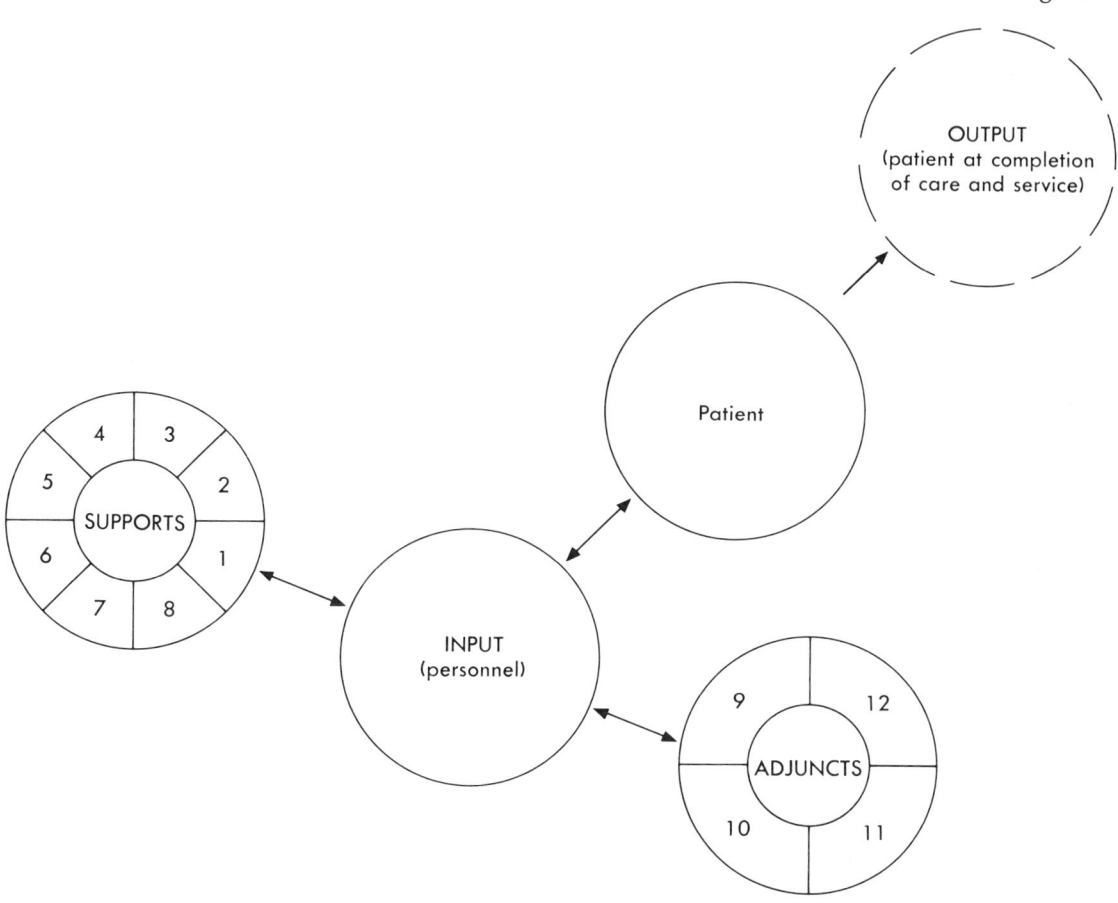

Fig. 5. The staffing process in a systems context. *1,* Classification of workers; *2,* recruitment; *3,* criteria for selection and placement; *4,* optimal utilization of personnel; *5,* staffing patterns; *6,* organizational behavior; *7,* communication; *8,* personnel evaluation; *9,* in-service education; *10,* personnel policies, contracts; *11,* equipment; *12,* legal aspects.

ministrative and clinical nurses, which corroborates the divisiveness sometimes found between these two groups and points out the absence of goal clarification and reconciliation.

It is interesting to note that in the 1970s we are still working on the findings of the 1950s and recommendations of the 1960s. It is clear that individual enterprises (either alone or in regional or local groups) that employ nurses have their work cut out for them in attempting to alleviate the nursing "shortage." It is also clear that the range of above suggestions falls within the staffing function of these enterprises.

FORECASTING

Job satisfaction surveys provide forecasting material from which staffing plans can be made and executed. Other forecasting materials include the annual statistical reports of the American Nurses' Association and the American Hospital Association; nursing and hospital journals, which give surveys and information about new services becoming available and trends in utilization, conservation, expansion, and contraction of existing services; state and local publications; and meetings that show regional and local applications of this information and these trends.

A significant illustration is the following quotation from the fall 1973 schedule of a junior college that offers A.D. and LPN programs. The college serves a county with 100,000 residents, and the schedule was mailed to each household.

> *Nursing*—Local hospitals are overstaffed this year with registered nurses . . . . Reduction in force procedures were implemented at both hospitals. One instructor is concerned that Clark is oversupplying the local market for nurses . . . . Salaries have gone up . . . thus attracting more and more aspirants. The situation may be similar to what happened to teaching a few years ago.*

The above quote presents a different picture, in view of nursing positions—mainly shift work and nursing home opportunities—advertised in the local newspaper. Where undesirable conditions prevail, distribution becomes a chronic problem, paralleling the shortage of physicians and nurses in underprivileged, rural, or remote areas. Nurses do not seem to want nursing home or shift work; and a survey of hospital nursing supply[3] corroborates the shortage of personnel for evening and night shifts, as well as shortages of specialized nurses for surgery, intensive care units, and emergency departments. However, as nursing homes continue to enter the mainstream of health care, work there should become more highly valued; and increasing shift-salary differentials may be the only solution to the shortage of nurses willing to take other undesirable jobs.

Another example of forecasting is the trend to return to active practice by nurses who live in areas with a depressed economy and whose husbands have lost jobs in the economic crunch. For example, massive layoffs in the aircraft industry have contributed to this trend in Seattle.

PERSONNEL ADMINISTRATION

Personnel administration is another term for the staffing function. Whereas the staffing function implies the wide range of activities involved in staffing an enterprise, personnel administration more aptly describes these activities. There has been great growth in this field since World War II, paralleling the growth in hospital and nursing service administration.

The American Hospital Association[4] describes a personnel department as follows:

> The foundation of a sound personnel program lies in the acceptance by management of its responsibility for creating an environment in which all employees can work together harmoniously and with coordinated effort, and in which each has an opportunity for self-expression, for achieving a sense of accomplishment, and for personal growth. Ideally, a sound personnel program fosters in the employee a feeling of responsibility for the work assigned, of satisfaction and security in his job, and of being an important part of the whole organization.

As personnel departments are introduced and flourish within health care facilities, they assume many responsibilities that were formerly carried out by other departments of the institution, thus relieving these departments of responsibilities not really theirs and providing excellent help in carrying out the staffing function. Nursing departments must be ready to shed those duties that can be more appropriately carried out by the personnel department and be receptive to the assistance and help that a good personnel department can provide.

There is justification for the systems approach so prominent today. By interlocking systems, a goal to meet the needs of new employees to become productive, satisfied workers as soon as possible is met by collaboration of personnel and other departments, including nursing, in establishing an outline or program using the essential elements of each to produce an overall program, deliberately divided departmentally but cohesive as a whole. Moreover, elimination or adjustment of trouble spots is more likely because of the interlocking systems view of the goal, even though the large percentage of nursing personnel involved may make this function seem to be solely a nursing project.

Pigors and Myers elaborate some specific areas in which the personnel department

---

*From Clark College Class Schedule, Vancouver, Wash., September 1973, p. 12.

provides the managers with certain services, including:

assistance in developing job descriptions, recruiting, screening, and testing candidates for employment, assistance in developing specific training programs, guidance in making performance appraisals, staff assistance in developing and administering a job evaluation program for setting relative wages and salaries for different jobs, and administration of employee benefit, service, safety, and health programs.*

They state that "personnel administration is a line management responsibility but a staff function."[5] It is carried out by line officers (directors, supervisors, and head nurses), with the resources, advice, and assistance of the personnel department. The staff function of the personnel department is essentially advisory, providing only those

*From Pigors, P., and Myers, C.: Personnel administration; a point of view and a method, New York, © 1963, McGraw-Hill Book Co., p. 34. Used with permission of McGraw-Hill Book Co.

direct services necessary to enhance the staffing function of the nursing department and its managers. Thus, nursing service management personnel are deeply involved at each level and in all phases of personnel administration; are guided, advised, and provided with alternatives and information; and are supported by the personnel department.

Nevertheless, one can see the unique position of the personnel department in the institution. No other department resembles it, because it interweaves its activities and functions with each and every department, though where public relations departments exist, they have a comparable function (see Chapter 17). Table 2 shows this interweaving comprehensively. It outlines the employment process in twelve steps, from the initial requisition for personnel through termination of an employee.

Table 2. Departmental–personnel department collaboration*

Department supervision (line)	*Personnel-employment specialist (staff)*
1. *Prepare requisition* outlining specific qualifications of employees needed to fill specific positions. Help create reputation that will attract applicants. [First step.]	**1.** *Develop* source of qualified applicants from local labor market. This requires carefully planned community relations, speeches, advertisements, and active high school, college, and technical school recruiting. [Second step.]
2. *Interview* and *select* from candidates screened by Personnel. Make specific *job assignments* that will utilize new employees' highest skills to promote maximum production. [Fifth step.]	**2.** Conduct *skilled* interviews, give *scientific* tests, and make thorough reference checks, etc., using requisition and job description as guides. Screening must meet company standards and conform with *employment laws*. [Third step.]
3. *Indoctrinate* employees with specific details regarding the sections and jobs where they are to be assigned—safety rules, pay, hours, "our customs." [Seventh step.]	**3.** *Refer* best candidates to supervisors, after physical examinations and qualifications for the positions available have been carefully *evaluated*. [Fourth step.]
4. *Instruct* and *train* on the job according to planned training program already worked out with Personnel. [Eighth step.]	**4.** Give new employees preliminary *indoctrination* about the company, benefit plans, general safety, first aid, shift hours, etc. [Sixth step.]
5. *Follow up, develop,* and *rate* employee job performance, *decide on* promotion, transfer, layoff, or discharge. [Ninth step.]	**5.** Keep *complete record* of current performance and and future potential of each employee. [Tenth step.]
6. Hold separation *interview* when employees leave —determine causes. Make internal department *adjustments* to minimize turnover. [Eleventh step.]	**6.** Diagnose information given in separation interviews, determine causes, and take positive steps to correct. [Twelfth step.]

*From Pigors, P., and Myers, C.: Personnel administration, ed. 7, New York, © 1973, McGraw-Hill Book Co., p. 35. Used with permission of McGraw-Hill Book Co.

CLASSIFICATION OF WORKERS
Licensure and education

Nurses are graduates of various kinds of education (hospital, junior college, or college programs), unified by common examination and mandatory licensure to work in health care institutions and independent services throughout the country. Some professional organizations are recommending a moratorium on licensure until some systemization of the myriad health care positions can be obtained. In education, there are such innovations as the external degree for nurses, by which examination is the sole criterion of eligibility for licensure. It is significant that the same criterion, examination only, has enabled occupational therapy assistants to acquire full professional status.

The range of occupations within the constantly expanding health field is astounding. We should try to appreciate the part played by nurses, with all the articulations and consequent interrelationships involved, if integration of these occupations is to be achieved in order to provide integrated nursing in which both excellence and reality are realized and brought into balance.

Concept of manpower

The vastness of the health field is shown by its place in the economy: it is preceded only by construction. One can begin to envision the many types of positions required to staff all the institutions and organizations within this field. Moreover, staffing needs multiply daily as concentration of new and old services develops, expands, and shifts. The problems of overlapping functions, licensure, and preparation are rampant and accompany this proliferation of workers who constitute health manpower.

World War II marked an important point in the staffing of nursing services. First, it began the transition from staffs composed mainly of student nurses to those composed mainly of graduate nurses and auxiliary workers, while students contributed less and less service as their educational programs were increasingly defined and refined. Second, as Yoder[6] points out, the human resources view of manpower began to supplement the human relations view held predominantly in the post–World War II years. One can only laud this shift in emphasis, because the relations component is never-ending, given the human condition. For this reason it can and often does become the overriding consideration in personnel work, to the exclusion of resources. Resources is more comprehensive and suggests the vast array of possibilities to enhance the fruitful performance of workers, including interpersonal relations, which are important to the smooth functioning of people in the organization who are charged with carrying the purpose forward. Moreover, a resource view may well correct and improve those conditions that give rise to problems in human relationships, for example, strengthening of the performance evaluation program or introduction of a hospitalwide correlated salary schedule.

Need for collegiality

Strauss[7] thinks that professional nurses should bring their co-workers (practical nurses and nurses' aides) into closer collegial relationship with themselves because of their devoted and valuable services in meeting nursing needs in collaboration with professional nurses. Team nursing in its ideal meaning and practice is an illustration of such cooperation. Such integration is found where there are long-standing personnel in continuing relationships, and additional opportunities could be found if we acknowledged the interdependence sufficiently. The divisiveness that gives rise to Strauss' suggestion may be another aspect of the divisiveness noted earlier between directors of nursing and their supervisors in one instance and their head nurses in another.

Categories of workers

Nurses' aides. During World War II nurses' aides (or assistants) were recruited in large numbers and were a stabilizing force in beleaguered nursing services. They remained after the war to continue to stabilize nursing services, which continued struggling to accommodate the nurse shortage while simultaneously trying to upgrade their services, become autonomous, and remain independent of nursing education. These auxiliary workers came mainly from lower economic and deprived racial groups. We will speak of their preparation in Chapter 13, In-service education. As their work became structured and uniform, their titles changed to such names as nurse assistant I, II, or III, reflecting their training, supervision, and experience.

Orderlies. Orderlies have been in nursing services a long time. Their duties largely concerned the intimate aspects of nursing care for male patients; the heavy work of transporting patients and equipment, for example, that required for oxygen therapy; and procurement and assembling of orthopedic equipment. Today, transportation is often centralized in an institution; orthopedic equipment is often under the aegis of the central supply department; and oxygen equipment is the responsibility of the inhalation therapist and frequently is built into the patient areas, thus eliminating the movement of heavy equipment.

Changes in the work of orderlies gives concrete evidence of the refinement of patient care over the years. They still minister to intimate needs and services for male patients, transport patients, and move and install heavy equipment, but they are vastly better taught and supervised.

Technicians. There is a growing number of technicians in nursing services. The 1965 position paper of the American Nurses' Association suggests that technician will eventually apply to graduates of diploma and associate degree programs, though this professional-technical problem is being reviewed. These technicians are essentially subprofessionals, thought not to have the broad background and depth of understanding of the professional, and are employed to do specific work competently and repetitively in increasingly complicated situations, even including those in coronary care units. Mastery of techniques is the distinguishing mark of the technician. It is vitally important in nursing services as patient care embraces more complicated technological devices. Technicians demonstrate the efficiency of functionalism.

There is a corollary here to personnel who are taught and are able to execute a complex procedure so that it will be done immediately and swiftly for the relief of the patient. For example, where there are numbers of patients who have had tracheotomies, it is more valuable to patient well-being if all personnel are able to suction these patients in an emergency, rather than leave a patient in distress while aides search for a professional person to do the procedure. Cardiopulmonary resuscitation is another example. The complexity of the procedure is acknowledged in the careful instruction and supervised practice of the people allowed to do the procedure. The repetition of the procedure provides the justification for permitting subprofessional personnel to carry out such complicated procedures. There are nurses' aides who in fact perform as technicians where they have worked a long time in a specific work situation. A few aides who regularly care for patients with cardiac disease can master the techniques necessary for the excellent physical and emotional care of these patients and may well be practicing at the technical level. The obstetrical department also offers considerable opportunity for the use of technicians, as do renal dialysis centers.

Ward clerks. Though not classified as technicians, in many ways the duties of ward clerks and even ward managers parallel those of technicians, that is, specific and circumscribed tasks or responsibilities intended to facilitate the work and conserve the time of the professional group. Ward clerks have assumed many clerical duties of the head nurse. They not only answer the phone, deliver mail, messages, schedules, and reports, and make out diet and other lists, but facilitate the scheduling duties of the head nurse by keeping notations of requests, meetings, and rotation of personnel. As they gain experience, some ward clerks can actually do the scheduling, at least in its essential form.

Ward clerks were forerunners of non-nurse personnel found increasingly in nursing offices. The clerical work involved in transcribing physicians' orders eventually became their work. Where standards were established for linen, stationery, drugs, and other supplies, these ward clerks could check the supplies against the standards and do the ordering.

Ward managers. The ward manager is an outgrowth of the position of ward clerk. This person assumes responsibility for all management of the unit, so that the head nurse can devote time and energies to the nursing component exclusively. Because of the added prestige, these managers are able to do much more interdepartmental work than the ward clerk or even the head nurse. Whereas the ward clerk makes and routes requisitions for repairs, additional supplies, and so forth, at the request of the head nurse, the manager assumes responsibility for these procedures, including followup when response to requests is not forthcoming. Liaison with other departments, such as housekeeping, maintenance, or dietary, becomes an important part of the duties of the manager. Though more closely advised by the head nurse, the manager may also do liaison work with professional departments, such as radiology and laboratory. A comprehensive study of the position of ward manager (Service Unit Management [SUM]) predicts an "irreversible trend toward some version of SUM in larger hospitals," noting that three hospitals had SUM in 1960 and an estimated 170 had it by 1970 [in Jelinik and associates[8]]. A subsequent study of SUM [in Munson[9]], identifying six critical stages in introducing the unit management system, points out the need to strengthen the nursing component of care so that the time released to nurses will be fruitfully used.

Alternatives to ward managers. It is questionable whether expansion of other departments, such as housekeeping, maintenance, and dietary, into direct supervision of patient areas would obviate the need for unit managers. For example, housekeeping supervisors do inspect the work of their employees in the patient areas, and it would be a short step to inspecting the patient units and service areas more comprehensively, making appropriate requisitions, overseeing, and following up on such repairs. In other words, if the work of each department were extended to its logical limit, would the long-standing involvement of the head nurse in monitoring, requesting, and following up on such deficiencies be obviated, thus also obviating much of the work of the unit manager? Adding positions may not be the best answer to carrying goals forward. Interdepartmental appraisal and action may provide not only an alternative but perhaps a better one in terms of economy and efficiency. Since the ward manager is essentially a middleman between hospital departments and the nursing unit, all alternate routes to efficiency of operations demand careful attention. Alternate uses of money are involved in the decision. The cost of employing unit managers should be weighed against other options, such as strengthening the interrelated departments by personnel and job analysis or greater standardization.

Licensed practical nurses (LPNs). Licensed practical nurses (or licensed vocational nurses) comprise a large and growing percentage of nursing service personnel. This large group of workers has been a mainstay of nursing services for at least three decades, and there is evidence that they have had a profoundly stabilizing influence on nursing services. Licensure was at first permissive, though there is persistent effort and some success on the part of practical nurses' associations in achieving mandatory licensure by all fifty states.

Licensed practical nurses suffered from underutilization for some time. Though they were paid more than nurses' aides, their duties were almost, if not, identical. Gradually this condition has been corrected, and they now are assigned duties well differentiated from those of aides or assistants. There has been a shift of duties from the RN to the LPN, more or less paralleling the shift of duties from the physician to the professional nurse. In many settings they assume charge responsibilities for shifts or particular specialized areas. There is always professional supervision, though it is sometimes tenuous or distant.

This group is characterized by a strong nursing orientation, though it may be that this characteristic is more visible now because the professional nurse has had to assume responsibility for the management of the care of large numbers of patients and the operation of increasingly complex procedures and equipment.

The National Association for Practical Nurse Education and Service, Inc., and its state and local affiliates, are well organized. In Washington State, while continuing to try to get mandatory licensure, the Association is seeking and getting contracts with hospitals governing employment and holds four educational meetings each year. This Association has a sophisticated code of ethics and a carefully thought out purpose, definition, lists of functions and vocational responsibilities.[10] A second national organization for LPNs is the National Federation of Practical Nurses. It is comprised of practical nurses only, whereas the National Association is open to others interested in practical nursing, such as professional nurses engaged in work with practical nurses.

Professional nurses. Professional nurses are the heart and head of the nursing service and are deeply involved in care, cure, and coordination. They are responsible for all ministrations for the comfort, well-being, and restoration to health of patients insofar as possible; for treatments, medications, and functions executed by the nursing staff, within the medical plan for the patients; and for seeing that all collateral professional services reach the patients and are synchronized around them. They have ultimate responsibility and supervision of all personnel serving patients within the nursing department.

Clinical specialists. The clinical specialist is a rising hope for the profession. These nurses can speed the day when comprehensive nursing practice will be the rule rather than the exception. The prevailing level of nursing care must be upgraded, and the assistance, coaching, teaching, and example offered by these specialists is a real boost to nursing services seriously trying to improve their practice.

A dimension of the work of specialist that has not yet received attention is the isolation and development of those commonalities applicable to specialties and nursing in general. If these commonalities were developed intensively, it might make the work of specialists more effective in raising the general level of nursing practice. It could parallel the direction clinical nurse education has taken in moving from clinical diseases to clinical conditions (found in one, several, or groups of diseases). An additional benefit would be incorporation of concepts of various several specialties into the development of these commonalities. The most obvious example is the inclusion of psychiatric–mental health concepts with medical-surgical or any other clinical specialty. Less obvious is the inclusion of means of detecting secondary psychological-societal elements that parallel or may interfere with recovery, such as alcoholism (see p. 208).

However, unless these specialists are equally well prepared in administration, they should remain staff persons (those who help other nurses by persuasion) rather than line people (supervisors). Change might occur faster in the latter position, because as supervisors they would have the power to insist on certain changes; but in the long run the power of persuasion will be more lasting. This does obligate the line person (head nurse or supervisor) to cooperate with the clinical specialist in the common goal of improved patient care (see also p. 71).

The preparation of clinical specialists is thought to be clinical work at the master's degree level, but this is not the only route. No less an authority than Reiter[11] tells us that one of her expert nurses did not have even a basic degree, but was self-educated.

Waite[12] reports a small hospital (84 beds) that has permanent specialized teams for treating patients with cancer and diabetes and for rehabilitation of those with stroke and respiratory diseases. The team members are selected because of interest, previous specialty experience, or both. Their preparation consists of reading and attending seminars and other educational experiences in their specialty. They enlist the aid of hospital services, such as dietary department, physical and inhalation therapists, and a part-time social worker, as well as outside services of the Visiting Nurse Association, Reach-to-Recovery, and the Cancer and Heart Associations, all of which provide the advantage of mutual and total nursing support. They prepare written manuals, descriptions, and procedures. An interesting offshoot is the formation of a fifth team on general patient care. Perhaps the commonalities of which we spoke are being or could be developed by this team.

We must not assume that such exciting clinical specialist development should be confined to the small hospital. It should be equally workable in any size institution. Moreover, there is the advantage of a grass roots feeling and consequent strength in developing one's own specialists.

The nurse practitioner is a nurse specialist of a rather specific kind. The pediatric practitioner was the first to be prepared. These nurses are found most often in outpatient departments, in practice with physicians, or working independently. They will probably become more visible in institutional care, especially long-term care, as the specialty grows. These nurses are prepared to care for patients with stabilized chronic disease. They draw on medical skills, such as the taking of histories, doing physical examinations, and other medical practices essential to fulfill their role. Because the work hinges so closely on medical practice, physicians are involved in the training of nurse practitioners. Protocols are established to cover specific activities derived from medical practice. These resemble in some ways standing orders for medical procedure found in coronary care units. All have been spelled out by physicians and nurses working intimately and cooperatively to meet patient needs. Patient teaching is an important part of the work of the nurse practitioner.

There is a growing number of experts in special care areas, such as coronary, intensive, and emergency care units, who work in these areas by personal choice, aptitude, or necessity. They have usually completed one of the three types of nurse education and either learn special skills on the job, go where they can learn the necessary skills in institutions where they are practiced expertly, or learn in adult education programs of community colleges. They are often as expert as physicians (more so than some) in the special skills needed.

Specialists must keep their general skills sharpened so that they can serve the total needs of patients as well as special needs. This is pointed out in an eloquent though popularized way by Slaughter,[13] who raises the question from the point of view of patients with coronary disease. While such patients need and appreciate the service of this highly competent nurse during the acute-care stage, will this efficient nurse be able to provide needed hope, first about whether they will survive and then how they will manage survival? Slaughter suggests the need for special preparation of specialists in the psychological care of patients, acquired more or less as they acquired their special coronary care skills. He presents the ramifications of the specialist-generalist dichotomy starkly but realistically when he poses the crucial question of whether specialists can also possess these collateral skills.

Volunteers. Volunteers in hospitals and nursing homes provide many services to both patients and staff. Fund raising is a big part of their activity. The duties are perhaps of a more general nature: providing amenities, delivering mail, staffing a message center, serving coffee, and supervising games and recreational activities in nursing homes. In some places, they feed, transport, and help patients walk. In a few nursing services, volunteers help with nursing care. High school girls, such as Candy Stripers or Future Nurse Club members, do most of such specifically nursing assistance duties. Volunteers are invaluable in rehabilitation centers where patients progress requires long-term consistent help in carrying forward the regime, and their services could be greatly expanded. Nurses with special skills and abilities or who are willing to acquire them also could be recruited as volunteers.

There is a growing practice of hospitals' offering services to the community. In those isolated instances where hospitals have introduced low-cost health care to senior citizens, nurses as well as others in the hospital and the community contribute their services. A hospital in Prosser, Washington [in Tolva[14]], provides systematic monthly low-cost medical examinations: they offer chest x-ray examinations one month, urinalysis the next, and so on, and send test results to the person's physician. Nurses employed there contribute as volunteers to an integrated hospital volunteer program. A part-time free clinic for the poor, operated by volunteer nurses, is another example [in Toms and Walker[15]].

Collaboration with the major health organizations in various programs and activities is another form of this professional volunteerism. For example, during February while the American Heart Association engaged in its public education and fund raising, St. Vincent Hospital in Portland, Ore., had an excellent display of educational materials, held a public seminar on heart conditions, and during visiting hours operated a clinic for 1 week, during which they checked the blood pressure of over 500 people and apprised personal physicians of notable elevations (see Fig. 13, p. 248).

It is a short step, though one that perhaps includes medical participation, to provision of free Papanicolaou tests to women, along with a display of materials and a public seminar, during a designated period in April, the education and fundraising month of the American Cancer Society. Nurses are essential participants in regional and other studies for cancer determination. One such is a current breast cancer detection demonstration funded by the American Cancer Society and the National Cancer Institute. In each of 27 cities, 10,000 women between the ages of 35 and 74 will be screened and followed up for 3 years, in an attempt to get the early diagnosis so necessary in cancer therapy.

People's clinics, which operate mainly in deprived areas, the increasing number of women's clinics, and senior citizens' clinics for diagnosis of glaucoma, high blood pressure, and so on, are interesting additions to the traditional volunteer role of the nurse in American Red Cross programs, such as operation of blood banks, prenatal instruction, and school programs such as immunization, health room management, and health education.

Volunteerism is really a cyclical activity: sometimes lay people volunteer and help nursing services, while nursing personnel are volunteering their services both within the institutional setting or in the community or are participants in volunteer programs. This reciprocal, growing volunteerism is helping to eliminate the monolithic nature of the hospital. Volunteerism thus becomes another institution in the community, of which nursing is a part.

Health educators. There is considerable proliferation of new occupations within the health field that affect the traditional role of nurses. These positions relieve nurses of some duties and responsibilities, while giving them new duties and responsibilities, but also put at their disposal additional workers whose contribution must be incorporated into the health care team for greater comprehension. An example is the health educator, who is an adjunct and extension of public health services and nurses.

Public health nurses are already familiar with the work of health educators. Institutional nurses must also have knowledge of the work of health educators in promoting community health by statistical, educational, and public relations means, so that institutional care can reflect, integrate, and reinforce the contribution of these workers, both directly and by enhancing the services offered by the public health nurse employed by the hospital. The presence of public health nurses on hospital staffs to help with patient referrals is a step in the right direction.

Conscientious objectors. A final category that has emerged lately is that of people who cannot be assigned to particular units or patients because of conscientious objection. Abortion is the principal area at present that necessitates selective assignment for the individual conscientious objector. In terms of staffing, this is important because neither urgency nor patients' needs can be used as reasons to violate such conscientious objection, nor can there be discrimination against these nurses in the selection and hiring process. This group will increase if and when the Antilife Movement extends into positive euthanasia (direct actions to terminate life, not to be confused with negative euthanasia, that is, removal of extraordinary life-support equipment or procedures from the terminally ill, which has always been practiced).

• • •

All personnel in the nursing service are deeply involved in care, cure, and coordination. Variously, they are responsible for ministrations for the comfort, well-being, and restoration of people to the highest degree possible; treatments, medication, and functions executed by the nursing staff within the medical plan for the patient; for seeing that all collateral professional services reach the patient and are synchronized around him; and for supervision of all personnel serving the patient within the nursing department.

CHANGING TITLES AND TERMS

Accompanying the fluidity within the health field is a trend to shifting nomenclature, or changing titles and terms. This trend has a serious effect on staffing. Alexander[16] uses the newer nomenclature.

We noted in Chapter 6 the change of title from nursing director to nursing coordinator and its attendant confusion. Also, directors and their associates and assistants are now called Nursing Service Facilitators and comprise a new Council of the American Nurses' Association (May 1973). These people are indeed facilitators; that is, they do make easy or less difficult the job of providing nursing services and care. Yet their primary function is responsibility and accountability for the satisfactory conduct of the nursing service to provide appropriate nursing care to the patients in an institution or agency. The essential nature of direction in discharging this responsibility, and accountability is misunderstood when director is changed to facilitator. The terms are simply not synonymous and only generate confusion if taken literally.

Another instance of name changing is the New York State Nurses' Association "New Position Descriptions in Nursing,"[17] which replaces the terms general duty or staff nurse, head nurse, and supervisor with nursing practitioner, associate nursing care coordinator, and nursing care coordinator. The reason given was that the "new legal definition of nursing practice in New York State (March 1972)" made the old terms "archaic" and "illegal."

According to this pronouncement, the term staff nurse implied that he or she was "not a fully independent professional practitioner." It is true that staff nurses are not fully independent professional practitioners in the institutional setting any more than are interns or residents. These nurses and physicians are accountable to the medical staff of the institution as well as to the institution itself; they function within the framework of the philosophy, practices, and policies of both jurisdictions while employed in that institution. If it were otherwise, it would be anarchic, not archaic. This is not to say that professional nurses do not practice independently within a given institution; professional nursing may be and most often is the same in the expectation of the nurse, the nursing service, and the hospital. If professional nursing is not viewed in the same way by the nurse, the nursing service, and administration, then the problem is one of reconciling the differences, not changing the name.

The titles of head nurse and supervisor have always implied a managerial component with consequent accountability for carrying goals forward. Calling these people associate nursing care coordinators and nursing care coordinators implies a coordinating function, which has a low accountability factor.

Stevens[18] has done an insightful critique of the New York State Nurses' Association's "New Position Description in Nursing." She speaks about two ways of looking at the "responsibility-authority structure." One is that "derived from the person's position in the organization," the other from "her position as a practicing professional." The New York position, which "opts for replacing administrative authority with professional authority in both job titles and job descriptions," loses "intelligibility for the client," understanding of "other managers in the health institution"; "shows such tendencies to underplay and softsell its own authority positions"; and uses job descriptions and some terminology in unusual ways.

Another proposed change in nomenclature that bears examination is the use of the terms distributive and episodic by the National Commission for the Study of Nursing and Nursing Education [p. 279].[19]

Distributive is defined as "that area of concentration in nursing practice which emphasizes prevention of disease and maintenance of health and is largely directed toward continuous care of persons not confined to health care institutions." Episodic is defined as "that area of concentration in nursing practice which emphasizes the curative and restorative aspect of nursing and which usually involves patients with diagnosed disease, either acute or chronic." These are only definitions of public health and institutional care or of preventive and therapeutic care. In fact, the terms episodic and chronic are contradictory, though chronic is included in the Commission's definition of episodic.

Communication is fraught with difficulties of all kinds without adding the confusion of name changing when it is illogical. Name changing will not increase the clinical component of traditional positions, for example, head nurse and supervisor. When comprehensive nursing care is known and practiced intimately and universally at all levels, upgrading of clinical competence will be achieved.

If greater precision is the result of name changing, then it is all to the good; if, however, it is related to the current cliché about the constancy of change or is done for its anticipated impact or for the sake of freshness, it may bring confusion and disorder.

Personnel in position
RECRUITMENT

The concrete job of staffing the nursing service is formidable and demanding. Recruitment of appropriate personnel to carry forward the ultimate goal of the department, that is, optimal and economical nursing care for a specific number of patients, is an important part of the staffing process. It is the means of enlisting workers for the enterprise, and ranges from the nurses' aide who enlists a friend to apply for a job at the same hospital to the most sophisticated advertising in national nursing journals.

Advertising

Advertising has changed over the last decade, from the most prosaic of advertisements to the most contemporary efforts of public relations personnel. One advertisement for a very famous institution has even evoked resentment because it suggests that it is one of the few places that really offers high-quality nursing care. The "girl meets boy" and "glamorous relaxation" themes of today supplement such enticements as reduced college tuition, inexpensive apartments, and day-care centers for the nurse's children.

Glowing descriptions of the opportunities one finds at X Hospital abound in journal advertising. Such blandishments are forgivable or understandable in a society inundated by advertising. Moreover, they keep the institutions thinking about a wide variety of incentives that they must attempt to provide if their credibility is to be maintained and new-employee bitterness is to be avoided, should the advertisement and the real situation not be essentially consistent.

Long columns of positions available are listed in journals that antedate the glowing advertisements and serve well the recruitment process. Newspapers of all kinds are used increasingly to recruit inactive nursing personnel who may begin thinking about returning to work when they find positions available so frequently in newspapers. Trends may be seen in these advertisements. For example, one hospital advertised for a lay person to manage the staffing work of a large nursing service. As well as a recruitment device, such advertising lets the community know that this institution is forward thinking in its utilization of staff.

The ultimate in newspaper advertising is to be found in a beautiful 16-page supplement in a major daily newspaper, which contained descriptive, pictorial, and discussion material in a sophisticated presentation that compliments rather than insults professional and public sensibilities.[20]

Job listings placed on employees' bulletin boards are another means of advertising. All personnel should know of job openings in the organization, for either their own purpose or the value of each person's sphere of influence in recruiting for the organization among family, friends, and so on.

Recruitment committee

DeVincenti[21] suggests and describes a recruitment committee with representative membership of nursing personnel and the personnel department, to formalize the efforts of all, prepare recruitment materials, and make recommendations to the director of nursing.

Recruitment at meetings

Recruitment is done at professional meetings. Opportunity and choice for the nurse takes precedence over taking promising personnel from others' staffs. Meetings of women's groups also provide recruitment sources.

Recruitment of the underprivileged

Recruitment of the underprivileged has been a special contribution of health agencies to society. Even before the days of the minimum wage, equal opportunity, federal and state controls, and so on, hospitals have been hiring handicapped and marginally employable persons, especially in inner cities, where large numbers of hospital beds were and remain today despite the flight of people and institutions to the suburbs. Thousands of nurses' aides and assistants avail themselves of these opportunities and represent a stable work force for the institutions. The accusation has been justifiably made that such personnel remain at the lower levels, and it is true that there is much to be done to get these workers up the career ladder by providing or finding for them incentives, financial assistance, and perhaps tutoring.

Though we have this creditable record in inner cities, it must be admitted that government efforts to improve the job situation of the underprivileged have had their positive effect on hospitals in regard to such employment. "Equal opportunity employer" on advertisements for nurses at least tells people that it has been thought about in that institution. State Fair Employment Practice laws and especially the Civil Rights Act of 1964 provide the legislation required to safeguard the rights of disadvantaged blacks, Spanish-Americans, Amerindians, and women. Surveillance of and guidance in hiring practices is made by the Equal Employment Opportunity Commission and the office of Federal Contracts Compliance and results in the continuing effort of affirmative action in seeing that the underprivileged have equal opportunity in the job market.

Recruitment of part-time employees

The recruitment of part-time workers continues but could be accelerated. The teaming of part-time personnel has not been developed fully. There are isolated cases where two nurses hold one head nurse position, but many more combinations might be developed that would give these people a greater feeling of participation in achieving the goals of the nursing service and increased sense of belonging, which would enrich the institution as well as the persons involved.

Float personnel, who have long stabilized nursing services, usually come from the ranks of part-time workers. They originally were sent anywhere there was an immediate need for personnel, because of absent staff, increased patient load, unexpected work load, and so forth. Float personnel reached their peak in organized groups known appropriately as "flying squads." This team approach provides the small group a mutual support factor.

Not all nurses are psychologically adapted to entering high-pressure or emergency situations, which often characterize the float situation. Recent studies on float personnel show opportunities for growth in knowledge and experience to be an advantage. Refinement of duties for this important group of nurses will help to meet their needs as well as those of the service required. Tailoring the assignment to the personnel is important. It is well worth the effort required in terms of worker satisfaction. Testing can ascertain personnel strengths and interests, but it cannot replace the effort to learn more about individual workers, in an attempt to put them in an appropriate assignment, or the skill of a supervisor at any level in observing these strengths and interests, which perhaps have not even yet been identified by the worker.

According to Thomas,[22] staff attitudes toward this category of nurses were less than satisfactory. We are gradually learning to respect individual differences. Greater effort toward increasing staff appreciation of strengths, difficulties, and nature of float nursing by counseling, in-service education, or any other means, would improve staff attitudes toward this group.

Another advantage of recruitment of part-time personnel is increased recognition and utilization of persons with special skills. An inactive nurse with knowledge and experience in team nursing—classic team nursing that requires a thorough grasp of comprehensive nursing care—could be hired on an hourly basis to do specific jobs or coach others in areas in which the particular nurse is especially proficient.

There is great need for research on a modest scale in all nursing services. The absence of nursing research personnel in any but large medical centers is another unmet need for which the part-time nurse could be sought. Additionally, instructors for the in-service education program can sometimes be found on a part-time basis, utilizing a specific specialty these nurses have or are willing to acquire.

Recruiting people for part-time positions requires imagination, willingness, and ability to search out nurses who have special skills and interests. It is an individualization aspect of recruitment that is so far underdeveloped.

There is a growing number of commercial sources for recruitment of temporary or part-time personnel. Manpower, Inc., the national agency that provides temporary personnel, has moved into the health field. It offers the potential employee temporary placement with choice of days and hours, top hourly rates, paid holidays and vacations, low-cost medical insurance, and free $1,000 accident insurance.[23] Another such source is Upjohn Homemakers, which operates in 175 cities and has expanded to provide temporary hospital staff from their long-time program of home health care and private-duty nursing.[24]

Geographic location

Geographic location plays an important part in recruiting. Whether the institution is in the inner city, suburbs, or rural areas often determines both the patient population and availability of workers.

Large public city hospitals, often associated with educational institutions, have a wide range of clinical practice and ready access to inner city personnel but limited access to professional staff because of travel time to residential areas or danger associated with the location of the hospital in deprived, high–crime-rate parts of the city. Such location often requires guarded parking lots, escort or even taxi service to public transportation, and so forth, as compensatory services to staff. Suburban locations have fewer security problems, a more congenial work location, and good parking facilities, but public transportation may be limited.

Proximity to universities or other professional schools, wherever they are located, usually provides staff from the ranks of working wives, but is accompanied by high turnover. In stable rural and city neighborhoods, nurses who are wives and mothers can be recruited on a full- or part-time basis to cover emergency situations, peak work times (such as 8 AM to 12 noon or 7 PM to 11 PM) or peak seasonal times (such as harvest time in agricultural locations, when accident admissions rise appreciably; in climates where inclement weather contributes to respiratory and circulatory conditions and accidents requiring patient hospitalization; or near resort areas, with their seasonal variations). The geographic location of the institution must be studied sociologically to determine both the assets and liabilities so they can be used or overcome expeditiously.

Long- and short-range incentives can be offered. For example, 20 years ago a hospital in a large metropolitan area offered salaries substantially higher than the going rate and quickly became the only hospital in the area with a waiting list of professional nurses. An institution that launches and continues a serious program to conserve professional time, maintain an open responsive climate, pay attention to individuality of staff members as well as patients, and encourage worker input in achieving goals will in the long run reap the benefits of a more stable staff. Strong or dramatic clinical areas or specialties will attract people with similar interests, as will colorful medical or nursing personalities with whom to work. The way in which employees reach out to the community and its activities will also affect staffing. And there is simply no replacement for the old-fashioned notion of a hospital's reputation as a good place to work and be cared for.

• • •

Recruitment is indeed a large responsibility, because it extends both into the community and into the heart of the nursing enterprise.

The vital part played by the personnel department greatly assists the nursing department. Once specific requests for personnel by number, kind, and description are made to the personnel department, it assumes responsibility for finding appropriate people for recruitment; interviews, tests, and checks references and work records of applicants; and assembles all data for the director of nursing service or a delegated colleague to review, interview, select, and place personnel in service. The personnel department and nursing service collaborate in orientation and on-the-job training. The nursing department evaluates the worker at specified periods, and the personnel department maintains such records. When an employee resigns, the nursing department does the exit interview, while the personnel department studies all the information so that its expertise can turn up patterns that show a need for change in policy and procedure in the work situation. There is a school of thought that advocates that the personnel department conduct the exit interview, in the hope that it will be a franker one than if it were conducted by the employee's department head. There is also the possibility that exit interviews do not produce frankness, because terminating employees fear that frankness, if it is derogatory, will be held against them in specific ways, especially in references required for future positions.

Another excellent device to help nursing departments and hospital personnel departments perfect their recruitment procedures is *ABC's of Nurse Recruitment* [in Hoffman[25]], a comprehensive condensed checklist that allows employers to see the whole recruitment picture.

CRITERIA FOR SELECTION AND PLACEMENT

Selection of nursing personnel has often been taken for granted; for so many years it embraced almost all applicants, because the need for personnel was so great. This becomes increasingly less the case as administrative practice and procedure, including the personnel function, are focused on and become operative. Societal factors affect the situation and are reflected in higher salaries, greater use of part-time workers, greater attention to special qualifications or attributes, geographic areas of high or low supply, increased public attention to the health care field, and so on. Moreover, there is the effect of the gradual refinement and growing sophistication in the health care field.

Selection interview

After the personnel department has compiled collateral material to the application, such as references, verification of data, and test results, the nursing service director or a delegated substitute will interview the applicant. The interview should cover all potential trouble spots in the projected employment, from both the organization's and the applicant's points of view.

Openness at the outset will prevent misunderstandings, confusion, and bitterness in the work relationship later on. For example, the time to be spent on evening and night shifts in proportion to day shifts should be clearly stated so that the nurse will know the specific ratios rather than the evasive information that staff nurses rotate regularly. Numbers and frequency of weekends off is another trouble spot requiring frankness and honesty. Deception of any kind must be avoided, though the temptation to evade is great in face of the difficulties of staffing unpopular shifts. Moreover, the applicant should not be placed in the position of having to ask such questions, including those of salary schedule. Such openness extends to a brief visit to random floors and units, where the nurse should have an opportunity to meet and speak privately to staff on duty, in conjunction with the interview. This content falls naturally into a description of the institution and its services.

Manfredi[26] discusses areas of content for the interview that are designed to bring out information necessary to both the employer and the employee, such as questions about family responsibilities, transportation, past-employment relations, unexplained lapses in employment, education, experience, and preferences for in-service needs. Observations relating to personal appearance, psychological responses, and so forth, are also part of the selection interview.

Position versus job choices. Cleland[27] points out correctly that there are opportunities within the occupation of nursing for positions in the career continuum, as well as jobs that provide personal and remunerative satisfactions, and stresses the need for clarity and precision in the minds of the applicant and the employer as to the specific choices open to them in selection and placement of personnel. She proposes that nurses choose whether they want a career position, with the consequent advantages of better hours but more home or extracurricular work and study, or a job that is perhaps self-limiting, contained, clearly defined, and with stated salary aspects. She speaks of bargaining from clear knowledge of what such options realistically entail and states that personal and professional goals must be reconciled in a meaningful way.

Educational objectives. Another area, which can properly fit in the interview stage and which is really a part of professional and personal goals, is the applicants' educational objectives. Even though applicants have opted for the "job" aspect, with immediate, circumscribed gains, there may be something in the current proliferation of educational opportunities that interests them. An applicant who has opted for the "position" aspect may appreciate the wide range of opportunities developing locally, regionally, and nationally as the career-ladder concept opens up and flourishes. The interviewer can open avenues for thought by being knowledgeable and positive about such career ideas.

Personal preferences and aptitude

Appropriate placement of personnel in positions that suit their personalities and attributes is a serious consideration in the relationship of the worker to the organization. We have not given proper attention to placement, partly because the work demands are so dominant and partly because personnel administration has not yet reached that degree of refinement in most nursing services.

Personal preferences often reflect aptitudes. Where they have been honored, experience has shown that there are persons who have sufficient patience to practice in long-term or rehabilitation services. Their tolerance for the frustration of being slowed down in the conduct of nursing care makes them especially suitable in these areas. In some people, manual dexterity or grace has made them especially valuable in the operating room; a fondness for abstraction can be met in the operating room also. Mechanical ability has been an asset to nurses working in coronary care or related units, where machines and equipment play a large part. There are persons who enjoy the float position—being "where the action is" at a given time and then moving on to other scenes of action. Early studies in comparison of medical and surgical nurses (in Lentz and Michaels[28]) demonstrated the interest of the medical nurse in the psychological aspects of nursing care and the surgical nurse's interest in swift completion of nursing care.

Testing

The use of tests to corroborate, question experiential observations, or identify latent talents in appropriate selection and placement of people is a route that could prove fruitful. Dunn and Stephens[29] categorize testing into general ability, intelligence, aptitude, skills (or psychomotor ability), interests, personality, and situational (or miscellaneous) experience. They list the more common tests in these categories. Expert help is necessary in establishing a testing program. Testing in nursing education can provide a model either to be copied or to serve as a base for examination. However, enthusiasm needs to be tempered by recalling the fallibility factor in testing and the phenomenal and often surprising potential of people.

Another facet of selection and placement of personnel is self-examination in a structured way. Reres[30] provides such a questionnaire, containing 73 items grouped under the headings of skills, temperament, communication skills, stamina, spirituality, role position preference, and cognitive skills. Such a device should inform both the employee and employer about placement.

• • •

Reconciling appropriate placement, determined either on the basis of personal preference, observation, or testing, with the immediate heavy demands for staff in nursing services remains difficult. Any movement, and it is hoped a growing movement, in that direction can only result in greater employee satisfaction and its sequel, improved nursing care. It is indeed worth the effort.

OPTIMAL UTILIZATION OF PERSONNEL
Fluidity in nursing

When one thinks of personnel in nursing service today, the fluidity of health personnel must be considered in order to avoid the pitfall of rigidity or uncontrolled movement. Movement of duties from the physician to the nurse continues not only with the expanded role of nurses as nurse practitioners, who give primary medical care in collaboration with a physician, as in the case of pediatric practitioners, and are permitted to diagnose (this is medical diagnosis, not to be confused with nursing diagnosis [Nurse Practice Act, State of Washington, 1973]), but concerns also the medical decisions made by nurses in coronary and intensive care units, albeit by prearrangement or protocol with the medical staff. Fluidity is also present within general medical units where licensed practical nurses are giving medications, again by prearrangement. Moreover, they are assuming charge duties in more and more institutions. This fluidity extends outward to include inhalation therapists, psychotherapists, teams that administer intravenous infusions, and so forth.

Efforts at ridding nursing of nonnursing functions require simultaneous reinforcement of the nurse in clinical practice by any and all means, such as recognition and acceptance of the problem, opportunities to strengthen nurses' own clinical performance, comparison with appropriate models, and improvement of their analytical skills.

A good example of action to end the dissipation of nursing by nonnursing duties is New York City's municipal hospital system.[31] Heartened by the passage of nurse practice legislation, supported by the New York State Nurses' Association, and having exhausted the study-recommendation route, these nurses now refuse to pass or collect meal trays, escort regular patients to and from other departments or on discharge, wash beds, go to the pharmacy, or check on x-ray films. Instead, they concentrate on comprehensive nursing care: checking patients more frequently, counseling them and their families, giving psychological support to women in labor, seeing patients in the admitting department to begin assessment and plans, turning patients every 2 hours, ascertainment of discharge planning in terms of instruction and referral, and so forth.

The essential point of these expansions for good order and management is prearrangement. The prearrangement must be thought through thoroughly so the responsibility assumed can be carried out competently, leaving nothing to chance and assuring that both the physician delegating the service or procedure and the nurse assuming responsibility for it accept and understand the whole transaction, with its obligations and duties.

Conservation of nurse time

In this fluid situation, interrelationships of positions, work, and departments occur with or without concomitant scrutiny and participatory decision making. There is abundant evidence that the dissipation of nursing time continues, albeit to a lesser extent. Inappropriate utilization appears in most nurse satisfaction surveys. Though part of the inappropriateness and underutilization may result from failure of the nursing department to clarify its goals, to assign work realistically, or to raise the sights of its staff, a substantial part comes from the long-standing haphazard relationship with other departments.

There is ample evidence that there is diffusion and confusion in the nursing role itself as a result of imprecise definition, nondescript management, wide range of clinical competence, nonanalytic nature of nursing, and the constant pressure of overwork. This diffusion and confusion complicate efforts to rectify the deficiencies, because there is evidence that nurses are uneasy when their work is finished. Nurses are not making significant efforts to rid themselves of obviously nonnursing duties. Absence of widespread practice of comprehensive nursing care may account for this reluctance, because consciously or unconsciously we may pursue duties that fill our time, though we suspect or know they are not our responsibility, rather than face the anxiety of having to fill the extra time with nursing care with which we are not yet familiar or willing to learn or practice. Norris[32] attributes this confused condition of nurses to "low self-concept" and the need for "rigid structuring of the patient's day":

> In their desperation to be useful, to be needed, to be busy and to do something familiar, they quietly take on many non-nursing functions that are bits and pieces of the functions of other departments. Thus we find nurses doing paper work and errands for a number of departments. Closely allied to this is another area where nurses step out of role at the suggestion or request of an authority figure.

Related to the need to conserve professional time in order to increase the quantity and quality of nursing care is the accountability factor. The more it is intensified, the more precise what is being accounted for must be.

There are budgetary implications too. The gradual refinement of budgeting requires precision in job positions within departments. Nursing does encompass the largest number of employees in the institution, but their work has always been swelled disproportionately by the absorption of work of other departments, resulting in budgetary distortion.

Intradepartmental conservation. In assuming nonnursing functions and responsibilities, ward managers and ward clerks offer excellent opportunity for intradepartmental conservation of nurse time.

We must sharpen our analytic prowess and apply it uniformly to past as well as present performance. For example, the simple device of using carbon sheets along with the physician's order sheet, perforated to allow sectional use, allows the copy of the original order for dietary, pharmacy, laboratory, radiology, or other services to be sent directly to each department for processing. It alleviates the laborious requisitioning that goes on in the nursing unit, thus reducing substantially the time spent on such duties by ward clerks or nursing personnel.

It was a long time before a concerted effort was made to upgrade the work of licensed practical nurses and differentiate it more completely from that of nurses' aides, though LPNs were always compensated at a higher level. This reluctance probably stemmed from the fact that delegating additional responsibilities to LPNs required stripping something from professional nurses. For example, administration of routine medication passed to LPNs much later and somewhat more reluctantly than it should have, and probably was transferred more in the interest of self-preservation than of appropriate delegation.

Interdepartmental conservation. The hospital administration position of assistant director in charge of patient services is often filled by a nurse. Nurses should have the same unprejudiced right that any other worker has to improve their personal condition. Such an administrative position places the nurse higher in the line of power and prestige, but usually takes a strong nurse away from nursing. This arrangement is not to be confused with the nursing service director, who is an assistant administrator by virtue of the responsibility borne for the essential service of the hospital, or because all department heads are assistant administrators, because here the nurse is retained in nursing.

Interdepartmentally we have been imposed on because nursing assumes continuous responsibility for patient care. Thus nurses perform many nonnursing functions because other departments are closed or "it has always been done that way." Night supervisors are still the night admissions clerks in some institutions. Often they are the hospital contact with the press, police, and so forth, as needed. On rare occasions they have declared a patient dead at the request of a physician and set in motion the postmortem care for the patient.

The evening or night supervisor as substitute pharmacist is still a familiar figure, though there has been a move in the direction of extending the hours of the pharmacy into the evening and even to 24-hour service to meet the needs of newly admitted patients, to prepare patients for the next day's procedures, and so forth. This pharmacy service carried out by nurses over the years has been potentially fraught with difficulties because of crossing professional lines. There may also be possible legal implications. Nowhere besides the pharmacy-nursing relationship does the professional pendulum swing so far at present, from the condition described above to almost total responsibility for drug administration by the pharmacy, from the physician's order to charting. It is an interesting phenomenon, demonstrating professional awakening in other departments as well as nursing.

Intravenous therapy is sometimes found under the direction of the pharmacy, though usually carried out by nurses. It is interesting to consider whether this procedure should have moved from physicians to the laboratory department, because vein penetration was and is part of the operating skills of laboratory workers.

Nurses have always absorbed a substantial portion of housekeeping duties, and, according to a recent survey [p. 43][3] a few hospitals of all sizes continue to have RNs clean discharge units. It is clearly the work of a comprehensive housekeeping department to see that all equipment is in order and operating. If this department assumed responsibility for maintenance as well as cleaning of patient units, nurses would be relieved of jobs such as checking, requisitioning, and rechecking.

In linen supply there has been considerable progress. Unit packs are commonplace, and it is not unusual to have linen supplies checked daily by housekeeping and a standard supply maintained.

Our assumption of dietary duties persists, though we have come a long way from the day when the head nurse served the food that had been brought to a unit kitchen and the staff set up and carried the trays. Nurses have been slow to relinquish the dietary department's rightful responsibility for carrying and picking up of trays. RNs still serve trays in a seventh to a third of hospitals.[3] Some nurses know first-hand, however, the satisfaction derived when the dietary department has been persuaded to pick up not only regular trays, but also those of patients with diabetes, weigh the uneaten food, and deliver replacements for the unused portions. There is an ultramodern continuation of nurse responsibility for dietary work in the use of new microwave ovens that are being placed in nursing units, in order that nurses can complete the final stages of cooking of food. However, care must be taken to have the dietary department follow through completely; such new types of equipment should not be allowed to be a camouflage for continuance of nurse exploitation.

Increased nurse responsibility

Few would object to the gradual transfer of medical duties to nurses as procedures become commonplace. Moreover, where ability to take histories and do physical examinations enhances nursing practice, there can be no objection to nurses doing these portions of the physicians' work. Perhaps, though, each item of transfer should be examined carefully to determine whether it fits into the nursing regime. There seems little doubt that primary care activities transferred to the nurse (for example, the pediatric nurse practitioner) are legitimate nursing functions. Such transfer increases points of entry into the health care field, which results in more patients seen, faster attention to their needs, and fewer complications. Rural, inner city locations, and long-term facilities are sites where primary care is likely to extend.

However, multiple entry points for patients as justification for increased nurse activity can be countered with the argument that nurses are again assuming medical responsibilities without attendant compensation; in a way, they are subsidizing physicians, as they have always subsidized them, the hospital, and the public. The problem is that the work relationship of physicians and nurses has never been clearly defined or accepted and is only beginning to reach a point of discussion, as a result of the recommendation by the National Commission for the Study of Nursing and Nursing Education [p. 289][19] for a National Joint Practice Commission, with state counterparts, to deliberate about "the congruent uses of the physician and the nurse in providing quality health care, with particular attention to: the rise of the nurse clinician; the introduction of the physician's assistant; the increased activity of other professions and para-professions in areas long assumed to be the concern solely of the physician and/or the nurse." It should be noted, however, that since 1964 there have been occasional national conferences of professional nurses and physicians, which certainly paved the way for present efforts in this direction.

This National Joint Practice Commission will deal with the realignment and readjustment of the nurse-physician work relationships that have resulted from the growth of knowledge, techniques, and skills. It plans two casebooks: one to demonstrate joint nursing-medical practice, and the other to show interprofessional continuing education efforts.[33]

Nurses in the emergency room. Emergency rooms and their staffs have changed greatly with the advent of the new specialty of trauma medicine, which derives from socioeconomic conditions, such as the increasingly heavy accident load carried by emergency departments as the country's highways, cars, and people's activities have proliferated. Emergency rooms are increasingly sophisticated, streamlined, and efficient in meeting greater and more complicated work loads. In many cases they are taking the place of former home visits by physicians, becoming an adjunct to both physicians' offices and people's homes so that medical needs are met more expeditiously. The acutely ill are often admitted to the emergency room, where preliminary examinations are done before the patients are sent to the patient areas. There may even be holding areas for patients who are not to be admitted but require some sort of care. Time is saved, diagnosis is made, and treatment is begun more swiftly in these comprehensive units. Triage nursing is a part of this new emergency room service. It consists of initial classification of patients as to their needs, with consequent placement within the department to get high-priority needs met first. There is often two-way communication between ambulance services and hospitals to facilitate swift service. Emergency departments are also greatly strengthened by the growing skills and preparation of ambulance personnel, now known as medical emergency technicians. Their preparation is often centralized in community colleges and consists of both basic and advanced work. It is a far cry from the original first aid instruction in its sophistication and quality.

Nurses as extenders of patient care. In the interest of cooperative effort to achieve comprehensive patient care, there is a legitimate use of nurse time and effort in assumption of duties of other departments. This is the coordinating function of nursing so that continuity is maintained and progress thereby hastened. Exercises enhancing the physiotherapeutic program, specific activities in occupational therapy, and attitude reinforcement of the psychotherapeutic regimes are examples of this kind of extension of work of special departments that can be carried out by nursing.

These reinforcements are as important and essential as those that nursing provides to intravenous or inhalation therapists. These latter two are more clearly accepted because they have been a part of nursing in the recent past. Nursing correctly assumes as much responsibility as its capabilities allow, in order to provide these special services where they are not available. For example, consulting with the patient and family in an effort to provide an appropriate recreational activity and assisting with its implementation and practice have physical and occupational therapeutic implications where such departments do not exist. Likewise nursing can, should, and has acted as an extender for the dietary department in teaching patients proper nutrition as well as specific therapeutic nutrition. This is essentially followup on teaching of the dietary department or reinforcement of the dietary instruction. Where there is no social worker, nurses can advise and assist patients in availing themselves of the various local or state resources, such as cancer or heart associations, health departments, or visiting nurses. Problem-oriented charting, where physicians and nurses combine and work cooperatively on mutually identified patient problems, is another collaborative effort.

Some of these examples may seem to indicate that nurses are doing the work of others, but they are also practicing comprehensive nursing. Again, to avoid exploitation, what is being done must be determined exactly: extending the services of another department by reinforcement or supervising practice, providing elemental services of another department where it does not exist, or both. Continuity of care is well within the province of comprehensive nursing care.

Nurses in extended-care facilities. With the tremendous growth in services and care to the aged and the effect of Medicare-Medicaid, not only on medical care but on the institutions and personnel providing it, there has been concomitant growth in geriatric nursing specialists, increasing numbers of nurses employed in extended-care facilities and nursing homes, and a marked movement of nursing homes into the mainstream of health care institutions. Long-term care has been strengthened and expanded essentially for the same reasons, all stemming from attention to the increasing numbers of older people in our society. Though offset somewhat by the closure of many tuberculosis and psychiatric facilities, the return of these patients to communities has meant increased use of nursing home space for them. All of these factors strengthen the long-term facility, open it to greater nurse scrutiny, and bring the possibility of discovering the real nature of nursing in them.

Nurses in utilization-evaluation programs. There are questions of nurse utilization in efforts to achieve maximum use of hospital beds and services. For example, there are nurses involved in the federally legislated Professional Standards and Review Organization (PSRO), an evaluation program for physicians who care for patients receiving Medicare-Medicaid. Is the work of these nurses really contributing to health care, or are they serving the medical profession exclusively in its review procedures? The same question arises about the work of nurse-coordinators where they function in quality assurance programs (not to be confused with nursing quality assurance programs) for hospitals to use in ensuring appropriate utilization of hospital facilities and the quality of medical care. These two particular evaluating systems (PSRO and QAP) do not have nursing components, though nurses sometimes function in them as nurse-coordinators.

With the extension of nursing into primary medical care, as in the case of pediatric and family practitioners, why not extension into utilization-evaluation programs, in the interest of health care for the public as opposed to medical care? Nurses, by virtue of their particular knowledge, are the only collaborators in health care able to participate in such programs. Moreover, such participation fosters physician-nurse communication and paves the way for the entry of evaluation of nursing care into such programs. We must examine all points of view and be certain that our contribution is appropriate nurse utilization and not another form of exploitation. Such deliberations are extremely complex, because of the traditional, current, and future relationships between physicians and nurses. Nursing must put its most knowledgeable and analytical nurses into such deliberations.

• • •

A clear definition of nursing is necessary so that we can eliminate the abuse of nursing that results from indiscriminate work assignment, while maintaining our responsibility as legitimate extenders of the care given by other departments or for cooperation and collaboration necessary to improve patient care. Clearly defined nursing care is also necessary so that the time released to nursing by elimination of nonnursing functions will be used fruitfully by nursing staffs who are willing and able to discharge increasingly comprehensive nursing care. It is important that growth in giving comprehensive nursing care parallels efforts to conserve professional time. Nursing care is not automatically enriched. Studies in Kansas [in New and associates[34]] and Iowa [in Aydelotte and Tener[35]] demonstrate factors of uneasiness and unchanged nursing care. It will require considerable effort to help nurses upgrade the quality of care given as their professional time is conserved.

STAFFING PATTERNS

Staffing patterns are the plans for providing appropriate numbers of different levels of nursing personnel to carry forward the goal of the institution and the particular units comprising it. The purpose of staffing patterns is appropriate coverage of the job to be done in the interest of the patients entrusting themselves to the institution and equitable utilization of workers in their interest. Concern for workers' interest redounds to the quality of the nursing care practiced.

Determinants of staffing patterns

There are many determinants in devising master plans for staffing patterns, because there are many variables surrounding patient populations to be served, including whether the institution is general or specific:

1. If general, does it include the standard clinical components? Do the standard clinical components include subspecialties, such as neurosurgery, heart surgery, or hemodialysis? Is the institution strengthening and enlarging its emergency department, outpatient department, or rehabilitation services?
2. If special psychiatric, does it include provisions for day or night care only in addition to regular care? Is it small and highly therapeutic; large, including therapeutic and custodial care; or one with emphasis on returning patients to their communities?
3. If long-term or chronic, other than psychiatric, is the institution largely therapeutic, restorative, custodial, or all three?
4. Does the institution embrace the progressive patient concept, with separation of patients by degree of illness (intensive, intermediate, or ambulatory)? Does it have a home-care component or an associated extended or long-care facility? Does it have a satellite clinic elsewhere in the community?
5. Is it one that has just merged with another institution in the community for management purposes in the interest of economy, or is it contemplating possible merger for the same reason? If so, will the services remain the same or be reallocated, for example, obstetrics in one and pediatrics in another or cobalt therapy in one and rehabilitation in another? Are there plans for distribution of services, in the interest

of maximum utilization, economy, or avoidance of duplication, by local or state health and welfare planning councils, by hospitals themselves, or by state regulating bodies?

The nature of relationships between institutions affected by consumerism and regulating bodies are primary determinants of staffing patterns.

Quantifying patients' nursing needs

Quantifying the nursing needs of patients is one of the first components to be determined in staffing. Types or methods of quantitative measurement range from primal experiential knowledge of nursing to scientific methods of industrial engineering, consisting of material and data systematically and carefully collected in collaboration with nursing staffs. These data reflect figures based on specific time required for each task, service, or treatment for a selected group of patients, recorded or observed a sufficient number of times to approximate an average that yields the total number of hours of nursing time needed for that particular category of patients. In general, the greater the arithmetical precision, the greater has been the influence of industrial engineering personnel, because they are singularly able to deliberate with and observe nurses in such a way that they can quantify activities, demonstrate patterns and trends, point out problem areas or bottlenecks, design graphic materials to display findings, and provide efficient forms for nurses to use. They sometimes meet with resistance because of the mathematical detail, but a nursing service will be richer for having utilized their methods. Thorough documentation accompanies work guided by industrial engineers, and they provide realistic measurement and data on which to base decisions and actions.

Using such precise measurement methods will make it easier to measure less tangible parts of nursing care as they become incorporated in increasingly sophisticated ways into general nursing practice. For example, psychological care, including "calming measures" and their numerical time measurement, is beginning to be described and quantified in procedure books, enabling methods of such nursing care to become more precise [p. 10].[36]

As long ago as 1959 Lentz and Michaels[28] in their research on comparative attributes of medical and surgical nurses raised the question of the time required by medical nurses to become familiar with, talk to, and generally interact with patients in order to provide the psychological care these nurses thought necessary. They pointed out that such nurses giving psychological support need more encouragement and emotional support than they ordinarily receive. This involves indirect quantification in terms of time allotment for nurse-superior communication if such support is to be forthcoming. They also asked if technical care and psychological care required the same amount of time. We still have not answered their question, although we are beginning to collect some data in this area, as indicated in the above example.

Between experienced nursing judgment and the skills of the industrial engineer, there are various classification systems that use essentially the same base, that is, division of patients into categories of illness, with care ranging from intensive to intermediate to minimal. There may be other categories within this range. O'Malley[37] uses the above three categories and allocates 6, 4.5, and 3 hours of care per 24 hours for each respectively. Warstler[38] proposes five categories of care: intensive, modified, intermediate, minimal, and self-care. Intensive care is confined to that in coronary care units. These categories are allocated 12, 7.5, 5.5, 3.5, and 1.5 hours per 24-hour period respectively.[39] Paetznick[40] uses a three-part classification for patient illness: critical, moderate, and convalescent.

Carter and associates[41] set forth an interesting variation of the three categories of self-, partial, and total care. They apply them numerically, 0 through 3, to each of five factors: ambulation and movement, feeding, bathing, elimination, and special nursing interventions. The number of points arrived at by this application then yields five patient types, which determines the number of personnel required.

Ott[42] carries a listing not only of the degree of illness in the usual three parts but of control of activity, behavior reaction, application of therapy, and teaching and rehabilitation, all of which are subdivided three times to allow for time estimation.

The modular scheduling technique in use in many high schools provides a model for refinement of scheduling by patient classification. This technique involves division of the school day, usually into 15-minute modules, which can be grouped to meet the requirements of a particular class. For example, some laboratory sessions require more than the standard 60-minute class time, so they are allowed five, six, or seven modules, making 75, 90 or 105 minutes available. Similarly with nursing care, additional modules could be added to the standard time allowed for a particular category. For example, toenail and foot care could be planned ahead, and a module added for that purpose when necessary. Similarly with patient teaching, time allotments could be measured in modules for components of specific teaching procedures.

Price[43] summarized several patient classification systems by purposes, underlying assumptions, the factors considered, techniques of data collection, resulting categories, and the use of the systems. She points out that all patient classification systems are developed according to current practice. This factor has significance especially for nursing services that are systematically increasing their quality of nursing toward the goal of comprehensive nursing care. However, current practice provides a base line from which to measure improvement in the quality of care as well as a base line of care itself from which components of comprehensiveness can be added systematically. Like any type of clinical analysis, it must be repeated periodically to ensure continuing reliability.

Price also points out the danger in generalizing from another's figures. There are many variables from institution to institution: for example, how well nursing has been stripped of nonnursing functions, and the corollary of how well dietary, housekeeping, pharmacy, and such departments are assuming total responsibility for their work; the degree of comprehensiveness of the nursing practiced; the physical arrangement; and the degree of study and simplification applied to nursing operations such as procedures and records.

One would be remiss in assuming that patient classification is complete, because there are variables in patient care itself. We have long acknowledged that, though patients may be in the minimal-care category, their needs for professional care in nonphysical ways may be considerable. Also, the amount of physical and therapeutic care varies considerably from one seriously ill patient to another. Another variable is age. We know that patients over 65 years require more nursing care time than those under 65. One approximate figure allows 22% more time for the older group; but this or any other figure can be validated, and calculations can be adjusted for the number of patients over 65 in a given patient population.

There is no reason to believe that these variables cannot eventually be quantified at least grossly, as existing quantifying classifications have been. (As noted, a sophisticated procedure book now contains a procedure that includes time allotment for calming measures.) Refinement of current classification systems will yield quantification where it does not now exist. Knowing the strengths and limitations of current systems is the first step in continuing the refinement process.

Quantifying nursing staff

Once the patient load has been analyzed, the same must be done with the existing staff, in order to achieve maximum utilization. The ratio of professional nurses to practical nurses to nurses' aides or assistants must be determined so that the distribution is effective in meeting goals and economical in conservation of resources. The quality of each person's preparation and orientation, as well as his or her grasp of the goals of the nursing service, the precise organization of the enterprise, and the supervision provided, all contribute to effective distribution and economic conservation.

There is evidence that patient satisfaction is related to the number of RNs on the staff. There is also evidence that the number of aides is related to patient satisfaction, assuming that there is adequate supervision and good preparation and orientation. In a tight staffing situation, the more auxiliary support the RN has, the better; when patient call lights and requests are responded to promptly, the patient's satisfaction increases, thus reducing the harassment of the overburdened RN.

A study done by Miller and Bryant[44] of twelve comparative ratios of workers, where nursing hours per patient did not go above 2.4, found that the inclusion of licensed practical nurses made the greatest single difference in quality of care.

In this regard the proportion of time given to each of the three shifts requires regulation: harassment has often plagued personnel on the evening shift and to a lesser degree those on the night shift. Battelle Northwest Systems Programs for Hospitals [p. 17][36] and others have found that approximately 45% of the total work load falls on the day shift, 37% on the evening shift, and 17% on the night shift. This provides a basis for distribution, or a check with which to compare the division of staff by shift. An approximate personnel mix arrived at similarly suggests that staff be divided as follows: professional nurses, including head nurse but not overall supervision, 30%; LPNs, 20%; and auxiliary personnel, including nurses' aides, orderlies, and ward clerks, 50%. Though a working day consists of 8 hours, an approximate figure of 6.5 hours represents actual work time after meals, breaks, personal time, fatigue, and unnecessary delays are accounted for.

At Harper Hospital in Detroit, the cyclical scheduling plan provides for the evening and night shifts first; if there is a shortage it is sustained by the day shift [in Morrish and O'Connor[45]]. This concern is edifying, because it is only recently that this kind of protection has been afforded these shifts. They have often gotten the short end of the nurse supply.

Carefully planned job descriptions and duty lists are necessary to maintain optimal utilization of personnel and to conserve resources. We have already noted reallocation of duties in order to even the work load and use staff more efficiently. The extension of ward clerks into evening and night shifts illustrates the effort to utilize personnel optimally, as does reinforcement of peak periods by part-time personnel.

Distribution by day in the week is a factor in staffing. The universal desire to be off on weekends coincides with the reduction of hospital activities at these times, though patient needs continue. For patient convenience (that is, where patients wish to have minor surgery, diagnostic tests, and such done on their free time), there are a few hospitals that are in operation 7 days a week, which necessitates a staff equal to resultant increased work load. Also, hospitals can be more heavily staffed on selected days, in order to provide time for in-service education, committee meetings, intensification of particular nursing components such as planning, teaching, or making rounds, or some other phase of the operation.

Seasonal distribution of staff warrants attention. In a personal interview, Mr. Ron Ellingson of Battelle Northwest Systems Programs for Hospitals suggested strengthening staff by keeping a full complement of patients and staff in selected units during lowered census in summer, while allowing other units to have fewer patients and staff. This provides stability of concentration of patients and personnel, rather than diffusion of work load and staff. The admitting office is part of such a plan.

Types of staffing patterns

Conventional staffing pattern (centralized-decentralized). The oldest and most common staffing pattern is the conventional, or traditional. It provides for the best possible allocation of staff to units, as determined by the person in charge of staffing, supervisors, and head nurses. Head nurses plan the staffing schedule within the framework of existing policies and personnel insofar as they can, and supervisors fill any vacant spots they can from their wider number of units. The staffing person in the nursing office then provides any additional personnel necessary, drawing on personnel in other units, the float list, the emergency telephone list, or an outside agency.

This system has both centralized and decentralized aspects. The schedule is made up initially in a decentralized (unit) way and sent to the supervisor (optional, depending on policies), and then is centralized in the nursing office. Complete decentralization is extremely rare; total responsibility must be centralized, or it will be so diffused that the cohesiveness and good order of the enterprise are jeopardized.

It cannot be assumed that the conventional system cannot be perfected; precision can be brought to it as to any other system. Indeed, it is constantly altered more favorably in the hands of administrators devoted to improving and measuring the quality of nursing care and the means of providing it. For example, the float concept (a centralized concept) has been in use a long time. It provides for filling in staff wherever they are needed. Outside sources, such as Manpower, Inc., provide emergency services for conventional use. One organization uses services of an outside agency that provides selected and oriented personnel on call for 130% of the average hourly rate [in Sauer[46]]. The part-time pairing of two persons to work as a team and do one job is another development of conventional staffing. Frequently the scheduling of RNs for the night shift is done centrally, in order to distribute fewer personnel as equitably as possible. Precise measurement of the nursing hours needed for a given patient population applies also in conventional staffing.

Cyclical staffing pattern. A cyclical staffing pattern is one that repeats itself on a 4-, 6-, 7-, or 12-week basis. Even more than the conventional system, it requires constant sufficient numbers of the appropriate mix of personnel to provide basic coverage; if it cannot do this fairly well, the system breaks down. It too provides for float personnel to fortify staffs where the work load is very heavy, where basic nursing hours per patient day are not being met, or where there are absences, illnesses, or vacations.

Price lists the following to be included in a complete cyclical pattern:*

1. Desired complement of personnel working each day
2. Categories of personnel
3. Shifts worked
4. Days off
5. Reduction in number and complement of personnel from weekday to weekends that is appropriate for the needs of the specific unit
6. Fair distribution of desirable and undesirable hours among all personnel
7. A means for controlling utilization of the ever increasing number of part-time employees for full and partial shift work
8. Improved utilization of a "float" staff to enhance flexibility within the schedule and equate staffing with fluctuation in patient care needs and staff absences

Warstler[39] and Morrish and O'Connor[45] describe in detail conversion to cyclical scheduling and stress the use of lay persons to manage the staffing after the system is established.

The 40-hour, 4-day work week. Another staffing pattern is the 40-hour, 4-day work week, with various advantageous groupings of days. However, there is the obvious disadvantage of fatigue when staff works

---

*From Price, E.: Staffing for patient care, New York, 1970, Springer Publishing Co., Inc., p. 102.

longer than an 8-hour day, which affects the workers and the care they provide patients. The psychic energy derived from the large block of free time offsets such fatigue only partially. A report by Morse[47] on 10-hour days in other organizations shows that the plan was abandoned by a police department, because of increased accidents in the last 2 hours of the shift; and a financial and business magazine, because employees were just not getting the work out. Moreover, labor groups protest it because it took 100 years to gain the 8-hour day from 10 or more hours a day; and a scientist associated with occupational safety and health holds that a 6-hour, 6-day week is best for worker efficiency. Nevertheless, the American Management Association predicts that movement is clearly in the direction of a 4-day or otherwise shortened week. As with any other pattern, essential staff is needed, because the plan is weakened if extra shifts must be worked.

A summary of some of the advantages as found in several institutions where the plan for a 4-day work week is partially installed is given in an *RN* review.[48] Advantages are that staff get more frequent weekends off; overlapping shifts provide better coverage for mealtimes and nursing care of long-stay patients; there are 16 working days less per year with full pay; and staff get extra pay for the ninth and tenth hours each workday. Also described is a system, in operation since 1969, in which nurses work three 10-hour shifts one week and four 10-hour shifts the next, with every other weekend free. The shifts are joined by the use of part-time personnel. Staff are paid extra for time over 8 hours, so that actually they are paid the equivalent of 77 hours' work for a 2-week period. Vacations and fringe benefits are computed on the 77 hours of work.

Larsen[49] describes conversion to a 10-hour day in a coronary care unit, using staggered hours to permit coverage and distribute fresh personnel more evenly. She stresses the need for sufficient staff preparation and coordination.

The 7-days-on, 7-days-off pattern. In this staffing pattern [in Cleveland and Hutchins[50]] personnel work a 10-hour, 7-day work week, with the next 7 days free. This plan really consists of two 24-hour staffs, one off duty and one on. The nurses are paid for 80 hours. There is no vacation or holiday time allowed, though 70 hours for sick leave are allowed per year. There is improved continuity of care, because the same staff may cover the whole of a patient's hospitalization. There is also improved communication between patients, physicians, and nurses, which permits them to work together more closely. The schedule has also strengthened the in-service program. After 1 year, the staff at Evergreen General Hospital, Kirkland, Wash., unanimously endorsed the plan.

Scheduling by teams. Froebe[51] suggests scheduling by teams. It is proposed that peak times, pressure, and cruciality can be better met by stable, continuing teams whose members support each other, share vital decisions, improve morale, and handle relief needs internally. It is an exciting idea that replicates those occasional informal cohesive unit staffs where longevity and familiarity have welded efficient and spirited cooperation. There are probably more of such units than we realize.

• • •

No matter what the staffing pattern or its modification, it must have ingredients of continuous coverage for patient care and equitable distribution of desirable and undesirable hours for staff satisfaction. Ever-clearer and improved personnel policies and greater precision in measuring patient needs and work distribution provide the base for experimentation and change in staffing patterns.

Master plan

After determination of the staffing pattern, a master plan must be developed for the nursing service that will show the staffing picture unit by unit, shift by shift, and week by week. In fact, there is always a master plan operative, though it may not be viewed as such. The base line for the master plan is the detailed description of staffing, as it exists and has existed, from current and past time sheets and records. It depends on existent personnel policies for information about length of work week; number and frequency of weekends off; shift rotation; number of consecutive work days allowed; and vacation, sick leave, and leave of absence allowances.

There will be separate categories. In addition to the normal complement of personnel by unit, there will be centralized staff in terms of a float pool (nonregularly scheduled part-time personnel) distributed on the basis of need, usually by the nursing office; nursing students of various kinds from either internal or external sources; and volunteers who give direct nursing care such as feeding and transporting patients, assisting with therapeutic exercises and activities in rehabilitation units, and discharging patients (63% in one institution[46]). All categories must be reducible to hours so that they can be included in arithmetical calculations. Nursing students present the greatest problem in this regard because of variations in experience and seniority, but ratios have been formulated that at least approximate useful time determinations. Another category is that of provision for relief for vacations, sick leave, and leaves of absence. This can be estimated from past experience and records: was extra personnel used or procured; was the staff spread thinner; were units closed; or how were such replacements made?

After such information has been assembled as a base line, its adequacy or inadequacy must be determined. Nursing hours per patient day will be available from back records that can be used to evaluate adequacy. Patient classification can be begun. Clinical analysis of units should be done periodically, because the compilation and study of figures may show change in clinical conditions present in a unit, though not readily visible even to the experienced eye. In addition to numerical estimation of staff requirements for a given unit operating on numerical patient classifications, experienced personnel can project a base line for staffing the unit lower than the one in use, *if* they can be assured of receiving help when they need it. Admissions of this kind are uncommon; people are wont to hedge their position in self-defense, in order to be ready for the "rainy day" rather than count on outside help when needed. Maintenance of an inventory of personnel willing to stay home without pay when the patient census is low and a plan for utilizing such an inventory help in stabilizing a master staffing plan.

From the base there can be steady progression to firmer positions by various means already discussed, such as refined personnel policies, more precise patient classifications, more precise mix of personnel so that each is used optimally, review of job descriptions to determine optimal utilization—in short, any administrative improvement that may result in a firmer and more realistic master staffing plan. Levine[52] found that nonfederal hospitals employ substantially more nursing personnel than do federal hospitals. Tighter administrative practices were thought to contribute to the figure for federal hospitals.

Calculation of nursing hours. There is some variation in the calculation of nursing hours. Conventionally, the hours of all personnel on the unit except the head nurse and ward clerk, exclusive of time used for in-service education, meetings, and so forth, are counted as nursing hours. This figure for 24 hours is divided by the number of patients, exclusive of those with private duty nurses, to yield the nursing hours per patient for 24 hours.

Another formula includes the head nurse and ward clerk. Where the head nurse is functioning at a high level—that is, her time is used clinically in guiding and helping personnel to give increasingly better nursing care by all means at their disposal, and even giving direct care occasionally for enrichment or demonstration—then including the head nurse in unit nursing hours seems appropriate. Where there is a unit manager, there would be no question about counting the head nurse in unit nursing hours. Ward clerks sometimes give some direct service, especially on evening shifts; however, usually they do not, and hence it is questionable whether they should be included in nursing hours. Perhaps a portion of time, rather than the whole 8-hour period, for the head nurse and ward clerk should be included in calculating nursing hours in this method. However calculated, a formula reflecting the real situation as closely as possible is desirable.

Monitoring is necessary. The weekly control chart is a statistical table that is of value in reviewing staffing by unit. It is used to record the weekly average nursing hours and shows the normal range for the particular unit. For example, O'Malley[37] found that 3.5 to 4 hours is considered the average for an intermediate medical-surgical unit. By plotting these averages weekly, one can quickly see the staffing range in terms of nursing hours over a considerable period. Staffing above the range of normal provides time to do extra things to strengthen the service. However, it is costly if such time occurs very frequently. Conversely, should it go below the range of normal with any consistency, remedial action of some kind—increased staff, reduced work load, or streamlined procedures—must be found.

The 6-month national comparison by region by Hospital Administrative Services (HAS) of the American Hospital Association affords a means of comparison for one's own data. Consultation service can accompany utilization of these data if so desired. Caution is in order in such comparisons, though; there must be the constant realization that nursing hours are far from standardized from hospital to hospital, and there is a great range in how effectively nurse time is conserved for purely nursing functions. Though the caution holds in the case of patient requirement hours and timed procedures, it is somewhat less than in the case of nursing hours, because patient requirements are based on clinical assessments of patients with particular clinical conditions, and the timed procedures are determined on averages of a sufficient number of practices. All such figures require periodic review.

Turnover rate. Another set of figures that affects the master staffing plan is the turnover rate. Instability, or high turnover rate, not only reflects low morale, but plays havoc with a staffing plan by regularly and frequently injecting changes. Moreover, because personnel are not always readily available, it adds periodic times of shortage over and above the chronic shortage of personnel while new personnel are recruited and oriented.

An American Hospital Association formula for separations (all severances from an organization) and resignations is:

$$\frac{S}{M} \times 100 = T$$

S, number of separations during a month; *M*, midmonth employment figure; *T*, turnover rate.

The number of resignations can be substituted for separations, giving the resignation rate.[53]

Methods of patient assignment

Related to staffing patterns and master plans is the assignment of patients. Patient assignment and nursing care can be stable only where the staff is stable. To increase and improve the nursing care, one must have not only insightful and well-prepared staff, but must keep as much continuity as possible in patient assignments, so that the care given can be built on a continuing relationship and yield more personalized and knowledgeable care. Primary nursing assignment is based on this continuing relationship; the concept of "my nurse" has therapeutic undertones.

Reduction in patient days is desirable because it frees beds, gets patients on the road to recovery faster, and reduces nursing care time, thus making continuity of care a greater necessity.

The functional method of assignment is probably the oldest. Its great advantage is getting a good deal of work done in the shortest possible time. Administration of medication remains largely on a functional basis, whether given by nurses or pharmacy staff. It is extremely efficient, but fragments nursing care.

Individual assignment, or the case method, is an ideal toward which we work. It offers the best opportunity to meet the total nursing needs of patients, which has been deepened and broadened by this intensive association. It is best exemplified by the private duty nurse and nursing students. The one-to-one relationship is the significant factor.

The *complemental nurse* gives nursing care that may begin in the physician's office, continue in the hospital, and go on when the patient returns home, or be operative any time during the course of the patient's illness. The nurse works as needed by patients rather than by set hours [in Wolford[54]].

Liaison nurses care for patients both while in the hospital and after discharge. They are a combination of clinical specialist and public health nurse. They see that comprehensive, integrated services are provided without interruption, wherever the patient is. They have a collateral function redounding to improvement of quality of the nursing staff by sharing with the staff and participating in their efforts to develop high-quality nursing care plans and giving that kind of nursing care [in David[55]].

One-to-one nurses become a particular patient's nurse when their relationship to and care for that patient qualify them for this special position. Their names are carried beside the physicians'. They are responsible for the patient's nursing care and discharge planning. Difficult patients respond to this type of assignment [in Berni and Fordyce[56]].

Nurse therapists plan all nursing care for patients assigned to them during hospitalization and coordinate the variety of services available in a rehabilitation center. They are charged with patients' comprehensive nursing care, though others may care for them too through the team nursing plan [in Martin and Associates[57]].

Primary care nurses[58–60] are assigned the long-range, total responsibility for nursing care of the patient. This nurse plans the care, revises it as necessary, and gives as much of it as the schedule allows. The primary relationship to that patient remains, even though the nurse is on the evening or night shift. Others carry out the plan and give care when the primary nurse is not on duty. The method of assignment is meant to strengthen nursing care planning by having one nurse responsible for it. In a study of complications in patients with kidney transplants, those receiving primary nursing care had a complication rate of 1.4 per patient, whereas those receiving standard nursing care had a rate of 4.6 per patient.[61] This is an impressive statistic in favor of the primary nursing care assignment method. Though not stated, it is assumed that there is reversion to the team plan when and if the patient's condition warrants alteration of the plan on another shift.

At the *Loeb Center for Nursing and Rehabilitation,* an extended care facility of Montefiore Hospital in the Bronx, New York, nurses plan and give direct comprehensive nursing care to a selected group of eight patients in one of the five sections of the center. There are no written care plans. The chart is the focal point of planning as well as record keeping. There is one messenger-attendant for every two nurses. Time is at the patient's disposal, especially for communication, which is influenced by Rogerian nondirective concepts.[62,63]

The *team method* of assignment was developed to meet the nursing needs of patients in nursing services dominated by several categories of nursing personnel. Team nursing has had wider national application than any of the other methods described. It too is dedicated to comprehensive nursing care. It relies on the nursing care plan to express this individualized nursing care and the team conference as the essential means of keeping the nursing care plan reviewed, revised, enriched, or maintained.[64-66] Team nursing has the advantage of involvement of all team members in planning, execution of plans, and evaluation of them. When all parts are working satisfactorily, this involvement provides job enrichment and job expansion to all workers, especially at lower levels on the team, which Myers[67] finds very important.

In investigating what is being done with team nursing, Kramer[68] found little relationship between comprehensive continuous care and team nursing. The mechanics of assignment is the problem. She thinks there has been goal displacement where rigidity of the mechanics has displaced the objective—comprehensive continuous nursing care. It is not known whether she thinks the team nursing in her investigations had at one time included comprehensive continuous nursing care. It is possible that the goal has never been present, rather than that it has been displaced. With no content to the nursing care conference and the nursing care plan, it is simply just another way to get the work done.

Donovan[69] proposes that all devices—the various assignment methods, nursing care plans, and conferences—will remain artificial and sterile until such time as comprehensive continuous nursing care is practiced completely and comfortably by sufficient numbers of nurses to make the devices come alive. These devices are only vehicles to facilitate the nursing care goals; they are not the goals themselves. The competence of the people using them is the crucial factor.

The patient assignment schedule is an important device in helping to get comprehensive continuous care to patients. Continuity of assignment is necessary, but is difficult to achieve with a 40-hour week, large use of float personnel, and staff movement in order to get the best coverage. The form of the schedule can help or hinder this continuity. It must provide for at least a week's assignment, with each day visible. This requires a large sheet so that not only is each day and each person's time schedule visible, including temporarily assigned relief or float staff, but also that there is enough room to list both current and incoming patients. It can be designed to fit whatever type of patient assignment method is in use.

It is a difficult job at best to assign personnel to patients. Attention must be paid not only to continuity but to appropriateness, so that the person with the requisite skills is caring for a patient needing those skills.

The job classification is not the sole determinant. Fortunately, there are many excellent nurses' aides who over a period of time have become very proficient in giving particular kinds of care, though their classification alone would not permit it. Such an assignment is a judicious one, but it is an example of respect for individual abilities of staff.

There are formidable deterrents to patient assignment methods. An important contributor to failure to embrace the team or any other method except the functional or efficient one has been the constant instability in staffing. Johnson and Campbell[70] speak realistically to the point of heavy assignments. They recommend acknowledging these times for what they are and working accordingly in a functional way to give safe and essentially therapeutic care. When staffing is better, individualized care can be given. Moreover, everyone will know which method is in practice and work accordingly. Open admission of and communication in such pressured times are necessary and far more fruitful than evasion or subterfuge. This would do much to reduce the frustration encountered when the time factor simply will not permit efforts toward comprehensive nursing care. However, if there is not simultaneous effort to know and practice individualized comprehensive care during those times when the pressure is reduced even temporarily, the ultimate goal will not be helped.

It is well to think about this realistic approach to assignments at any time. However, if it is accompanied by efforts to bring specific measurement to the work assignments and schedules, it should ultimately make the workers fit the work load, or vice versa, more appropriately so that there will not have to be such frequent shift to the functional in order to care for patients without undue strain.

Need for clinical enrichment

Thought and attention to clinical enrichment by any means—good supervision, direction, in-service education, and so forth—is imperative if staffing is to be productive. There is ample evidence that we are dissipating the nursing hours we now have available, not only in doing the work of others but by mediocre nursing, instead of filling every nursing hour with sophisticated and knowledgeable nursing care. The nursing care plan and nursing conference are important tools to help us achieve this improvement; they constitute the means by which we direct the nursing care given. Change of shift reports also contribute to comprehensive nursing.

ORGANIZATIONAL BEHAVIOR

The staffing function seems to be related to what Argyris[71] calls organizational behavior. This "organizational behavior contains two basic components . . . the individual and the organization . . . when fused give birth to the social organization." He recommends knowing the properties of each component. He later elaborated on the notion of organizational behavior when he helped three organizations to improve their humanistic practices in pursuit of a healthier state.[72]

Workers as individuals

We have spent some time on the formal organization; now let us think about the individual. Each person is unique and complex. Each person also has the capacity to change. This change is growth when it is positive. It is of concern not only to individuals but also to those whose function it is to help people become happy productive workers or willing and able participants. The notion of "becoming" is crucial because it points up the ongoing quality of growth. Maslow [p. 3][73] is a strong proponent of the growth factor in individuals. To do his best work, the truth seeker will do better if he is "psychologically healthy," living in an improving culture, and having access to psychotherapy. There can at least be a society where mental health concepts are more commonly and widely known and aspired to.

Self-actualization. Maslow [p. 149][73] describes self-actualizing people as those whose basic needs for food, shelter, security, acceptance, and love have been met, enabling them to live and work fruitfully and comfortably.

Gross[74] prefers self-development to self-actualization, or even self-fulfillment or self-realization, for the reason that the latter three suggest "overtones of predestination" or "working out some predetermined pattern." Growth is perhaps more consonant with development than actualization. These differentiations may seem superfluous, but if they help us see people even a little more realistically, they are valuable.

Gross says "the behavior of people is at the very heart of the administrative process. The study of administration depends upon, or is part of, nothing less than the study of man." He has an interesting summation of bases of the nature of man:

1. The purposeful behavior of human beings is motivated by a multiplicity of interests.
2. Human beings are always part of some specific group environment.
3. Conflict is an inevitable part of human nature.
4. Human beings are unique personalities.
5. A large part of human behavior is irrational or nonrational.*

---

*From Gross, B. M.: The managing of organizations, New York, 1964, The Free Press, p. 319.

It is well to remember that when one has achieved a goal, it is no longer a motivator. There will be various goals achieved along the way to self-actualization or self-development, which will be succeeded by other goals. Pursuit of goals is a dynamic, not a static process.

Negativism. There is a negative, arbitrary, and self-defeating side of human personality. While the human personality can be enriched through conscious self-growth and effort, people are still faced with character defects of some proportion and intensity that make the self-improvement process difficult. Acknowledging such negative elements may be an early requirement in effort toward self-awareness.

In this regard Dubos[75] reports that at a UNESCO meeting held in 1970 "specialists on aggression unanimously rejected the theory of instinctive human aggression [p. 57]." This is an amazing piece of information to ponder in our aggression-ridden culture. In self-analysis, one is forced to look at self, relationships, and background for causes and effects of aggressive characteristics and not to the self-excusing notion that aggression is innate. Moreover, it forces one to consider both the desirable as well as the pejorative sides of aggression. Dubos helps us in such personal appraisal (or any kind of appraisal) by telling us that "objectivity is misleading when it does not take subjective feelings into account [p. 61]." Objectivity in its purest sense is difficult when dealing with ourselves or others; so this proposed incorporation of subjective feelings is not only useful but comforting in searching for objectivity. For example, in appraising aggressive tendencies, people look to their upbringing. Those who are chronic overreactors stimulate aggressive tendencies in those around them. The overreactive response is found especially in families. The subjective reaction to overreaction helps explain behavior and also helps to ameliorate aggressive tendencies when people decide to carefully watch their responses to overreactors in order to curb their own overreactions.

Dubos's statement also indicates the complexities of trying to be objective and suggests a large gray area as opposed to stark black and white as persons grope toward objectivity in our complex society and institutions, especially in relation to themselves and those with whom they commonly relate, such as family members or co-workers.

Valusek is perhaps franker:

> Until such time as the majority of persons in our nation come to understand that we, ourselves, cause ourselves, it will be impossible to relate more effectively to others, to reduce hatred of others, to reduce hatred for self, to reduce unnecessary violence directed toward other individuals, groups, or organizations, to reduce the hatreds which destroy both ourselves and those toward whom we express hatred.*

Hatred is not a common or popular notion, and we tend not to admit our feelings of hatred in a personal way. The above statement from a current educational publication gives us courage to look into ourselves honestly when we observe that Valusek thinks hatred is a common feeling. Hatred of self and others, or some degree of it, may be in us individually or collectively, because our interpersonal relationships are often criticized by colleagues and co-workers as well as patients and the public. Hagen and Wolff[76] wonder "how nurses can view the patient as a suffering human being and treat him as an individual while, at the same time, completely neglecting to treat other individuals as human beings." Is there anyone who has never used imaginary "occupational rush," or its newer name, task interference, to cut short or avoid giving services or time to patients? The generosity to look into rooms with open doors to greet patients, while knowing full well the risk of being summoned to do something for the patient and the consequent interruption in work, is an illustration of overcoming or reducing latent or real hatred.

---

*From Valusek, J.: On humanizing education, Educational Horizons, Fall 1973, p. 4.

Like Dubos, Valusek goes on to more optimistic concerns. He tells teachers that they must accept themselves as "decent human beings, in spite of . . . faults," so that such awareness can color the relationship of teacher and pupils favorably. Moreover, he tells teachers that they are the most important resource in the classroom. There is surely a corollary here to nurses, where nurse-patient relationship is akin to teacher-pupil relationship. In the former we call it therapeutic use of self. It requires self-awareness to use oneself in this way to promote the patient's progress, not only by ministrations but by personality too. To show understanding of the difficulties involved in maintaining a rigid diet forever by acknowledging that there will be breaks in it from time to time is to show a humanness that may encourage the patient to persevere when tempted to break the diet regime at a later time or to start again when he or she succumbs. To bring all possible supports to bear when dealing with a harassed colleague is likewise therapeutic use of self.

To see error as how it affects people, rather than as an occasion for reprimand, is a reflection of personality as well as good professional behavior. For example, to see a 24-hour delay in a series of radiographs of the gastrointestinal tract because the patient ate breakfast by mistake as more anxiety about the possibility of cancer to the patient and assembled family, rather than an occasion for bearing the annoyance of the physician, is to combine self and practice appropriately. It is part of becoming more sensitive, which increases humaneness. Rubin[77] describes activating compassion as the most powerful antidote to self-hate.

Games people play. The notion of "games people play" and the concept of transactional analysis in both interpersonal and managerial behavior have serious implications for the nursing enterprise.[78-82]

Political activity. The work of the American Nurses' Association in activity related to contract procurement, its recent formation of a political arm growing out of the efforts of Nurses for Political Action, and the efforts of the American Academy of Nurses to inject nursing into the Professional Standards Review Organization (PSRO) project all attest to the political effectiveness of nursing.

Nurses as women. The influence of the Feminist Movement on nursing cannot be denied: we have the efforts of university faculty nurses to right long-standing prejudices, the effort of *Ms* magazine to illumine the plight of nurses, and the growing interest of women in their own health care.[83,84]

• • •

The organizational behavior resulting from the fusion of the individual and the organization will be altered substantially and essentially for the good wherever there is growth and increased awareness of nurses as persons. The studied attention personhood has received from psychologists and other experts, the wide involvement of nurses in political activity, and movements such as Women's Liberation are bound to leave impressions on the nurse. Self-knowledge and societal knowledge seem to be increasing. The nurse is immersed in both by education and experience. However, growth and awareness do not come automatically, but require considerable effort and patience to acquire the equanimity and peace that accompany growth and awareness. The ancient Greek admonition to know oneself is still valid today if it is pursued as means to the good life and not as an end in itself.

COMMUNICATION IN STAFFING

One can scarcely think of the staffing function, or personnel administration, without considering the communication component; it is all-pervasive where so many people are required to achieve the goal of optimal nursing care for patients. If administrators at all levels were to count and analyze the intercommunications of one day, they would find there is considerable range in purpose, nature, and quality of communications.

Routine conferring face to face with colleagues up and down the hierarchical line, laterally with immediate staff, interdepartmentally, with patients, their families, and the general public constitutes a good part of a day. This routine conferring is likely to be essentially extemporaneous and geared to the current demands of the work situation, or routinized but still growing out of the work situation. It can be clinical or administrative, that is, with patients or co-workers.

Interviewing

There will be points or areas in routine conferring that must be taken further or selected for particular exploration, refinement, or exposition. These selected areas for deliberation usually result in an interview. Because of fear of formality, self-consciousness, or simply disinterest, these encounters are referred to as talks, conferences, or not named at all. However, they do constitute interviews, an activity to which considerable attention has been given by all concerned about one-to-one communication in our society.

Interviewing is an encounter for a specific purpose between two persons, and ordinarily includes a tentative plan that allows for leeway in achieving the purpose. It is usually scheduled, though it can be immediate; and should be conducted in an appropriate place for physical comfort, though auditory privacy is the only absolute for an appropriate place.

The burden of responsibility rests with the interviewers to establish and maintain a climate of acceptance, respect, warmth, and objectivity, because they are in charge of the encounter. Their own degree of maturity is important. Interviewers should recognize their own biases, even though they are still struggling to overcome them, so that they will not unduly color reactions or responses. They should be unobtrusive so that the persons making a case or presentation can do so comfortably and in their own way. They must be as tolerant and nonjudgmental as possible. Responses that include questions should assist the interviewee to see the situation or problem as clearly and accurately as possible, including the ramifications and alternatives. These responses should incorporate or return tangential comments to the mainstream and provide only that amount of probing necessary to help the interviewee gain insight, see alternatives, or make choices. The interviewer must imply no blame, not argue, and show sympathy for the situation or predicament. This is no easy job; interviewing requires skills and knowledge, though intuition and even luck can play a part.

There are differing points of view on note taking during an interview. Whether notes are taken during or after the interview, they are thought necessary for continuity and followup. Notes taken during the interview must be only skeletal and solely for keeping key points in mind during a long interview. The interviewee must give consent for the use of a tape recorder, and such a device may have an inhibiting effect.

The more calmness and sincerity on the part of both the interviewer and interviewee, the more fruitful the encounter will be. Carl Rogers, a master in the art of interviewing, regards the sincere interest of the interviewer to be more important than the technique.

PERSONNEL EVALUATION

One of the most difficult parts of the staffing component of administration is personnel evaluation, the regular written review of a person's character and competence as they are displayed in the work situation. Performance is measured, not potential, though growth is acknowledged. It is rooted in the present or immediate past, that is, the length of the evaluation period. The evaluation is usually performed by one's immediate supervisor, with or without collaboration of the next-level manager; and sometimes there is a self-evaluation report to which the superior reacts, or occasionally colleagues on the same level evaluate one's performance.

Personnel evaluations are done so that management will have some regular formal way of ascertaining whether employees are performing satisfactorily in meeting the needs of patients (or carrying forward the goals of the enterprise). They become part of the employee's permanent record and are used as bases for termination, demotion, promotion, transfer, subsequent references, regular salary increases, or merit pay. They are also used for counseling and guidance. Collectively, they may show general strengths and weaknesses that can be used in supervision, in-service education, staffing readjustment, policy reformation, goal clarification, or some other phase of administration or element of nursing care.

Objectivity

There is something awesome about personnel evaluation. The prime difficulty is that people are reluctant to commit to writing anything but satisfaction and praise. On this difficulty hinges the fear of subjectivity. For the conscientious person, there are bound to be feelings of inadequacy. There is an innate reluctance to make the judgments necessary to evaluate personnel. This reluctance may be beneficial: if it increases a sense of responsibility, there will be a greater attempt at objectivity. There is also fear of damaging a person by an unfair evaluation. People have been judged unfairly, with consequent harm to them, and untold and often unknown (to the rater) damage has been done individuals by hasty or ill-conceived evaluations. Only the strongest protest; others bear the brunt and suffer silently. While it is true that the great majority of workers fall within the satisfactory category, a sufficient number do not. The greatest care and conscientiousness must be applied in writing evaluations. This care and conscientiousness can bring a discernment in evaluating the satisfactory that can isolate discrete strengths, thus making the evaluation more valuable and useful to the one being rated.

There are ways in which objectivity can be increased. Of prime importance is the establishment of clear standards for both simple and complex jobs to be done by each category of workers as they proceed toward optimal nursing care for patients. The standards must be known by the worker and the supervisor so that there is a common understanding of them for both job achievement and employee evaluation. The orientation program should provide employees an opportunity to become familiar with the standards operative in the enterprise as they are spelled out in instructions, procedures, and policy manuals.

Also related is the anticipatory guidance inherent in the supervisory process, whereby workers are alerted to the expectations of the supervisor and the goals of the institution and enterprise by which all are judged. In short, one may expect to know precisely what he or she will be held accountable for and judged against.

Common understanding of behavior

There are additional criteria that should govern the evaluating procedure and are incumbent on supervisory staff charged with personnel evaluation. The first is the need for a common understanding of what constitutes appropriate behaviors within the categories of performance in operation in a particular institution. Time must be spent by the whole staff in reviewing such behaviors, reconciling differences, and preparing specific illustrations of behavior that have been reduced to a common denominator. Moreover, new supervisory staff must be made acquainted with the results of this common deliberation. This group deliberation and decision is the best means of safeguarding the integrity of the evaluation process within an organization. For example, illustrations of resourcefulness that sometimes looks like aggressiveness in the negative sense can be weighed against each other so that a common view of these behaviors is held. Independent judgment of behavior is dangerous if it is not tempered by group exploration of its meaning and consequent common acceptance. Erratic rather than consistent evaluation will ensue unless this safeguard is provided. Personnel have a right to expect uniform application of what constitutes specific attributes or faults in a given organization, from unit to unit.

Likewise, evaluators within an enterprise must give the same weight to performance; that is, while they may agree that a behavior is satisfactory or unsatisfactory, they may not agree on the relative importance of such behavior. For example, in weighing importance of an untidy bedside table with a point of essential care, such as correct positioning of a patient for maximum respiration, the correct positioning is more crucial to good nursing than is the state of the bedside table. This is a simplistic but essential application of the Flanagan critical incident technique, in which an attempt is made to determine the critical requirements of a job by studying large numbers of examples of extremely good and extremely bad behavior, in order to evaluate success or failure in a particular job [in Hardin[85]].

Bailey[86] used the critical incident technique in her investigation of nursing effectiveness. She found considerable variation in response from nurses, physicians, and patients.

A study done by Research and Study Service of the National League for Nursing [in Tate[87]] sought to find what the head nurse group, because they were closest to the actual work being done, regarded as essential traits. Approximately 280 head nurses considered the list of traits and illustrations of each trait until consensus was reached. These traits were knowledge and judgment, conscientiousness, skill in human relations, organizational ability, observational ability, reaction under pressure, communication skills, objectivity, and flexibility. Because insufficient illustrations could be found and agreed on, communication skills were placed under skill in human relations, and reaction under pressure was placed under knowledge and judgment. Difficulty likewise was found in illustrating flexibility and objectivity. Such variation and diffusion demonstrates the deterrents to nursing definition of which we have spoken. Tate's work culminated in a nonchecklist performance evaluation device.[88] One can see not only the need for but the difficulties involved in arriving at commonly accepted illustrations of desired behavior.

Sources of help in personnel evaluation

Exposure to and deliberation about sufficient numbers of varying behaviors is necessary for the common understanding of the raters of items for evaluation and their relative weight, not only to arrive at consensus but to supply substantial amounts of illustrative materials to the raters. These can be developed by the group itself or found by examination of the literature and reports of others' work.

A detailed and itemized list of behaviors is found in The Slater Nursing Competencies Rating Scale.[89] This is a seven-page scale on a five-point grading system, and contains 84 items grouped under psychological, individual and group, physical, general communication, and professional categories. Each of the 84 items is elaborated by three to five illustrations.

A short though significant list comes from the insightful work of Norris [p. 102][32] in the field of psychiatry. Implicit in this list is a good deal of knowledge of the psychiatric milieu and its nursing care and of what self-knowledge consists.

Copious material for review can be found in Hagen and Wolff.[76] There are hundreds of lists of effective and ineffective behavior actually collected from working people for each level of administration. Moreover, because the material deals solely with administrators, it carries the sober reminder that, while one may be a rater, he or she will also be rated.

As the monolithic nature of hospitals gives way to participation in the total community, goals for hospital administrators include new behaviors that demonstrate such community participation. Likewise, nursing service administrators should demonstrate behavior that shows concern for the hospital as a part of the community. Participation in the work of other community agencies, such as the American Red Cross and health and welfare planning councils, show such concern.

Bidwell and Froebe[90] describe the development of an evaluation instrument to accompany an organizational switch from the traditional to a unit manager–clinical nurse system. It uses Bloom's hierarchy of performances in the cognitive domain, reduced to three categories each for a two-track system of clinical practice and administration. The three categories —knowledge and comprehension, application and analysis, and synthesis and evaluation—are then spelled out by illustrations for three levels of practitioners in each of the two tracks.

Personnel evaluation forms

The form is to personnel evaluation what the care plan form is to nursing. It suggests possible areas for evaluation that are deemed essential for all hospital workers, including nurses, because more and more frequently one form is used by all departments in an institution. Often one hospital's evaluation form is adopted by another; but all forms should be periodically reworked or modified.

After an evaluation form has been filled out, the rater should discuss it with the employee who was rated. There should be space on the form for written comment by both the superior and the employee, perhaps with the direction to "comment freely" or "comment in favor of or against the rating," so that negative responses may be included more commonly and comfortably. This will lessen the trauma that can accrue to those who feel they have been rated unfairly or incorrectly, though it will not eliminate reticence to speak up against felt injustice.

The evaluation form should also have space for the signatures of the rater and successive supervisors in the line of responsibility for the evaluation. Accountability goes two ways in personnel evaluation. It is designed to account upward for the appropriate performance of the employee to those responsible for the enterprise; it also should be designed to protect the integrity and reputation of the workers and consequently be accountable to them. This protection for the worker is the reason annual performance appraisals are sought by negotiating bodies such as state nurses' associations. This accountability is extended to those who might represent workers, such as unions, civil service commissions, the American Civil Liberties Union, or professional associations. It demands not only a carefully executed and maintained evaluation system, but minds that are open to all possibilities, including error. There is usually space provided for illustrative material, especially for extraordinary performance in either direction.

Other usual items on the form include evaluation of the way the work is performed, the personal qualities of the worker, and so forth. These may be accompanied by a scale that constitutes the actual evaluation. A serious problem that arises with use of a scaled form is that, for example, dependability and personal appearance or punctuality and job knowledge may be listed together. These items are very different in terms of ultimate qualifications or cruciality. For this reason, some personnel evaluation forms (systems) have numerical values attached that discriminate among the items or groups of items listed. Punctuality and personal appearance would have a smaller number than job knowledge or dependability, because they are less critical. Even though a worker was rated high in each item, the total score would reflect numerically the greater importance of certain items in the total evaluation of performance.

Nonchecklist form. An interesting departure from the customary listing of characteristics and competencies for evaluation is seen in the nonchecklist form (see Appendix A, pp. 253-254). This structure relies more heavily on the observation powers of the rater. There are no lists, but places for description of exceptions to satisfactory performance, recommendations for removing these exceptions, and any commendations that are in order. The purposes of the evaluation are listed. This form is especially appropriate in evaluating the long-time employee whose performance is satisfactory and when repetition of the same listing year after year seems redundant. Moreover, it allows opportunity for any exceptions that might occur as a result of professional arrest, stagnation, or any other reason. It has the possible advantage of the stimulation that may derive from a break with the checklist routine, requiring the rater to make more independent judgments.

Professional Performance Interview Schedule. This schedule (see Appendix A, pp. 255-258) is a companion to the nonchecklist form and is optional at the request of either rater or ratee. It resembles a checklist in that it has five parts, each with varying numbers of descriptions. It is confined to the rater and employee and is not put into the personnel file. This optional interview form would be exceptionally helpful in evaluation of new employees or in a new rater-ratee relationship. This combination report allows more flexibility in the evaluation system while providing detail and specificity if such is wanted by either party. It reduces the potential for rote found in checklists.

Management by objectives appraisal

There is a kind of performance appraisal concerned with managers at all levels in the management by objectives concept (see Chapter 5). In this case, rather than be totally concerned with desirable characteristics, appraisals are made on how well nurses achieved the objectives they set for themselves, in conjunction with superiors, at the beginning of the accounting period. It puts an achievement component into the appraisal system, because it insists on some predetermined objectives that must be measurable at least sufficiently to do the performance appraisal at the end of the accounting time. In both cases, end results are the criteria against which personnel or their work is judged. For example, to revert to the short-term goal of a 6-month appraisal of current nursing practice compared with the ideal that is possible, one would expect head nurses to carry out such examinations in units with their staff in particular reference to the kinds of conditions the patients had. These examinations should not be done in isolation but as part of the servicewide examination, with all its advantages. Implied too is the collegial relationship in which each medical head nurse might assume responsibility for patients with a particular condition or a discrete part of such an analysis in the interest of economy of effort, though still responsible for measurable outcomes. Other examples would be installation of a primary nursing assignment system, strengthening team nursing, strengthening patient admission notes, increased staff knowledge of a particular condition, or determination of standards of care for a particular type of patient—all with predetermined measurable outcomes.

Self-evaluation

In an insightful and forthright critique of conventional performance appraisal systems, Rieder[91] supports the two previous points of view: elimination of checklist forms and use of the management by objectives concept. Citing the McGregor theory (see p. 14) of people in which creativity, the need to achieve, the notability of high standards, and the innate capacity for self-discipline abound, he proposes periodic talks, not interviews, in which people are encouraged to set goals or objectives for themselves and are freely offered any necessary help from superiors. Notations are duly made and added to after each subsequent talk. Such notations then form the basis for appraisal during the annual review. Inherent in such a system is the ongoing collegial, coaching, helpful support and understanding of th evaluater. Attention is always centered on the work to be done or goal to be achieved and not on the person doing it. It also allows for deterrents, complications, and difficulties that may accompany a person's goals or work. This system seems to view people as human beings with strengths and weaknesses rather than as composites of characteristics. It builds on strengths rather than the uniform optimization of characteristics.

Evaluation by peers

Peer review is a term used in various types of evaluation. One specific meaning is the review of performance by one's peers; for example, staff nurses are reviewed by other staff nurses instead of by the superior accountable for the unit, which is the common practice. Safeguards for fair appraisal are equally applicable to peer review as to any other type of evaluation.

Gold and associates'[92] account of an attempt by clinical specialists to evaluate their own work supports the needs identified earlier to overcome reluctance in judging oneself or others and to have established criteria for clinical effectiveness.

Supportive data

An ongoing problem in personnel evaluation is scarcity of observations on which to assess performance. Without supportive data, the rater may be insecure in the assessment or tend to use the "halo" effect, wherein impressions though scant are generally good. The opposite occurs where bad incidents are remembered while good ones are not, resulting in a bad evaluation.

Being cognizant of such traps helps to avoid them, but there is only one really good way to evaluate, and that is to have sufficient observations of all kinds recorded and dated over the whole grading period so that there is evidence for judgments made.

When this method is used thoroughly, patterns can be seen in accumulated observational data. Moreover, such systematically gathered observations provide the base for periodic conferences with the worker between formal evaluations, as part of the supervisory process. Such conferences are especially important where the work of the employee is less than satisfactory, because they verify that the employee was informed and counseled about any discrepancies in performance or attitude, based on substantial observed data.

There are occasions when behavior has been so flagrantly bad that a specific warning, including possible sanction, should be given the employee in writing, again based on specific detailed material. Such actions constitute the disciplinary function. Disciplinary action requires all the safeguards of other kinds of personnel evaluation, including adequate evidence, record of interviews (including warnings), and well-known job descriptions and standards. It also requires careful attention to possible attenuating circumstances, counseling prior to sanctions, and sanction alternatives such as transfer or demotion as well as discharge. Where unions or professional associations are involved, such data and conferences are important for the record.

We must develop the habit of keeping records of these observed behaviors, customarily and conveniently, so that we have data on which to judge when the evaluation procedure comes due. Notes can be made and later transferred to a more permanent record, to facilitate such data collection.

• • •

While admittedly difficult, personnel evaluation can be rendered more satisfactory and sound if within the enterprise there is common understanding and recognition of attributes, common study of the ranges of possible behaviors, a well-developed form that provides maximum recognition for crucial components of personality and work performance, and ongoing data collection of observed behaviors. It is a duty with such inherent danger and importance that the best effort should be cultivated to make it as fruitful and foolproof as possible in assessing each person's contribution to goal achievement.

REFERENCES

1. Report of the National Advisory Commission on Health Manpower, Washington, D.C., 1967, U.S. Government Printing Office, p. 23.
2. Benton, D., and White, H.: Satisfaction of job factors for registered nurses, J. Nurs. Admin. 11(6):55-63, 1972.
3. The nurse supply; shortage or surplus? Part I. RN 36(6):34-44.
4. Hague, J., editor, and Johnson, M., consulting editor: Practical approaches to nursing service administration, vol. 6, Chicago, 1967, American Hospital Association, Division of Nursing, p. 1.
5. Pigors, P., and Myers, C.: Personnel administration; a point of view and a method, New York, 1973, McGraw-Hill Book Co., p. 25.
6. Yoder, D.: Personnel management and industrial relations, ed. 6, Englewood Cliffs, N.J., 1970, Prentice-Hall, Inc., p. viii.
7. Strauss, A.: The structure and ideology of American nursing; an interpretation. In Davis, F., editor: The nursing profession; five sociological essays, New York, 1966, John Wiley & Sons, Inc. p. 107.
8. Jelinik, R., Munson, F., and Smith, R.: SUM (service unit management); an organizational approach to improved patient care. In Aydelotte, M.: Nurse staffing methodology, Washington, D.C., 1973, Department of Health, Education, and Welfare, no. 73-433, pp. 152-155.
9. Munson, F.: Crisis points in unit management programs, Nurs. Digest 11(3):36-44, 1974.
10. Declaration of functions of the licensed practical/vocational nurse, New York, 1969, National Association for Practical Nurse Education and Service, Inc.
11. Reiter, F.: The nurse clinician, Am. J. Nurs. 66(2):274-280, 1966.
12. Waite, P.: Specialty nursing teams in a small hospital, RN 37(2):35, 1974.
13. Slaughter, F.: Can a nurse be angel and "robot" both at once? Family Weekly, June 30, 1974, pp. 4-8.
14. Tolva, D.: Prosser medical plan for elderly catches attention here, Vancouver, Wash., The Columbian, January 27, 1974, p. 28.
15. Toms, K., and Walker, S., Sr.: A free clinic for the working poor, Nurs. Outlook 21(12):770-772, 1973.
16. Alexander, E.: Nursing administration in the hospital health care system, St. Louis, 1972, The C. V. Mosby Co., p. 199.
17. News, Am. J. Nurs. 72(12):2135, 1972.
18. Stevens, B.: A second look at "new position descriptions in nursing," J. Nurs. Admin. 111(6):21-23, 1973.
19. National Commission for the Study of Nursing and Nursing Education: Summary report and recommendations, Am. J. Nurs. 70(2):279, 289, 1970.
20. The University of Chicago hospitals and clinics, Chicago Tribune [Supplement], March 24, 1974.
21. DiVincenti, M.: Administering nursing service, Boston, 1972, Little, Brown and Co., pp. 302-303.
22. Thomas, B.: Job satisfaction and float assignments, J. Nurs. Admin. 2(5):51-59, 1972.
23. Advertisement (Manpower medical services), Vancouver, Wash., The Columbian, June 13, 1974.
24. Advertisement, RN 37(5):37, 1974.
25. Hoffman, R.: ABC's of nurse recruitment, Am. J. Nurs. 74(4):682-683, 1974.
26. Manfredi, C.: The interviewing and selection process, Supervisor Nurse 5(5):26-27, 1974.
27. Cleland, V.: Role bargaining for working wives, Am. J. Nurs. 70(6):1242-1246, 1970.
28. Lentz, E., and Michaels, R.: Comparisons between medical and surgical nurses, Nurs. Res. 8(4):192-197, 1959.
29. Dunn, J., and Stephens, E.: Management of personnel, New York, 1972, McGraw-Hill Book Co., pp. 129-130.
30. Reres, M.: Assessing growth potential, Am. J. Nurs. 74(4):670-676, 1974.
31. Optimal utilization of personnel; New York City nurses ditch non-nursing functions, Am. J. Nurs. 72(12):2135-2138.
32. Norris, C.: Administration for creative nursing, Nurs. Forum 1(3):96, 102, 1962.
33. Memo from the Editor, RN 37(4):1, 1974.
34. New, P., Nite, G., and Callahan, J.: Nursing service and patient care; a staffing experiment, Kansas City, Mo., November 1959, Kansas City Community Studies, Inc., no. 119, p. 74.
35. Aydelotte, M., and Tener, M.: An investigation of the relationship between nursing and patient welfare, Iowa City, 1960, University of Iowa Press, GN4786 and GN8570.
36. Battelle Northwest Systems program for hospital nursing; a personnel utilization plan, 1970, pp. 10 and 17.
37. O'Malley, C.: Application of systems engineering in nursing, Am. J. Nurs. 69(10):2155-2160, 1969.
38. Warstler, M.: Some management techniques for nursing service administrators, J. Nurs. Admin. 11(6):25-34, 1972.
39. Warstler, M.: Cyclic work schedules and a non-

nurse coordinator of staffing, J. Nurs. Admin. **3**(6):45-51, 1973.
40. Paetznick, M.: A guide for staffing a hospital nursing service, Geneva World Health Organization, 1966, p. 18.
41. Carter, J. H., and associates: Standards of nursing care, New York, 1970, Springer Publishing Co., Inc., p. 80.
42. Ott, L.: To make a good assignment, New York, 1963, National League for Nursing, no. 20-105, p. 10.
43. Price, E.: Staffing for patient care, New York, 1970, Springer Publishing Co., Inc., pp. 82-92.
44. Miller, S., and Bryant, W.: A division of nursing labor, Kansas City, Mo., 1965, Kansas City Community Studies, Inc., p. 94.
45. Morrish, A., and O'Connor, A.: Cyclic scheduling, J. Nurs. Admin. **1**(5):49-54, 1971.
46. Sauer, J.: Cost containment—and quality assurance, too. Part I. Hospitals **46**:78-93, 1972.
47. Morse, J.: Second thoughts on the 4 day work week, Portland, Ore., The Oregonian, December 23, 1972.
48. Four-day work week? Oh, those long weekends! RN, **35**(1):42-45, 1972.
49. Larsen, C.: A four-day week for nurses, Nurs. Outlook **21**(10):650-651, 1973.
50. Cleveland, R., and Hutchins, C.: Seven days' vacation every other week, Hospitals **48**(15):81-85, 1974.
51. Froebe, D.: Scheduling by team or individually, J. Nurs. Admin. **21**(10):650-651, 1973.
52. Levine, E.: Nurse staffing in hospitals, Am. J. Nurs. **61**:65-68, 1961.
53. Hague, J., editor, and Johnson, M., consulting editor: Practical approaches to nursing service administration, vol. 7, Chicago, 1968, American Hospital Association, Division of Nursing, p. 2.
54. Wolford, H.: Complemental nursing care and practice, Nurs. Forum **3**(1):8-20, 1964.
55. David, J.: Liaison nurse, Am. J. Nurs. **69**(10):2142-2145, 1969.
56. Berni, R., and Fordyce, W.: Behavior modification and the nursing process, St. Louis, 1973, The C. V. Mosby Co., p. 91.
57. Martin, N., King, R., and Suchinski, J.: The nurse therapist in a rehabilitation setting, Am. J. Nurs. **70**(8):1694-1697, 1970.
58. Manthey, M., and associates: Primary nursing, Nurs. Forum **9**(1):65-83, 1970.
59. Ciske, K.: Primary nursing; an organization that promotes professional practice, J. Nurs. Admin. **4**(1):28-31, 1974.
60. Robinson, A.: Primary nurse; specialist in total care, RN **37**(4):31-35.
61. RN News Caps: Added benefit of primary care nursing, RN **37**(6):5, 1974.
62. Isler, C.: New concept; more care as the patient improves, RN **27**(6):58-70, 1964.
63. Brown, E.: Nursing reconsidered; a study of change, Philadelphia, 1970, J. B. Lippincott Co., pp. 157-165.
64. Lambertsen, E.: Nursing team—organization and functioning, New York, 1953, Columbia University Press.
65. Newcomb, D.: The team plan, New York, 1953, G. P. Putnam's Sons.
66. Kron, T.: Nursing team leadership, Philadelphia, 1961, W. B. Saunders Co.
67. Myers, M.: Every employee a manager, New York, 1970, McGraw-Hill Book Co., p. 63.
68. Kramer, M.: Team nursing; means or end? Nurs. Outlook **19**(10):648-652, 1971.
69. Donovan, H.: Is the delivery system or health care the crucial problem in nursing service? J. Nurs. Admin. **1**(2):4-5, 1971.
70. Johnson, B., and Campbell, E.: It's time to be realistic about the work load, Am. J. Nurs. **66**(6):1282-1285, 1966.
71. Argyris, C.: Personality and organization, New York, 1957, Harper & Row, Publishers, p. 229.
72. Argyris, C.: Management and organizational development, New York, 1971, McGraw-Hill Book Co., p. xi.
73. Maslow, A.: Motivation and personality, ed. 2, New York, 1970, Harper & Row, Publishers, pp. 3 and 149.
74. Gross, B. M.: The managing of organizations, New York, 1964, The Free Press, p. 328.
75. Dubos, R.: A god within, New York, 1972, Charles Scribner's Sons, pp. 57 and 61.
76. Hagen, E., and Wolff, L.: Nursing leadership behavior, New York, 1961, Columbia University Press, p. 152.
77. Rubin, T.: Compassion and self-hate; an alternative to despair, New York, 1975, David McKay Co., Inc.
78. Berne, E.: Games people play; the psychology of human relationships, New York, 1964, Grove Press, Inc.
79. DeLodzia, G., and Greenhalgh, L.: Recognizing change and conflict in a nursing environment, Supervisor Nurse **4**(6):14-25, 1973.
80. Levin, P., and Berne, E.: Games nurses play, Am. J. Nurs. **12**(3):483-487.
81. Meininger, J.: Success through transactional analysis, New York, 1973, Grosset & Dunlap, Inc., pp. 214 and 262.
82. Jongeward, D., and associates: Everybody wins; transactional analysis applied to organizations, Menlo Park, Calif., 1973, Addison-Wesley Publishing Co., Inc.
83. Cleland, V.: Sex discrimination; nursing's most pervasive problem, Am. J. Nurs. **71**(8):1542-1547, 1971.
84. Kushner, T.: The nursing profession—condition critical; and Johnson, B.: A day in the life of Diane Adler, RN, Ms Magazine, August 1973, pp. 72-81.
85. Hardin, C.: Critical incident—what does it mean to research, Nurs. Res. **3**(3):108-109, 1955.

86. Bailey, J.: Critical incident technique in identifying behavioral criteria of professional nurse effectiveness, Nurs. Res. 5(2):52-64, 1956.
87. Tate, B.: Evaluation of clinical performance of the staff nurse, Nurs. Res. 11(1):7-9, 1962.
88. Tate, B.: A method for rating the proficiency of the hospital general staff nurse, New York, 1964, National League for Nursing, no. 19-1122.
89. Slater, D.: The Slater Nursing Competencies Rating Scale, Detroit, 1967, Wayne State University College of Nursing.
90. Bidwell, C., and Froebe, D.: Development of an instrument for evaluating hospital nursing performance, J. Nurs. Admin. 1(5):10-15, 1971.
91. Rieder, G.: Performance review—a mixed bag, J. Nurs. Admin. 4(3):20-24, 1974.
92. Gold, H., and associates: Peer review; a working experiment, Nurs. Outlook 21(10):634-636, 1973.

CHAPTER 8
DIRECTING

In the definition of directing, one finds words such as regulate, dominate, and determine, which suggest power and authority. These are words that may be suspect in contemporary society (especially the word dominate, because it connotes an antiegalitarianism that is unpopular for some good reasons, though this unpopularity may stem from negative rather than positive uses of the term or misunderstanding of what is involved). Equality of opportunity, not of achievement, is the crucial but sometimes confused point. Achievement may start with equal opportunity, but beyond that is dependent on other factors: personality, native endowment, timing, and such.

Authority is another unpopular word in contemporary society. "Doing one's own thing" suggests, if not in fact means, avoidance of authority of some kind. The connotation of authority derives either from abuses of it, which are frequent enough (for example, denial by hospital administrators of workers' rights to organize on their own behalf), or misunderstanding of the nature of authority in achieving the goal and maintaining good order. Accountability for this goal is an essential and inherent part of direction, because it places emphasis on the goal to be achieved and not on the person directing.

RELATIONSHIP BETWEEN DIRECTION AND SUPERVISION

Newman[1] is very explicit about the function of direction, pointing out first that it can be taken for granted because it is so much a part of administration. Its real and important function is to implement plans that further the purpose of the enterprise. This implementation requires directing of personnel.

Newman goes on to describe the qualities to be found in good direction. Directions must be reasonable, complete, clear, and consultative; that is, ideas and reactions to a proposed direction should be sought out in advance from those who will have to carry it out, so that it will receive intelligent, cooperative obedience. Giving essential information in advance of a proposed direction or surrounding an actual one is not too time consuming when weighed against the good effect obtained.

These directions are given in several ways: verbal directions in face-to-face encounters, sometimes incidental though more often in planned counseling sessions and the like; and written directions in the form of policy and procedure manuals, written standards of care, job analysis and job descriptions, nursing care plans, and such.

Newman also makes a clear distinction in the relationship of direction to supervision. He states that "direction is a part of supervision," and describes supervision as "the day-to-day relationship between an executive and his immediate assistant; and it is commonly used to cover the training, direction, motivation, coordination, maintenance of discipline, and minor adjustment of plans to meet immediate situations that take place in the executive-subordinate relationship [p. 372]."[1]

Correlated to the day-to-day contact is the day-upon-day contact demanded in followup and follow through, which requires maintaining contact with the past and present over a period of time to make sure the job gets finished. It may require review, encouragement, or more direction in the process. The more complex the organization and its purpose, the more necessary is such followup activity.

Supervisors

The supervisor usually holds the middle position in the hierarchy, between the director of nursing, associates and assistants, and head nurses. The supervisor is responsible for two or more units, a floor, or department, depending on size of the institution and degree of specialization.

Just as the administrative process cuts across all positions in the nursing hierarchy, so does the supervisory process. They are not separate and equal, as is often stated. Wherever and whenever nurses have responsibility for the work of others, these processes are operative. Their work is deeply involved in all facets of administration, which includes supervision. This pervasiveness of the supervisory process in each position in the organization must be acknowledged, for failure to do so leads to devisiveness and confusion.

In writing about the dilemma of the position of supervisor, Stevens[2] suggests a division of the work of the supervisor into three positions: Supervisor A, a coordinator of patient care services; Supervisor B, coordinator of nursing personnel and staffing; and Supervisor C, coordinator of nursing systems. The head nurse would then deal with each in a particular category of need. This proposal is in opposition to the premise held in this book; namely, that goal determination and achievement are the province of each administrative level—director, supervisor, and head nurse—in concert, and that the centrality of this theme is crucial to success in goal achievement. Within this framework, Stevens's three classifications for the supervisor would better suit assistant directors.

NEED FOR CLINICAL COMPETENCE

Sufficient clinical competence is needed at each level to evaluate, teach, and direct the activities of subordinates. In one point of view, administrative and clinical competence vary inversely through the hierarchy: the director of nursing has the greatest administrative and the least clinical competence, the head nurse has these skills reversed, and the supervisor has equal components of each. This position is questioned by Donovan[3]: "The relative clinical competence of the supervisor and head nurse is open to doubt. I would dread to be the supervisor whose clinical competence was less than that of my head nurses, at least in the aggregate, although it might be less in specialized areas."

Certainly both competencies must be present sufficiently to know what is appropriate and correct in each category. One weakness in the supervisory level has been the degree of clinical competence, which may be the greatest contributor to the confusion so often found at this level. One finds the words administrative and clinical sometimes modifying the title of supervisor; both are redundancies or are added in an attempt to strengthen or emphasize that particular component of the supervisor's work where it is deficient. Apropos of this clinical component for administrators, there is a point of view that proposes that administrative personnel should engage in clinical nursing care, to guard against incompetence growing out of disuse of practice. Reinforcement for maintaining clinical competence at all levels is shown in a rehabilitation institute where all professional personnel, including the director of nursing, assume responsibility for planning nursing care for at least one patient.[4] This practice clearly supports the sound theory that "anyone giving clinical support to nurses needs to keep up in order to question patient care, and be secure in backing up the nurses who identify really important patient problems [David[5]]."

A corollary to this periodic return to clinical practice is intershift change, so that supervisors can keep abreast of the clinical and administrative behaviors peculiar to the evening and night shifts. Such experience can only result in more sensitive and knowledgeable performance of duties in one's regular assignment within the nursing organization and his or her relationship to the work of colleagues at other times and places, in the continuous effort to meet the nursing needs of patients.

We have singled out the administrative position of supervisor for consideration and sometimes blame, implied if not explicit, probably because that is where administrative and clinical skills can or should achieve some kind of equilibrium. However, other administrators (top management and head nurses) also frequently fail to meet their obligation to achieve greater clinical competence. It is not enough to dispatch others to upgrade their clinical competency if administrators at all levels do not aspire to personal growth in clinical competency too. This practice is hollow and has an insidious effect on nursing practice; it may be the greatest deterrent to giving comprehensive nursing care to patients by satisfied, productive workers in manifold possible ways.

The overriding reason for clinical incompetence at any level goes back to our inability to internalize what we practice, that is, to be comfortable practicing comprehensive, continuous nursing care. If the alleged clinical incompetence of the supervisor leads us to see the universality of the allegation, we are one step further in the search for a definition of comprehensive nursing. Present knowledge of nursing is far greater than that part of it that is practiced every day in the aggregate. This knowledge is not being used and internalized by a sufficient number of nurses, including administrators at all levels, to make the significant difference.

NEED FOR STANDARDS

Another reason for our dissatisfaction and confusion, again deriving from the supervisor as middle management, is the absence of standards of nursing care to be used in directing and helping people to give improved nursing care. Though we have procedure and policy manuals to give us concrete criteria for measuring procedural nursing care, we have not had standards of general or specific care, other than those acquired from our education and experience, to use as a base in guiding others.

This observation can be countered by pointing to all the educational efforts devoted to teaching and upgrading nursing care in past decades. These prodigious efforts and their success cannot be denied; nor can we deny the maintenance of standards by the complete and thorough examination and licensure system. Yet standards have been conglomerate and diffuse, except for the specificity of licensure examination.

The American Nurses' Association has recently spelled out standards of nursing practice in general as well as in particular clinical areas and has launched a program for certification of members in clinical competency in particular clinical areas. This national certification program will ensure a high degree of competence, whereas examination for licensure ensures minimal competency. It is noteworthy that these proficiency examinations for certification will operate from the base of the Standards for Nursing Practice of the America Nurses' Association 1973.

Justification and need for such development of standards of nursing care is found in the summary and recommendations of the Survey of Hospital Nursing Services. An overwhelming number of respondents (nursing service directors) thought their time should be spent in developing standards for the nursing care of patients and their families. Moreover, at the time of the Survey only those directors in hospitals with 24 or fewer beds were establishing written standards of nursing care [Aydelotte, p. 18].[6] Small hospitals undoubtedly demand that the director of nursing do many jobs closely involved with direct nursing care. One assumes that these directors of nursing surveyed intended to include supervisors and head nurses, if not also staff nurses, in such development of standards.

These standards for clinical practice of the five ANA divisions—community health, geriatrics, maternal and child health, medical-surgical, and psychiatric and mental health—were formulated within the following guidelines:

> Acceptable to those importantly concerned, as proper and adequate for the particular purpose
> Reasonable and attainable
> Specific to a division but broad enough to encompass the practice of its sub-groups
> Inclusive of the significant factors in the division's practice that make it different
> Built upon an operational definition of the nursing practice of that division*

A standard, then, supplies a definite rule, principle, or measure established by some authority; whereas a criterion may apply to anything used to test quality, whether formalized as a rule or principle or not. The distinction between standard and criterion is noteworthy because the terms are increasingly used interchangeably. The difference seems to be essentially one of tightness or structure on the part of the standard.

Standards as base for direction and control

Though standards are used primarily for evaluation by providing a rule or principle with which regular practice can be compared and judged, they are highly directional because the same information provided for evaluation provides directions for performance. Standards are being established concurrently with the refining of audit procedures. What is sometimes called mandatory or directional charting, necessary to offset discrepancies before they occur or to be picked up later in the audit procedure, is a base for clinical entity nursing care standards. Simultaneous formation of standards of care and audit procedure demonstrates cohesiveness and coherence, because both are tied to nursing care and contribute to its improvement. Direction and control, of which evaluation is a part, are the two sides of the "standards coin." Also, standards reduce the number of verbal or written directions necessary to carry the goal forward.

Though representative of the best thinking on a particular subject, standards must be reviewed regularly to incorporate new information, equipment, and insights that develop continuously as nursing, medical, and other related sciences advance.

Greenough[7] suggests that "standards for nursing practice be specifically worded in terms of action and behavior which are visible and measurable." This use of action and behavior strengthens both the direction and evaluation components. Specificity is evident in nursing procedure books, but is equally applicable in other instances, for example, the expected content of a nursing admission note or the data base in problem-oriented medical recording, service to family of a terminally ill patient, and so forth.

Greenough also suggests that standards be arrived at collectively, so that input is allowed by those who will have to comply with them. This is an application of consultative management.

She speaks of nursing care as comprising clinical nursing practice and nursing services, the latter being the facilitating services composed of administration, supervision, and teaching. Both nursing practice and nursing services require standards of operation.

Nicholls[8] makes an insightful distinction in standards for nursing care. She uses the ends-and-means concept. Patient outcome or objectives are ends standards, whereas means standards are the plans for achieving these patient objectives. She goes on to describe three criteria for standards: they must be stated in terms that are clear and unambiguous, be within the realm of possibility of all concerned (patients, personnel, and institution), and be capable of measurement.

A necessary ingredient of standards is

---
*American Nurses' Association: Standards for practice being written, Am. J. Nurs. **68**(10):2155, 1968.

that they can be broken down sufficiently to describe the actual components of the care to be given (for direction) or that has been given (for evaluation). This breakdown of the general standard must be done; otherwise the component parts are left to the individual practitioner's view of the care or the issue, rather than to the specific standard requirements of a given institution.

Carter and associates[9] have developed several very detailed categories of standards of nursing care. Items in each category are called indices of care. The medical-surgical clinical standards comprise 97 items in 14 categories; the nursing record (chart), 29 items in 9 categories; and the nursing care plan, 32 items in 10 categories. These standards represent a vast array of possibilities for nursing care that constitute direction of care and potential for evaluation. This work for general medical-surgical patients could be expanded to preoperative, operative, and recovery room care, as has been done for the obstetrical patient. It could also be the base for specific addenda to cover a variety of particular medical or surgical conditions, either by groups or individually based on clinical analyses showing the frequency of clinical conditions.

RELATIONSHIP OF GUIDELINES AND STANDARDS

Guidelines for care are related to standards, because they lay out the requirements for a specific type of care in sufficient detail to direct the practitioner and also supply the means to evaluate the care given. Useful models often come from rehabilitation nursing, where nursing care is so uniformly well developed that such standards, in terms of guidelines or detailed descriptions, are available for care of patients who have had ostomies or patients with spinal cord lesions, among others.

Though purposes for the use of standards may vary, as in the case of evaluation with its consequent direction for counseling, in-service education, supervision, and so forth, the best current thinking on how to do things or how to behave to achieve the objective for which the standards were compiled is implied. Direction is inherent in them. In addition, the multiple utilization of standards provides cohesiveness that helps to keep the prime purpose (comprehensive nursing care) of the standards and the enterprise in which they are developed in the minds of the personnel for whom the standards are provided and who may have contributed to their formation.

MANUALS AS DIRECTION

By describing in detail exactly how policies and procedures are to be carried out, manuals direct workers. This kind of direction prevents confusion and permits precision in the work flow necessary to carry out specific tasks. The direction inherent in manuals ensures economy of time, effort, and material, because these factors were considered in its compilation and descriptions. Also, the direction given in manuals has been refined and rethought by the very act of committing it to writing, and subsequent rewriting or revisions will carry additional refinement.

Procedure manuals

The Joint Commission on Accreditation of Hospitals (JCAH) specifies four uses for the procedure manual[10]:

To provide a basis for training programs to enable new nursing personnel to acquire local knowledge and current skills.
To provide a ready reference on procedures for all nursing personnel.
To standardize procedures and equipment.
To provide a basis for evaluation and study to ensure continued improvements and techniques.

Procedure manuals were probably the first standards in nursing as it developed in the post-Nightingale period. They have advanced substantially since the days when it took seven pages to describe care of the body after death. Streamlining procedures so that they are easily assimilable has been a steady progression. The principal change has been one of eliminating extra words or sentences so that the points are more visible. Use of strong verbs to denote the steps or actions is another development. Much has been learned from instructions in the commercial world, which in turn has benefited from the advice of psychologists and comparable specialists. Liberal use of diagrams and precautions helps to keep the instructions direct and exact.

There are nursing manuals that include the approximate time required for a procedure to be carried out. These time specifications are generalized and allow for some leeway, but are quite exact in that the procedures have been thoroughly examined and observed a sufficient number of times to ensure reliability. Industrial engineers have assisted with or overseen time designations for these procedures.

Procedure manuals have been simplified over the years as more and more procedures are accomplished with equipment from central supply. Although central supply usually assumes responsibility for this equipment, arrangements are usually carried out by a procedure committee. There is room for expansion of the procedure manual to elements of nursing care not usually considered procedures, such as psychological and teaching care. For example, home equipment and the procedure for teaching patients to give their own insulin could accompany the usual insulin administration procedure. Preoperative instructions such as showing the operating and recovery rooms, describing administration of anesthetic, teaching proper breathing, and static and active exercises for postoperative use could become a part of the procedure manual. Expansion into such a well-established practice as the use of the procedure manual fortifies and facilitates the utilization of new material.

Policy manuals

The JCAH spells out six areas in which there shall be policy statements[10]:

Noting diagnostic and therapeutic orders
Assigning the nursing care of patients
Medication administration
Charting by nursing personnel
Infection control
Patient safety

Many other areas are of concern to the nursing staff. There is a tremendous amount of information in the heads of personnel and in writing in various forms and diverse places within a nursing service, which should be organized and put in the policy manual so that all might benefit from and have easy access to it. For example, while a group of supervisory nurses were discussing weaknesses in patient teaching, including the need to have medical staff approval for specific instructions, it came to light that in fact the job was well begun: five or six specific protocols had been established, including medical staff approval, and were in use in various departments. Had they been collected and placed in a policy or procedure manual under patient teaching and instructions, they would have received more uniform attention in practice and provided a base for inspiration and expansion of a part of nursing care universally acknowledged to be weak.

The difficult job of converting vague content (as in patient teaching and instruction) to concrete, easily usable material can be helped by formalizing collection of existing material in a policy manual. A related point can be made that seldom do we start anything from scratch; investigation and probing often turn up much material that contributes directly to whatever we are pursuing. It is often a matter of seeing relationships and having a certain dedication to the concept of growth upon growth.

Interdepartmental relationships are best spelled out in written policy. These policies contain the information that nurses need to know in order to coordinate a patient's care departmentally. Sometimes procedural-type instructions, such as preparation of a patient for x-ray or laboratory examinations, are carried in the procedure manual, though they may be contained in the policy manual. In establishing these stated interdepartmental relationships, personal contact with the departments is necessary in order to explore what should be known by the nursing staff about each department in order to coordinate and cooperate in interdepartmental service to patients. This kind of exploration is often the first step in breaking down the isolationism of departments, including nursing. Such exploration may then be maintained on a continuing basis.

The location and specific means of procurement of all kinds of equipment and material should be included in the policy manual.

The administrative policy manual becomes the repository for all instructions, memoranda, and information, which can be catalogued and stored as presented or modified in such a way that they fit into an existing category within the manual. Moreover, because instructions, memoranda, and information may supercede other material, there is often replacement of the old by the new. This requires careful attention so that the manuals remain uniform and up to date. A person or a committee must be assigned to preside over this incorporation of information to guarantee the desired uniformity. There can be a separate provisional manual for such materials until their assimilation plan has been decided and formalized. The need for currency requires a loose-leaf form that accommodates change.

The administrative policy manual also becomes the storehouse for all ongoing deliberations when they have been finalized. The disaster plan for a hospital, along with the plan for synchronization with other parts of the community, is an example. The protocol for contacting clergy, policy regarding contacts with the media, and many other subjects are part of the administrative policy manual. In short, all policy necessary for the nursing staff to work knowledgeably and effectively may be part of the policy manual.

OPERATIONS ANALYSIS

Operations analysis contributes to the direction of the enterprise secondarily, but significantly. It is the scope and arrangement of activities, assessments, or views used to examine something; it is a way of seeing the whole by examination of parts.

The range of operations is large, embracing all the activities we consider in the various parts of managing the nursing enterprise as it works toward its goal. Operations analysis is likewise broad. Its contribution to directing the nursing service lies in the influence such analysis has on the ingredients of direction, such as standards, guidelines, and procedure and policy manuals.

Operations analysis is a staff position; that is, it is a study-recommendation position dependent on persuasion, by means of data assembled, to get its points across. It is line personnel (in concert with the analyst) who accept, reject, or modify the proposal and put it into practice.

Roy[11] points to an inherent problem for this staff person. The analyst is engaged in examining the work of others, though as an observer and not as a practitioner. There is the implication of criticism in the very nature of analytical work. These factors can generate irritation and distrust in those observed. So human relations skills should be an important part of the analyst's personality. The quality of his or her work will depend not only on the acuity of observational, analytical, and projectional skills, but equally on ability to maintain good relationships with the workers who are being observed. In addition, the analyst should be involved in the early implementation stage, so that insight and knowledge can contribute to overcoming the usual difficulties encountered in early stages of any endeavor.

Because operations analysis is relatively new to hospitals, the work of the analyst should be explained in advance as well as concurrently to reduce the potential anxiety and irritation of persons in the operational part of the enterprise. Recognition of the unspoken fears of elimination of positions and workers is necessary so that the plan for provision for the worker in case of such elimination can be presented. Fear of elimination is often accompanied by fear of change in habits and routines. This too can be exteriorized and discussed in the hope of reducing such fears.

Operations analysis is related to ergonomics—"an interdisciplinary science, involving functional anatomy, anthropometry, physiology, psychology, physics, and engineering . . . ergonomics is concerned with fitting the job to the worker [Larkin[12]]." The effect on personnel of changed sleep patterns in shift work and a longer workday in the 4-day workweek staffing pattern are potential areas of concern to the ergonomist. Though so far ergonomics is an obscure activity in the health field, the implications for it are clear enough. It is a good illustration of the need for a new science, albeit deriving from and drawing heavily on other sciences, to meet the complexity of the times in which we live. It also demonstrates order in the collectivization of scientific data.

Operations analysis is related to systems analysis, because it shows relationships between each of the parts to each other and to the whole, respects the input, sees that nothing is lost or diverted as the input and the parts of the system interact, and shows either a steady or disordered state. They share precision and relationship awareness.

Operations analysis is related to research, too, because it uses some of the same tools, at least the scientific method whereby the observations, analyses, and subsequent data are collected and arranged with as much precision and accuracy as possible and discrepancies are carefully noted. Too, it is like tightly controlled problem solving.

Most hospitals do not as yet have operations analysts on staff, but use the services of these people in a consulting capacity, either on a retainer or fee-for-service basis, or both. The American Hospital Association and its state affiliates provide such a service at no charge to member hospitals. In this regard it is interesting to note that management engineering as a staff function is recommended and described in an official hospital planning guide.[13] It also is contained in job descriptions for hospitals.[14]

Early nursing study

One of the early major nursing studies [Wright[15]] used industrial engineering theory and practice exclusively. It was a comprehensive study of four institutions and included thorough descriptions, analysis of work loads, personnel, patient population, and attitudes and expectations of personnel and patients, with a view to improving patient care in a time of general shortage and imminent expansion. All was carried out with strong industrial engineering support, guidance, and assistance. The prime direction found necessary to implement the findings of the study was the need for education. It is interesting to note that in-service education was formally introduced as a result of the study; today it is commonplace. Work simplification and job analysis, in which essentially all personnel engaged, had a profound effect on all phases of the nursing enterprise: staffing, work patterns and procedures, and so forth.

Another innovation was the assignment to the ward clerk of the job of transcribing physicians' orders and making consequent requisitions, among other duties, with final check remaining with the professional nurse; this too is now commonplace.

These illustrations from an important early work serve to remind us of the gradual refinement of the nursing service enterprise over the years, not only for encouragement in continuing the job and as a base for subsequent growth, but also for recognition and reminder of the operations analysis component that contributed data and findings, both suggesting and supporting such beneficial changes.

Consultant services

Consultation can take many forms, depending on the needs of the institution and the services available; but all are aimed at operations analysis within the institution, whether accompanied by specific assistance or not.

For example, Hospital Administrative Services of the American Hospital Association[16] compile sophisticated semiannual regional statistical summaries by clinical, departmental, size, and type categories for use by its member hospitals. It also offers consultant service in utilizing these summaries. An illustration of how these data provided an administrator with figures to use in determining whether another person should be added to the staff by request of a department operating within its budget, or whether other means of meeting the work load were indicated, demonstrates use of these figures [Hansen[17]].

The Commission for Administrative Services in Hospitals (CASH),[18] serving member hospitals in California, is another organization that provides services rooted in industrial engineering to hospitals. Their manuals, covering areas such as procedure, staff utilization, and quality control, use such theory and practice, with much enrichment to the nursing services in the hospitals served.

CASH grew out of the work of the Hospital Council and Blue Cross of Southern California. It and Community Systems Foundation (CSF) in Michigan are the oldest of the centralized engineering teams serving groups of hospitals regionally. It has served as the model for most subsequent such organizations and services.

The CASH concept operates in different parts of the country under various names and sponsorship. Battelle Northwest Systems Programs for Hospitals serves member hospitals in Oregon, Washington, and Idaho and is sponsored by the respective state hospital associations. Its objectives are wide ranging as well as penetrating:

1. To assist hospitals to maintain or improve the quality of their service
2. To improve the effective use of health care resources (manpower, facilities, etc.) within the Northwest
3. To strengthen and improve control of the costs of patient care
4. To direct research and special studies which will identify and/or clarify current needs related to health care facilities and services, e.g., shared services, transportation and allocation of resources
5. To direct and perform long-range studies in order to forecast local and area health care needs within the Northwest
6. To alert hospitals, hospital associations and the general public to trends, improvements, problems, and possible solutions related to health care within the Northwest by collecting, evaluating and disseminating relevant data and study results
7. To help hospital management keep abreast of new developments, techniques, and methods
8. To help increase the skill and overall productivity of health care personnel by developing and assisting hospitals to implement educational and training programs
9. To help hospitals introduce technical innovations by stimulating needed research and development
10. To cooperate where possible with agencies concerned with health and planning in the Pacific Northwest and in the nation*

Since nursing comprises the largest portion of hospital employees, it is frequently given opportunities to use such services, which are also a resource for the director of nursing who might be under various pressures from hospital administration, other departments, or staff. These consultants can give objective help in eliminating or reducing such pressures. It is often a matter of sorting out the issues involved and reducing them to concrete manageable proportions.

An excellent and well-documented account [O'Malley[19]] of improvements in nursing services of a CASH member hospital tells of successful efforts to keep nurses nursing by stepped-up use of ward clerks, broader work distribution to avoid peaks, a concrete staffing and budget plan, and a quality assurance program. O'Malley

---

*From Battelle Northwest Systems Program for Hospitals: Systems research/development/evaluation, Portland, Ore., p. 2.

makes the sage observation that the CASH consultant can only suggest means, analyze, and guide; it remains for the nursing staff to identify problems, implement data procurement, and make resultant changes.

The Battelle Northwest service is a four-part program aimed at consistent, sophisticated collection of data to provide a quality assurance plan (controlling); a nursing personnel utilization plan (staffing); custom studies geared to individual institutional needs and shared service studies, equipment utilization, and floor layouts; and ongoing training in the form of workshops, printed material, and so forth. Lest these sound too formidable, the Battelle Northwest Staff meets with nurses to help them isolate problems and propose possible solutions. It is always the nurses who provide the material and make the decision for implementation. Institutions, including nursing departments, have the ongoing advantage of access to these management engineers, who are continually studying the institutions and services in their sophisticated, mathematical, systematic, and coordinating way.

DERIVATIVES OF OPERATIONS ANALYSIS

Operations analysis is the framework for considering job analysis and work simplification. It includes analysis of the positions and work extant in an organization at a given time, their interrelationships, and all other relationships (for example, the organizational structure or educational components) contingent on achieving the goals of the enterprise. Comprehensiveness of subject to be analyzed characterizes operations analysis.

Job analysis and work simplification are more circumscribed analytical endeavors. They may be accomplished through operations analysis by an outside consultant, other direction from outside the organization, internally with direction and assistance from the personnel department, or as a do-it-yourself project.

Job analysis

Job analysis is described as "the systematic process of collecting and making certain judgments about all of the pertinent information related to the nature of a specific job.... It is a dynamic process—an ongoing effort to assure an accurate and reliable basis for personnel management decisions."[20] The job analyst is listed and described in the standard hospital job description text.

Job analysis has not kept pace with the proliferation of jobs in the health field. There is a great need for such analysis, first vertically and then laterally. Only in such comprehensive analysis can alignments be made and duplications and gaps exposed and adjusted. As noted, there is an effort at moratorium of additional licensures until precision is brought to this conglomerate group of health care workers. With each group developing individually, and no attempt at lateral synchronization, extension of confusion and waste develops. The waste occurs not only in the work situation, resulting in increased cost to patients, but affects training programs and their costs too. With overall analysis of what each group does, there could be pooling of educational programs in the interest of economy of resources and faculty. The core concept is slowly growing, not only for levels of nursing but for all paramedical and other health care workers. Growth in this direction will reduce costs. Moreover, it will work to the advantage of all practitioners if they learn partly together, because it should develop mutual appreciation not possible in isolated vertical educational arrangements.

In a study done at the University of California at Los Angeles on 18 different health occupations (bioelectronic monitoring, biomedical photography, dental auxiliaries, medical laboratory technology, nursing, radiologic technology, respiratory technology, medical office assisting, business office services, social services [medical], orthotics, engineering maintenance, food services, medical records, pharmacy services, ward administration, gastroenterology technology, and purchasing for hospital care facilities), Barlow[21] found that there was considerable duplication of tasks and a common scientific base for most of the curricula. On the intraprofessional aspect, it was found that 60% of nursing tasks are done by all nursing personnel. As a result, 36 modular units of instruction for entering workers in nursing were prepared.[22]

It will take considerable effort in using job analysis to bring cohesiveness and order out of the vast and still developing number of health care positions. One is cautioned to choose job titles carefully. They should be short but descriptive, have a natural sound, and be consistent in the usage of certain key words.

Job analysis provides greater precision in hiring, placement, and transfer or personnel; allows greater opportunity for using talents; gives direction to in-service education and safety and health programs; contributes to work simplification; and provides a base for job and employee evaluation.

The standard questions—what, how, why—apply, accompanied by skills involved. Specificity is essential. Special requirements must be spelled out. Precision in language and observation is necessary. We have not been thorough in this; for example, we have not taken into consideration problems that result from working alone (for the professional worker) or nearly alone or from seldom acknowledged pressure times and locations. To these two factors can be added such standard ones as knowledge, training, judgment and initiative, responsibility for accuracy, cooperation and contact, responsibility for supervision of others, responsibility for confidential data, and physical effort [Dunn and Stephen[23]]. These can be weighted so that the more crucial factors count for more than the less crucial. For example, physical effort would be weighted considerably less than judgment and initiative or responsibility for management of others.

The standard methods of job analysis are by questionnaire, interview, experience, or observation (steady or sample). Verification of job analysis is an additional safeguard whereby the analysis is checked against a similar job that has not been completely analyzed. Exceptions and additions show up in this process. Because of the variety of times (shifts) and places (critical care unit to long-term care facility), this comparative process is useful.

Job analysis illumines and specifies the work of the enterprise, making the direction of workers clearer and less onerous because the work then is systematized and plain for all to see. This illumination helps use time, effort, and energy economically and opens the way for conservation of professional time. It is an ongoing task, because periodic surveillance is necessary.

Job descriptions

Job descriptions flow from job analysis. Job specifications are the requirements for the job, and are therefore part of the description, which also includes other parts of the job, such as work content and accountability. Pigors and Myers[24] define the job description as "a word picture (in writing) of the organizational relationships, responsibilities, and specific duties that constitute a given job or position. It defines a scope of responsibility and continuing work assignments that are sufficiently different from those of other jobs to warrant a specific title."

The revised job descriptions for hospitals[14] break down the job description into the following parts: job duties; machines, tools, equipment, and work aids; education, training, and experience; worker traits; and job relationships and professional affiliations. Worker traits are broken down into five parts: aptitudes, interests, temperaments, physical demands, and working conditions. The job description should be verified with the worker, supervisor, and those connected with the job, before finalization. The draft would be prepared from all existing information about the job.

Job descriptions are useful not only for recruitment, placement, and transfer, but also for guidance, direction, and evaluation of personnel. They also help to reduce conflict, frustration, and overlapping duties. They are essential for working relationships with outside bodies such as unions and professional organizations. They support the worker and are an important part of job satisfaction.

An interesting addition to job descriptions is combination, whereby several jobs are meshed to achieve a purpose. This brings precision and coordination where specialized skills and timing are necessarily synchronized. An example is the three-nurse resuscitation team developed in the trauma unit of Cook County Hospital in Chicago.[25] Each of the three nurses on this team is a qualified trauma nurse who can perform all parts of the work of such a specialist. The three experts work in precise unison to achieve the purpose.

Job evaluation

Job descriptions form a base for wage and salary administration. Job evaluation flows from and is a necessary part of such administration and is contingent on accurate and current job descriptions. The equity one hopes to achieve by detailed comparisons of jobs, both within a department as well as in relation to other departments, rests on the job description.

Job evaluation compares factors of considered jobs under several categories, such as skill, effort, responsibility, and job con-

Table 3. Relative weights for job factors in hourly rated jobs and salaried jobs in comparable job evaluation plans*

Hourly rated jobs		Salaried jobs† (clerical, supervisory, and technical)	
Factors	Percent of total points	Factors	Percent of total points
Skill		1. Education	25
1. Education	14	2. Experience	31.25
2. Experience	22	3. Complexity of duties	25
3. Initiative and ingenuity	14		81.25
	50	4. Monetary responsibility	6.25
Effort		5. Contacts	6.25
4. Physical demand	10	6. Working conditions	6.25
5. Mental-visual demand	5	(For supervisory jobs, additional points are added for "types of supervision" and "extent of supervision," with other percentages reduced correspondingly.)	
	15		
Responsibility			
6. For equipment or process	5		
7. Material or product	5		
8. Safety of others	5		
9. Work of others	5		
	20		
Job conditions			
10. Working conditions	10		
11. Hazards	5		
	15		
Total	100		

*From Pigors, P., and Myers, C.: Personnel administration, ed. 7, New York, 1973, McGraw-Hill Book Co., p. 371. Reprinted by permission of McGraw-Hill Book Co.
†Note the greater percentage weights for "education" and "experience" for salaried jobs. The higher weight for "complexity of duties" as compared to "initiative and ingenuity" (for hourly rated jobs) and the lower weight for "working conditions" for salaried jobs.
Source: Computed from tables in manuals prepared by the Industrial Relations Department of the National Electrical Manufacturers Association, New York: Job Rating Manual, Definitions of Factors Used in Evaluating Hourly-rated Jobs (1946 ed.), and NEMA Salaried Job Rating Plan: Definitions of Factors Used in Evaluating Clerical, Supervisory and Technical Positions (1949, reprinted in 1956).

ditions for hourly rated jobs. Salaried jobs are broken down into education, experience, complexity of duties, monetary responsibility, contacts, and working conditions. Table 3 shows such categories with weights to allow numerical comparisons within categorical comparisons.

It is interesting to compare the revised *Job Description and Organizational Analysis for Hospitals and Related Health Services* of 1970 with the original done in 1952. It not only documents certain changes in the 18-year period, but can be counted a historical record. Management engineering as a part of hospital administration does not appear in the original, though job analysis does. Data processing likewise is missing in the early issue. In-service personnel (director and instructors), surgical technician, and ward services manager appear in the 1970 revision only. There are 14 listings under technical services in the revision that do not appear in the original. The intravenous therapist can be found in neither, which is an odd omission. The revised edition is 200 pages longer than the original. It should be noted that both editions were prepared in cooperation with the American Hospital Association.

Job simplification

Job simplification is another form of job analysis, requiring step-by-step examination to locate areas of weakness or awkwardness and waste of time and effort. Asking why, what, where, when, who, and how helps to analyze the five steps: selecting the job, breaking the job down, questioning the job, developing a new method, and implementing improvement, all in the interest of improving patient care and hospital activities while reducing costs.

The job to be improved may take too much time, involve unnecessary work, make poor use of skills, require too much chasing around, have an inefficient work distribution, waste materials, have unnecessary hazards, or require heavy physical effort. The most common changes are elimination, combination, change of sequence, and simplification.

Use of a flow process chart is a common method of examining a piece of work for possible simplification. Fig. 6 shows a proposed change in the handling of medication cards. It will reduce the distance traveled by 50 feet and the time saved by 30 seconds per operation when medication cards are stored adjacent to the nurse's desk instead of in the medication area. This procedure for analyzing a piece of work moves through five symbolized steps: operations, transportations, inspections, delays, and storage. It is a dramatic illustration of economy of time and effort effected by a mundane change.

Bennett's[26] ten principles of motion economy are useful and applicable in job simplification. They consist of motions that are productive and bring achievement closer; that are simple, curved rather than straight, and rhythmic and smooth. Equipment and material are in easy reach and prearranged, using gravity and combination (half red–half blue pencil) where possible. Workers are in as easeful and appropriate posture and environment as possible and their hands are relieved as much as possible by other parts of the body, as in the use of foot pedals in treatment rooms.

While formulas to be followed and step-by-step description, examination, and evaluation are essential ingredients of job simplification, insightful observation that pinpoints the problem is also valuable. This is called process analysis and grows from the habit of awareness of internal and external relationships occurring within one's jurisdiction. It is really a state of mind that generates the process. The following examples show the method.

Fig. 7 represents a three-corridor nursing unit, with rooms on all sides to accommodate about 30 patients. In the middle is a long, narrow utility service room and medication area, which was accessible only from the far corridor. Because there is only one entrance to the unit, staff had to go around to the far corridor to work in the medication area. An insightful head nurse suggested that another doorway to

PRESENT METHOD ☐ PROPOSED METHOD ☑

FLOW PROCESS CHART

PAGE 1 OF 1

SUMMARY

	PRESENT	PROPOSED	DIFFERENCE
○ OPERATIONS	7	7	0
⇨ TRANSPORTATIONS	5	3	2
☐ INSPECTIONS	1	1	0
D DELAYS	3	3	0
▽ STORAGES	2	2	0
DISTANCE TRAVELLED	75 FT.	25 FT.	50 FT.
TIME SEC.	120	90	30

JOB USE OF MEDICATION CARDS ON NURSING FLOOR

Subject Charted MEDICATION CARD

CHART BEGINS IN CARD BOX

CHART ENDS IN CARD BOX

CHARTED BY L. OLSEN DATE 6/12/62

	DESCRIPTION OF EVENT	OPERATION / TRANSPORT / INSPECTION / DELAY / STORAGE	QUANTITY	DISTANCE IN FEET	TIME	NOTES
1	MEDICATION CARD IN MEDICATION CARD BOX	▽				ON TABLE NEXT TO NURSE'S DESK.
2	CARD TAKEN FROM BOX	○				OCCURS APPROXIMATELY
3	CHECKED WITH KARDEX	☐			30	50 TIMES EACH DAY ON EACH FLOOR.
4	CARRIED TO MEDICINE CABINET	⇨		25	15	
5	PLACED ON TRAY	○				
6	WAITS WHILE MEDS. ARE POURED	D				
7	CARRIED TO BEDSIDE WITH MEDS	⇨	VARIES			
8	WAITS WHILE MEDS. ARE GIVEN	D				
9	PLACED IN NURSE'S POCKET	○				
10	CARRIED BACK TO DESK	⇨	VARIES			
11	REMOVED FROM POCKET	○				
12	PLACED ON DESK	○				
13	WAITS WHILE MEDS. ARE CHARTED	D			45	
14	PICKED UP FROM DESK	○				
15	PLACED IN MED. CARD BOX	○				ON TABLE NEXT TO NURSE'S DESK.
16	REMAINS IN MED. CARD BOX UNTIL NEXT MED. IS GIVEN	▽				
17		○⇨☐D▽				
18		○⇨☐D▽				
19		○⇨☐D▽				
20		○⇨☐D▽				
21		○⇨☐D▽				
22		○⇨☐D▽				
23		○⇨☐D▽				
24		○⇨☐D▽				

Fig. 6. Job simplification as determined by use of a flow process chart. (From Bennett, A.: Methods improvements in hospitals, Philadelphia, 1964, J. B. Lippincott Co., p. 31.)

this service–medication area be made on the entrance corridor, so that there would be access from two sides. This was accomplished, resulting in great saving of staff time and energy. It is possible that this had occurred to someone before but had not been explored or implemented. Such possibilities for improvement exist in our new modern hospitals as well. However, newness should reduce inefficient construction, especially if nurses are involved in the planning stages.

In stage one of the procedure for a gallbladder x-ray film series, films are made of

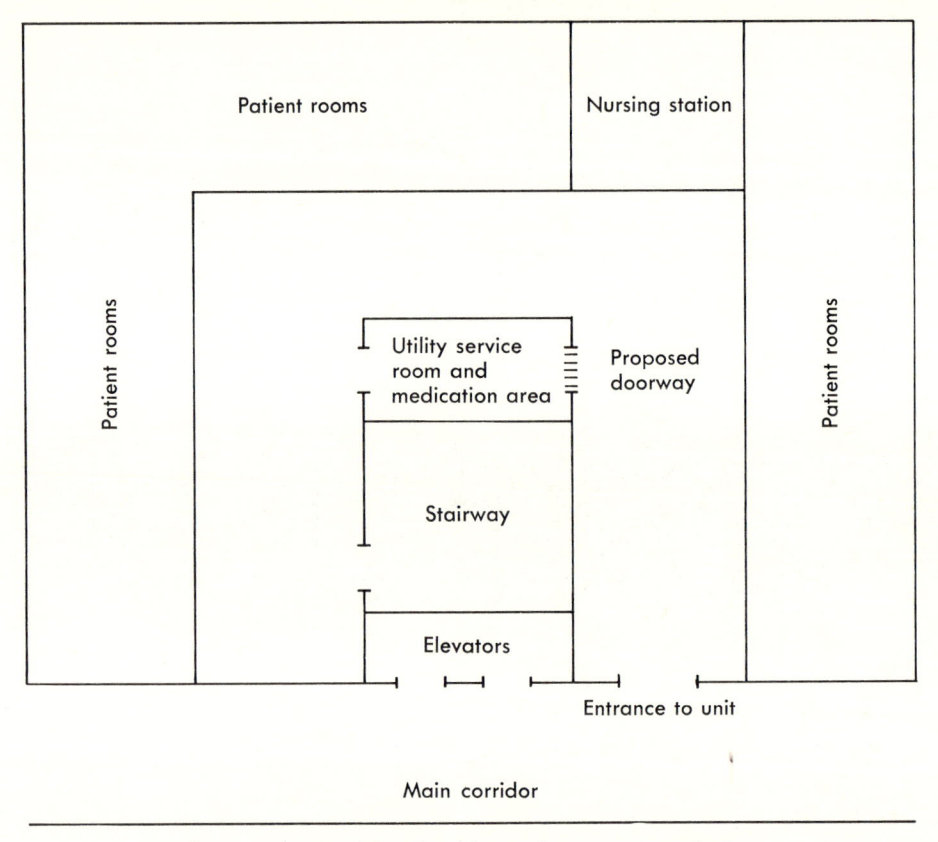

```
┌─────────────────────────────────────────────────────────────────┐
│                                  ┌──────────────┐               │
│         Patient rooms            │Nursing station│              │
│                                  │              │               │
│              ┌───────────────────┴──────────────┐               │
│              │                                  │               │
│   P          │   ┌─Utility service─┐            │   P           │
│   a          │   │  room and       │ Proposed   │   a           │
│   t          │   │  medication area│ doorway    │   t           │
│   i          │   └─────────────────┘            │   i           │
│   e          │                                  │   e           │
│   n          │         Stairway                 │   n           │
│   t          │                                  │   t           │
│              │                                  │               │
│   r          │         Elevators                │   r           │
│   o          │                                  │   o           │
│   o          └──────────────────────────────────┘   o           │
│   m                          Entrance to unit       m           │
│   s                                                 s           │
└─────────────────────────────────────────────────────────────────┘
                          Main corridor
```

Fig. 7. Job simplification through process analysis.

the patient's gallbladder before ingestion of a fatty meal. The routine was to have the patient return to the unit, have the fatty meal, and then return to radiology at the prescribed time following the meal so that further x-ray films could be made. This involved two transportation trips and order and procurement of the fatty meal (now a drink). Another insightful nurse wondered why the fatty meals could not be procured in the radiology department and the patient kept there in an appropriate waiting room until time for the next films. This would eliminate the two trips, the ordering and procurement of the fatty drink, and midmorning intrusion on a busy dietary department preparing lunch. It took some months, persistence, and patience to bring about the change, but eventually the radiology and dietary departments were conditioned to consider the proposal; work out the internal arrangements, such as provision for refrigerator storage for daily supply of fatty drinks delivered to radiology and estimation of probable number needed; and establish requisition and delivery systems.

Another means of examining work for efficiency and economy of time, effort, and money is to collectively list all the areas or as many as can be identified that are deserving of deliberation and do a systematic review from that point, with consequent revision, realignment, or whatever is indicated. CASH has such a list, composed of 44 items for possible improvement of work distribution, procedures, and conservation of time. In conservation, for example, there is use of wash-and-dry towelettes for premeal and bedtime use. Scheduling baths over the whole day is another suggestion. In the interest of patient sleep, probably the sickest, those needing frequent attention, or those receiving Communion in Catholic hospitals could be bathed before 7 AM. It is also possible that some patients could be bathed at bedtime or even during the night if a sedative is to be repeated or treatment given. Baths can be scheduled around visiting hours.

There are suggestions that discharge and admitting times be made earlier, though this would add to the complaint that hospitals are run for staff rather than patients, because patients' hospital time would be increased.

An excellent item aimed directly at nursing care is to pass the sedatives later in order to reduce the need for repeating them. Related to this is the need to plan the night medications so that the longest period of rest possible is arranged for the patient. Medications that need to be considered principally are those given every 4 hours. For example, giving the midnight dose at 11:30 PM and the 4 AM one at 4:30 would extend the rest period by 1 hour. Reviewing and adjusting all the medications for a patient at one time would greatly enhance patient rest and comfort. As nursing care plans become a reality, such deliberations will become commonplace.

There are also items bearing on physical plant and equipment, such as automated beds, to make the patient more self-sufficient, and telecommunication between patient, nurse, and desk or communication center, to reduce walking time and expedite service.

Work measurement is a corollary to work simplification that is sometimes used to describe examination and change in work flow or pattern. In fact, measurement is a built-in part of the job simplification process. It is part of the analysis that must precede review, revision, reformulation, realignment, or maintenance of the work under examination.

NURSING CARE DIRECTION

Direction of nursing care itself is secondarily provided by nursing care plans, nursing care conferences, and patient care conferences. These are the vehicles for all manner of instructions, guidelines, and suggestions for care pertaining to a particular patient. These procedures continuously subject the nursing care of a particular patient to scrutiny; measure it against existing standards; and review possibilities for strengthening, correcting, or individualizing those standards for the particular patient.

Nursing care plans

Nursing care plans are commonly committed to card format. There is considerable evidence that these plans do not reach an acceptable level where they do indeed contain a plan of care for the patient; rather, they list physicians' orders to be processed.

From the literature, Cuica[27] has done a thorough review of history and use of the nursing care plan over the last 20 years. He found three phases of development: "communication, assessment and diagnosis and multidisciplinary approach." After analyzing a substantial sample of nursing care plans, he found them used essentially for communication of such items as "medications, treatments, monitoring of vital signs, intake and output, and diagnostic studies." He sees the need for "staff development programs . . . utilizing personnel who are capable of developing nursing care plans and who can provide leadership and guidance."

In considering the nursing care plan as a means of directing nursing care, Kramer[28] has made a significant proposal that patients and their families be included with nursing staff in planning their own care. This proposal would be a redundancy if we were anywhere near the practice of individualized nursing care. She confirms the findings of Cuica that nursing care plans as they exist are hollow and scant; and thinks goals have been displaced by procedure, generating the present impoverished state of nursing care plans.

Findings of the Survey of Hospital Nursing Service [Aydelotte, p. 40][6] also support those of Cuica and Kramer: no directors of

144 Framework for study of nursing service administration

GOOD SAMARITAN HOSPITAL AND MEDICAL CENTER
REHABILITATIVE SERVICES

NAME _____

CODE: I – INDEPENDENT; A – ASSIST; D – DEPENDENT

AMBULATION

ASSISTIVE EQUIPMENT:

TRANSFER
  TYPE:
  METHOD

ACTIVITIES OF DAILY LIVING
  BATH   TYPE:
         SCHEDULE
  TEETH/DENTURES
  HAIR
  SHAVING
  MAKE UP
  FEEDING
  DRESSING
    UPPER BODY
    LOWER BODY
  ADL PROBLEMS

BED ACTIVITIES (INCLUDE SLEEP, PRONE LYING, TURNING SCHEDULE, EXERCISE, ETC.)

BOWEL PROGRAM
  PREVIOUS PATTERN
  PRESENT PATTERN
  NEEDS

BLADDER PROGRAM
  RETENTION CATHETER SIZE
  DATE CHANGED
  TOC (TRIAL OFF CATHETER) DATES
  IRRIGATION ☐   INSTILLATION ☐
  NEEDS

PROBLEMS:
  #1 SKIN
  #2 MUSCULATURE:
  #3 COMMUNICATION:
  #4 VISION & HEARING:
  #5 BEHAVIOR:
  #6
  #7
  #8
  #9
  #10

APPLIANCES: (CIRCLE THOSE APPLICABLE)
  SPLINTS
  BRACES
  COLLAR
  LIFT
  TRAPEZE
  SWIVEL BAR
  BALKAN FRAME
  DEMEDCO MATTRESS
  DEMEDCO CUSHION

PATIENT GOALS:

P.T. CURRENT LEVEL:
  GOALS:

O.T. CURRENT LEVEL:
  GOALS:

NURSING – SHORT RANGE GOALS:

LONG RANGE GOALS:

TEAM CONFERENCE:

SOCIAL INFORMATION:

DISCHARGE PLANNING
  DESTINATION: DATE:
  ADDRESS:
  REFERRAL:
  HOME CARE PLAN:
  OUTPATIENT THERAPY:
  EMERGENCY HELP CARD: DATE:

EXTENDED LOA DATES

CODE: N – NEEDS, H – HAS BEEN TAUGHT
H/N – HAS BEEN TAUGHT, NEEDS REPEATING
(CROSS OFF ITEMS NOT APPLICABLE)

TEACHING

	DATE	PATIENT INITIAL	DATE	FAMILY INITIAL	CODE

SKIN
  INSPECTION & MIRROR ISSUE
  PREVENTION & TREATMENT OF PRESSURE SORES
  POSITIONING
BLADDER PROGRAM
  CATHETER CARE
  CATHETER IRRIGATION
  CHANGING CATHETER
BOWEL PROGRAM
  SCHEDULE & METHOD
DIET
MEDICATIONS
  PURPOSES & PRECAUTIONS
TRANSFERS
SAFETY PRECAUTIONS
BOOKLETS
  STROKE
  SCI
  OTHER

LAB, X-RAY, TESTS

DATE	TEST	DONE	DATE	TEST	DONE

Form No. 5109 Rev. 8.21.72 J.B.

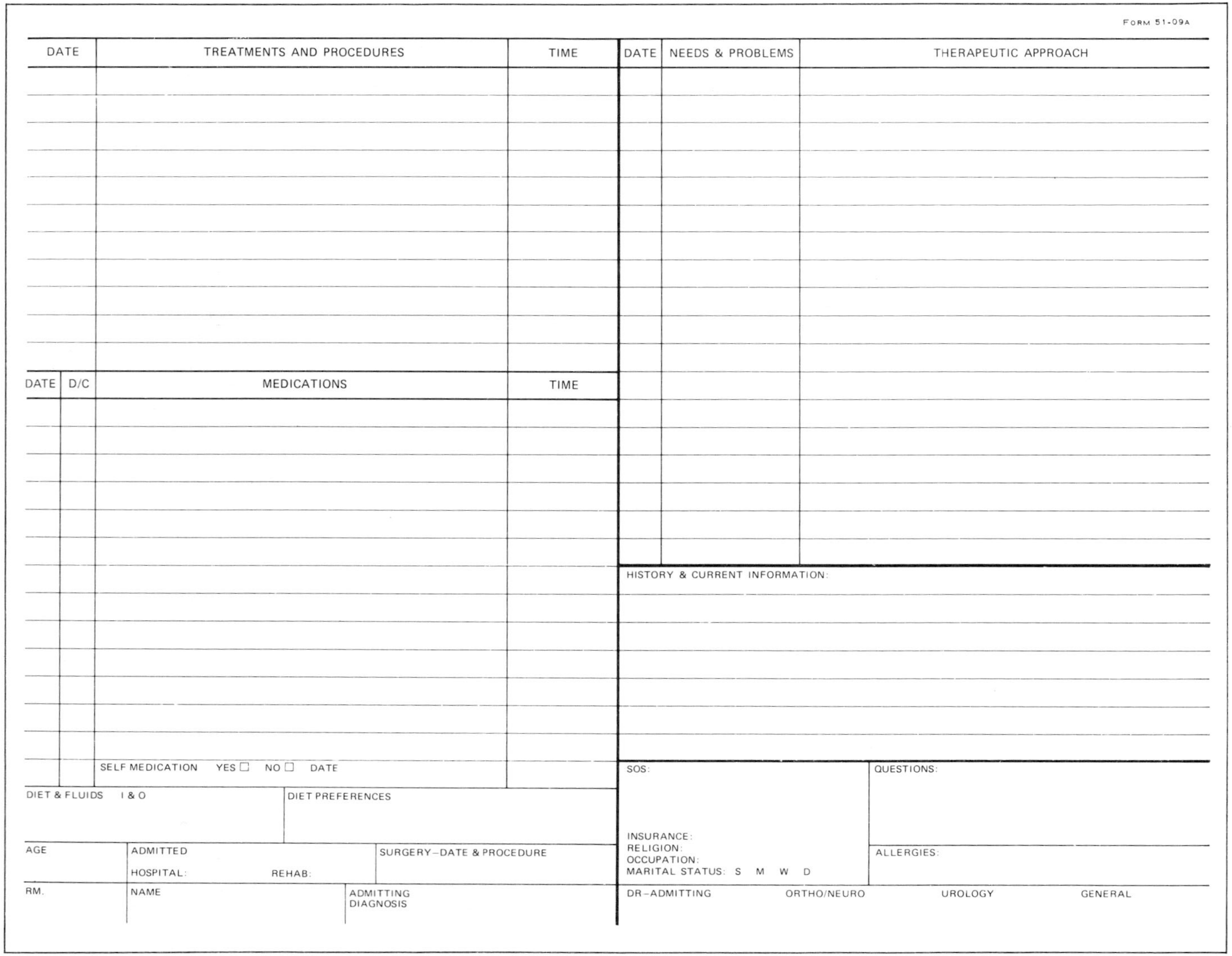

FORM 51-09A

DATE	TREATMENTS AND PROCEDURES	TIME

DATE	D/C	MEDICATIONS	TIME

SELF MEDICATION YES ☐ NO ☐ DATE

DIET & FLUIDS I & O

DIET PREFERENCES

AGE

ADMITTED

HOSPITAL: REHAB:

SURGERY–DATE & PROCEDURE

RM.

NAME

ADMITTING DIAGNOSIS

DATE	NEEDS & PROBLEMS	THERAPEUTIC APPROACH

HISTORY & CURRENT INFORMATION:

SOS:

INSURANCE:
RELIGION:
OCCUPATION:
MARITAL STATUS: S M W D

QUESTIONS:

ALLERGIES:

DR–ADMITTING ORTHO/NEURO UROLOGY GENERAL

Fig. 8. Nursing care plan. (Courtesy Good Samaritan Hospital & Medical Center, Portland, Ore.)

nursing reviewed nursing care plans periodically except in hospitals with 24 or fewer beds. It can be argued that this is not an appropriate duty of directors of nursing; yet how else can they be certain the goals of the nursing service are being carried forward if they do not review this crucial adjunct to nursing care while they are making nursing care rounds? Two areas that need study derived from this Survey: (1) how to improve the leadership in nursing services in order to meet the nursing needs of patients and their families, and (2) the function and identification of nursing services as related to nursing care plans and the care they express.

Consonant with the thesis of this book, the problem is viewed as one of getting nursing personnel to practice internalized, continuing comprehensive nursing care universally, through definitive and knowledgeable goal setting and appropriate direction by clinically-oriented and competent nursing service administrators aided by a staff-development program, with clinical specialists using internal and external clinical resources to raise the nursing practice level. The nursing care plans, as well as similar service or procedures, will remain depressingly undeveloped until such time as all or the majority of nurses (including significant numbers of administrative personnel, especially supervisors and head nurses) are practicing comprehensive nursing care competently, steadily, and comfortably. A good test of the plan's usefulness is to visualize it as would a float nurse, new to the unit and in the middle of the night. This test is useful in getting all staff to commit a patient's care to the written care plan rather than keeping it in their minds.

The form for the nursing care plan is very important. Fig. 8 shows a plan from a rehabilitation institute. Frequently in such a setting, comprehensive care is practiced continuously and comfortably. With modification as necessary, this plan has specific application to any other site. It should be noted that cards are of standard $8\frac{1}{2}'' \times 11''$ size, obviating the squeezing and abbreviation required with smaller cards as the nursing care plan is expanded. Patients in such institutes are there on a long-term basis, so time is available to develop such fine plans; however, care must be taken so that lack of time is not used as a reason for not proceeding with such detailed nursing care planning in other settings.

A useful item to include on the nursing care plan is the patient's social history. It takes only a few lines to provide such an entry, yet it is invaluable to the staff to know something of the patient's occupation, family constellation, and so forth, in planning for care. Also on the nursing care plan, common observations and possible or anticipated symptoms of a patient with a particular disease can be included for the convenience of quick review by personnel (for example, hypo- and hyperglycemia in the case of a diabetic patient).

Related to this practice of listing crucial or salient points in a given pathological condition on the nursing care plan is the practice of maintaining a file on each common pathological condition, to be taken out and attached to the nursing care plan for a patient with that condition, for the purpose of expediting the necessary care by making easy reference possible for the staff. Brevity is important. The review of signs, symptoms, and complications, usual medical plan, and comprehensive nursing review, all in point form, would suffice. Such formulations constitute standards. These reviews or guides could be worked up and kept centrally by the in-service department, nursing office, or central supply.

A corollary of the above practice is one of formulating standard care plans that provide all essential information and an efficient base for individualizing particular patients' care when they are admitted. This idea also comes from a rehabilitation institute [Cornell and Carrick[29]]. Standard nursing care plans are computerized and stored in the computer, ready for individualized use as a patient's data became available. Print-outs of care are available daily or as data are changed. Patients participate in these nursing care plans. There are master print-outs containing this information, in addition to privileged information for the staff. There is also a chronological composite print-out that becomes the day's work schedule.

Retention of the nursing care plan in the permanent record deserves attention. Usually there is no provision for keeping it, but where it has been developed conscientiously and knowledgeably, it contributes to the total record of the patient's care, as do parts of the chart. When changes are made in the care plan, the previous entry should not be erased; rather, a line should be drawn through the entry to denote discontinuance.

The health care plan shown in Fig. 9 is another guide to help staff think comprehensively, not only about nursing care but other therapies available to a particular population for which nursing often assumes overall, if not particularized, supervision. This plan addresses itself essentially to the long-term patient and requires quarterly review of goals and plans of component parts of health care for the institutionalized patient. It could, however, be adapted to short-term care, in an effort to think directionally about and treat the patient comprehensively in today's complex health care locations.

Adjuncts to nursing care plans. There are and can be adjuncts to the nursing care plans to facilitate their implementation. For example, in some instances medications or treatments are contained in a separate card file, or there may be a separate dietary file, which should include the original diet order sent to the dietary department for full processing. One-time procedures that constitute the day's work, such as preoperative care, medications, and laboratory tests, can be shown on a card, sheet, or blackboard. Intake and output measurements, treatments, patients receiving therapy outside the department, or any other category common to the unit or service, may be listed on such a work sheet. The daily work sheet assists in error control, expediency, and efficiency. It may be accompanied by a board with tags showing location of patients at all times.

Fig. 10 (Activities of Daily Living [ADL]) shows an extension of the nursing care plan found at the patient's bedside for the staff's information and benefit. It brings precision to the physical care because of its detail and evaluation by the occupational therapy department.

Another accessory of the nursing care plan is the nursing history, which in fact precedes the nursing care plan and gives direction to it. Nursing histories have developed considerably over the years, and are an expansion or extension of the traditional admission note on a patient. Excellent examples of nursing case histories are included in Little and Carnevali's definitive work on the nursing care plan. A programmed instruction unit for taking a patient's history is contained in the *American Journal of Nursing* (February 1974).

New and associates,[31] in their report of a staffing experiment in which they found substantial lack of communication between the patient and health personnel, propose as an antidote that graduate nurses conduct the admission interview so that they will gain personal knowledge of the patient, thus enriching the ensuing nursing care. The patient could be simultaneously oriented to hospital and nursing routines and procedures.

Before or while data are becoming part of the nursing care plan, there is an assessment (and/or diagnosis) stage. Bonney and Rothberg[32] have set up an excellent model in great detail for this phase of nursing care or nursing process, with 14 pages in outline form devoted to collection of data, assessment, and nursing diagnosis, therapy, and prognosis. It is accompanied by a numerical scoring system that helps in determining diagnosis and therapy and in identifying patient strengths and weaknesses.

The first National Conference on the

Fig. 9. Health care plan.

HEALTH CARE PLAN

Patient's Name _____ Facility _____
Age _____ Dr. _____ Date of Admission _____

Dept.	Second Quarter	Third Quarter	Fourth Quarter
Nursing Service	Progress: ↓ – ↑ ↑ ↑ Modified Plan: _____ _____ _____ _____ _____ Short Term Goals: _____ Long Term Goals: _____	Progress: ↓ – ↑ ↑ ↑ Modified Plan: _____ _____ _____ _____ _____ Short Term Goals: _____ Long Term Goals: _____	Progress: ↓ – ↑ ↑ ↑ Modified Plan: _____ _____ _____ _____ _____ Short Term Goals: _____ Long Term Goals: _____
Physical Therapy Restorative Service	Progress: ↓ – ↑ ↑ ↑ Modified Plan: _____ _____ Short Term Goals: _____ Long Term Goals: _____	Progress: ↓ – ↑ ↑ ↑ Modified Plan: _____ _____ Short Term Goals: _____ Long Term Goals: _____	Progress: ↓ – ↑ ↑ ↑ Modified Plan: _____ _____ Short Term Goals: _____ Long Term Goals: _____
Dietary Service	Current Diet: _____ Problems: _____ Treatment Plan: _____	Current Diet: _____ Problems: _____ Treatment Plan: _____	Current Diet: _____ Problems: _____ Treatment Plan: _____
Occupational Therapy Service	Progress: ↓ – ↑ ↑ ↑ Modified Plan: _____ _____ Short Term Goals: _____ Long Term Goals: _____	Progress: ↓ – ↑ ↑ ↑ Modified Plan: _____ _____ Short Term Goals: _____ Long Term Goals: _____	Progress: ↓ – ↑ ↑ ↑ Modified Plan: _____ _____ Short Term Goals: _____ Long Term Goals: _____
Pharmacy Service	I have reviewed the patient's drug regimen and noted the following: _____ _____ DATE SIGNATURE	I have reviewed the patient's drug regimen and noted the following: _____ _____ DATE SIGNATURE	I have reviewed the patient's drug regimen and noted the following: _____ _____ DATE SIGNATURE
Psycho-Social Service	Progress: ↓ – ↑ ↑ ↑ Modified Plan: _____ _____ Short Term Goals: _____ Long Term Goals: _____	Progress: ↓ – ↑ ↑ ↑ Modified Plan: _____ _____ Short Term Goals: _____ Long Term Goals: _____	Progress: ↓ – ↑ ↑ ↑ Modified Plan: _____ _____ Short Term Goals: _____ Long Term Goals: _____
Activities Department	Progress: ↓ – ↑ ↑ ↑ Modified Plan: _____ _____ Short Term Goals: _____ Long Term Goals: _____	Progress: ↓ – ↑ ↑ ↑ Modified Plan: _____ _____ Short Term Goals: _____ Long Term Goals: _____	Progress: ↓ – ↑ ↑ ↑ Modified Plan: _____ _____ Short Term Goals: _____ Long Term Goals: _____
Other			

I have reviewed the above Health Care Plan and authorize its continuation or modification as follows:
_____
_____

_____   _____
Date   Physician's Signature

Fig. 9, cont'd. Health care plan. (Courtesy Patricia A. Cruise, Geriatrics Health Services, Inc., Portland, Ore.)

```
                      NAME _____  DATE _____

                            REHABILITATION INSTITUTE OF OREGON
                                  Activities of Daily Living

                          ■  Solid colored square - Independent
                          ◩  Diagonal half colored square - Partially independent
                          ☐  Blank square - Dependent


            HYGIENE                                    DRESSING, UNDRESSING
     ☐ Wash face, hands                          ☐ Shorts, panties
     ☐ Bed bath                                  ☐ Bra
     ☐ Brush teeth                               ☐ Girdle
     ☐ Shave, make-up                            ☐ Slip-over garment
     ☐ Comb, brush hair                          ☐ Buttoned shirt, blouse
     ☐ Clean, trim nails                         ☐ Slacks
     ☐ Use hankerchief                           ☐ Hose, socks
     ☐ Shampoo hair                              ☐ Slippers, loafers
                                                 ☐ Tie shoes
     ☐ Adaptive devices                          ☐ Braces, prosthesis

            EATING
                                                 ☐ Adaptive Devices
                                                        TRANSFER ACTIVITIES
     ☐ With fingers                              ☐ On, off bedpan
     ☐ With spoon                                ☐ On, off toilet
     ☐ With fork                                 ☐ In, out bathtub
     ☐ From glass                                ☐ Wheel chair - bed, and back
     ☐ From cup                                  ☐ Manipulate wheel chair
     ☐ Use knife                                 ☐ Operate elevator
     ☐ Adaptive devices
```

Fig. 10. Checklist for activities of daily living. (Courtesy Good Samaritan Hospital & Medical Center, Portland, Ore.)

Classification of Nursing Diagnoses was held in 1973 and reported by Gebbie and Lavin.[33] The following list shows 34 tentative nursing diagnoses determined by the conference. Several of these, such as altered self-concept and anxiety, are elaborated. It is recommended that the list be explored and deepened by using the medical record system, essentially as the physician does, to get classification and retrieval for evaluation and study.

Tentative list of nursing diagnoses*
  Alterations in faith

---

*From Gebbie, K. M., and Lavin, M. A.: Classifying nursing diagnoses, Am. J. Nurs. **74**(2):251, 1974.

Altered relationships with self and others
Altered self-concept
Anxiety
Body fluids, depletion of
Bowel function, irregular
Cognitive functioning, alteration in the level of
Comfort level, alterations in
Confusion (disorientation)
Deprivation
Digestion, impairment of
Family's adjustment to illness, impairment of
Family process, inadequate
Fear
Grieving
Lack of understanding
Level of consciousness, alterations in
Malnutrition
Manipulation
Mobility, impaired
Motor incoordination
Non-compliance
Pain
Regulatory function of the skin, impairment of
Respiration, impairment of
Respiratory distress
Self-care activities, altered ability to perform
Sensory disturbances
Skin integrity, impairment of
Sleep/rest pattern, ineffective
Susceptibility to hazards
Thought process, impaired
Urinary elimination, impairment of
Verbal communication, impairment of

It is possible that the current effort to classify nursing diagnoses would bear fruit faster if the traditional systemic organization of medicine were operative. For example, on cursory categorization, and disregarding overlays, among the above 34 tentative nursing diagnoses seven involve the neurological system, four the gastrointestinal, two each the respiratory, circulatory, and musculoskeletal, and one the urinary system; four involve psychological state; and two concern pain. This unevenness might yield to systemic categorization.

Roy[34] sees a system of classification of nursing diagnoses as instrumental in the development of the science of nursing, as a means of differentiation of nursing from the work of other health professionals, as criteria for determining nursing skill in diagnosis, as a source of explicit information about nursing for legislators and the public, and as specific justification for payment for nursing services. The homogeneity and precision to be found in such a classification of nursing diagnoses would bring comparable specificity to deliberation, implementation, and measurement of nursing care on the part of practitioners.

Conferences. The nursing care conference, a corollary to the nursing care plan to which it should contribute, is another directional activity that, if recognized and acknowledged as such, will energize nursing care. The nursing service administrator must continually point out the relationship between conferences and nursing care so that collateral effort is seen in direct relationship to patients. Team conferences, where staff practicing comprehensive nursing care deliberated, evaluated, changed, or continued the nursing care plan, were early and fruitful forms of the nursing care conference.

The nursing care conference, whether unit-, area-, or servicewide, is essentially a scheduled meeting to review nursing care of one patient or a group or a category of patients, preparatory to evaluation and decision making about that care. Frequently one person is charged with the review and another may be charged to contribute findings from the literature, outside resources, or another department(s) of the hospital. Occasionally, patients may participate in and contribute to the conference. If the purpose is to be served and the time justified, such conferences must redound to improved immediate or future nursing care plans for patients.

The patient care conference has the same purpose, characteristics, and effect, but others besides nurses are participants in the conference. Representatives from other departments of the hospital who contribute to the care of particular patients, outside and related resource or contributing agencies, and occasionally patients participate in the patient care conference. Again we can use practices in long-term settings as models, particularly those in rehabilitation centers where patient care conferences are well established.

Both nursing and patient care conferences contribute much to the direction of nursing care, though they vary in direct relationship to nursing care planning. They are particularly effective where nursing care is comprehensive and continuous, and constructive where growth toward comprehensive nursing care is occurring. They at least provide a vehicle that encourages exploration where nursing care is not yet being examined and studied.

PHYSICAL PLANT IN DIRECTING

The physical plant in which nursing is practiced provides direction to nursing care. Utilization of old plants, renovation or reconstruction, and plans and implementation of new facilities all dictate to some degree the way nursing care will be practiced. More correctly, they direct the work of personnel functioning within the confines of a particular institution.

Long wards with multiple beds are a thing of the past, but two- and four-bed units are not. Though we talk of individualized nursing care, we violate the concept by use of these units without really thinking much about it. Nursing care cannot be individualized where all care rendered is heard and smelled, if not seen, by a patient in an adjacent bed. Yet conversion to the single unit is slow, perhaps because the luxurious private-unit model prevails, while efficiency-economy single units, resembling cubicles because space for essential equipment is all that is allowed, are less common.

We have justified the two- or four-bed physical arrangement on the basis that patients are company for each other. This may be partially true, but nowhere else in our society are strangers forced to live so intimately with each other. We have even suggested that they help each other! Likewise, we have been slow to introduce day rooms, sitting rooms, or dining areas in patient units, where the socialization we expect in the multiple unit could be carried on more appropriately. Such facilities need not await new construction, because space could be found in ingenious ways if we felt a commitment to providing such facilities. Moreover, the newer modes of partitioning could be used to supplement the traditional curtain, thus increasing the privacy of patients.

Proximity to patients remains very important in giving nursing care, as the specialized units of coronary and intensive care demonstrate. In new construction, there are directional characteristics of many kinds, for example, the circular unit that provides a core center from which staff serves and observes patients more efficiently, with a minimum of walking. There are other ways by which new construction has facilitated, if not actually directed, nursing care. Piped oxygen and suction equipment at bedsides, pneumatic tube systems, and electronic monitoring systems all provide precision and efficiency in delivering care and reducing the tension level of staff.

Friesen plan. The Friesen plan [35-37] deserves comment because it is a combination of physical plant and division of work designed to enhance nursing practice by putting personnel and equipment nearer the patient. Indeed, it may be the ultimate in proximity—and the ultimate in invasion of privacy. All supplies, including medication (in a locked compartment), chart, nursing care plan, or whatever is needed for the care of the patient, are kept in a two-way cupboard opening into the patient's room and into the hallway. Regular and routine delivery of needed items, including medication, is made directly to these individual stations; nursing station medication and supply centers no longer exist. All nursing activity is individualized around the patients and the supply-service cupboard in their rooms. The unanswered question here is what inroads this centralized and localized activity has on the patients' privacy, peace, and quiet. A floor plan in which there is a vestibule for dressing and toilet facilities (such as found in motels) would provide a buffer area between patient and work area, affording some privacy.

PATIENT DISTRIBUTION IN DIRECTION

Progressive patient care, or the distribution of patients by degree of illness, is a prevalent and useful arrangement for providing nursing service. Such distribution consists of (1) units for critically ill patients (those who require coronary or intesive care), (2) intermediate care units for the stage following care in the first category, or the usual hospital units, (3) units for patients who are ambulatory, or self-care units, (4) units for patients needing long-term care and/or rehabilitation, and (5) home care service operated by the hospital [Abdellah and Strachan[38]].

There is a growing need for a unit, in close approximation to the critical or coronary care unit if possible, where patients who are out of the critical stage may be followed more closely than in the intermediate unit but less closely than in the critical care unit, allowing a longer stabilization period for these patients. Other candidates for this unit are patients who need more nursing care than is usually provided in the intermediate care unit, such as frequent positioning or closer observation, as well as those who are incontinent. This type of unit is known sometimes as a definitive observation care unit. Where it exists, intermediate or general care becomes the third category.

Intermediate care is the traditional and continuing standard nursing care in hospitals today. Intensive care units are commonplace for care of critically ill patients. Self-care is less common, but growing as the benefits in terms of economy to patients or their insurance representatives and conservation of nurse time become more apparent. Adjuncts to self-care units are holding areas near emergency departments, where patients can remain until it is determined whether they can be discharged or must be admitted. A comparable facility is one provided for 12-hour admissions, from which the patient is discharged in the evening after minor surgery or a procedure requiring short-term hospitalization.

Long-term care and rehabilitation are usually administered outside the hospital in extended care facilities, nursing homes, and rehabilitation institutes, though some are an integral part of a hospital. Medicare-Medicaid programs have provided considerable stimulus to this type of facility.

Home health care is the least-used component of progressive patient care, though it is becoming more frequent. It is found that older patients with long-term diseases are good subjects for such care. The first such plan was developed in the 1940s at Montefiore Hospital in New York City. It permitted patients to be cared for at home by having personnel take their services and equipment to the patient. It conserved scarce hospital beds, while providing greater patient satisfaction by allowing them to remain at home. This plan was followed by a program sponsored by Associated Hospital Services of New York (Blue Cross).

Brown[39] found that where there is a home health service, referrals to a visiting nurse service are more frequent because staff are oriented to selection, evaluation, and referral of such patients. Brown's account of extension of hospitals into home health and satellite outpatient clinics, the expanded role of nurses, and cooperative health agency efforts is descriptive, interesting, and exciting.

Patient distribution, then, directs the staffing function by its need for specialized kinds of nurses in specific numbers to meet the needs of patients categorized in useful and coherent ways. In short, the extended role of nurses and the clinical analysis of their services dictate or give direction to the nursing enterprise.

Total patient care consists of five or six elements of progressive patient care, plus the widest possible range of clinical or outpatient services to the patient population.

An important consideration is the number of clinical services available. Modified progressive care refers to any combination of or addition to these elements in a given institution. It describes total patient care based on the categorized needs of the patient population.

REFERENCES

1. Newman, W.: Administrative action, ed. 2, Englewood Cliffs, N.J., 1963, Prentice-Hall, Inc., pp. 371-385.
2. Stevens, B.: The problem in nursing's middle management, J. Nurs. Admin. **11**(5):35-38, 1972.
3. Donovan, H.: What is supervision? Nurs. Outlook **5**(6):373, 1957.
4. Letters, J. Nurs. Admin. **1**(5):6, 1971.
5. David, J.: Personal correspondence, March 15, 1974.
6. Aydelotte, M.: Survey of hospital nursing services, National League for Nursing, 1968, pp. 18 and 40.
7. Greenough, K.: Determining standards for nursing care, Am. J. Nurs. **68**(10):2153-2155, 1968.
8. Nicholls, M.: Quality control in patient care, Am. J. Nurs. **74**(3):458, 1974.
9. Carter, J., and associates: Standards of nursing care; a guide for evaluation, New York, 1972, Springer Publishing Co., Inc.
10. Accreditation manual for hospitals, Chicago, 1974, Joint Commission for Accreditation of Hospitals, Nursing Services Section.
11. Roy, R.: The administrative process, Baltimore, 1965, The Johns Hopkins University Press, pp. 73-82.
12. Larkin, J.: Work study, New York, 1969, McGraw-Hill Book Co., p. 13.
13. Administrative services and facilities for hospitals, Washington, D.C., 1972, U.S. Department of Health, Education, and Welfare, pp. 46-48.
14. Job descriptions and organizational analysis for hospitals and related health services, Washington, D.C., 1970, U.S. Department of Labor, Manpower Administration.
15. Wright, M.: The improvement of patient care; a study at Harper Hospital, New York, 1954, G. P. Putnam's Sons.
16. Hospital Administrative Services: Six-month national comparison for period ending June 30, 1973, Chicago, 1973, American Hospital Association.
17. Hansen, W.: Documentation valuable, Oregon Hospitals **XX**(12):3, 1974.
18. Commission for Administrative Services in Hospitals (CASH), Santa Ana, Calif.
19. O'Malley, C.: Application of systems engineering in nursing, Am. J. Nurs. **69**(10):2155-2160, 1969.
20. Job analysis, Washington, D.C., 1973, U.S. Civil Service Commission, Bureau of Intergovernmental Personnel Programs, BIPP 152-32, p. 3.
21. Barlow, M. L.: The UCLA allied health professions (USOE grant no. 8-0627), Los Angeles, 1968-1972, University of California.
22. Wood, L. A., editor: Nursing skills for allied health services, Philadelphia, 1972, W. B. Saunders Co.
23. Dunn, J., and Stephen, S. E.: Management of personnel, New York, 1972, McGraw-Hill Book Co., p. 290.
24. Pigors, P., and Myers, C.: Personnel administration, ed. 7, New York, 1973, McGraw-Hill Book Co., p. 248.
25. 1-2-3 Resuscitation, Am. J. Nurs. **73**(6):1010-1011, 1973.
26. Bennett, A.: Methods improvements in hospitals, Philadelphia, 1964, J. B. Lippincott Co., pp. 97-98.
27. Cuica, R.: Over the years with the nursing care plan, Nurs. Outlook **20**(11):706-711, 1972.
28. Kramer, M.: Standard 4/nursing care plans ... power to the patient, J. Nurs. Admin. **11**(5):29-34, 1972.
29. Cornell, S., and Carrick, A.: Computerized schedules and care plans, Nurs. Outlook **21**(12):782, 1973.
30. Little, D., and Carnevali, D.: Nursing care planning, Philadelphia, 1969, J. B. Lippincott Co., pp. 66-97.
31. New, P., and associates: Nursing service and patient care; a staffing experiment, Kansas City, 1959, Community Studies no. 119, p. 77.
32. Bonney, V., and Rothberg, J.: Nursing diagnosis and therapy, New York, 1963, National League for Nursing.
33. Gebbie, K., and Lavin, M.: Classifying nursing diagnoses, Am. J. Nurs. **74**(2):250-253, 1974.
34. Roy, Sr. C. A.: Diagnostic classification system for nursing, Nurs. Outlook **23**(2):90-91, 1975.
35. Kraegel, J., and associates: A system of patient care based on patient needs, Nurs. Outlook **20**(4):257-264, 1972.
36. Germaine, A.: The nurse, the patient and Friesen, Supervisor Nurse **2**(3):27-32, 1971.
37. Downs, R.: Nursing in a Friesen hospital, Supervisor Nurse **2**(3):39-43, 1971.
38. Abdellah, F., and Strachan, E.: Progressive patient care, Am. J. Nurs. **59**(5):649-655, 1959.
39. Brown, E. L.: Nursing reconsidered; a study of change. Part II. Philadelphia, 1971, J. B. Lippincott Co., p. 268.

CHAPTER 9
CONTROLLING

Controlling the enterprise is an essential part of administration; indeed, it is difficult to envision a more precarious situation than one where it is not known whether the operation is satisfactory or economical, the workers are performing appropriately, and the objectives are being achieved. Moreover, there are gradations of achievement (or lack of it) that make evaluation more difficult and the need for control more imperative.

Control has come relatively later to the hospital setting than it has elsewhere in the community, because hospitals are less competitive organizations (the public has little choice about using their services) and are cloaked in considerable secrecy because of their specialized nature. Nonprofit and often philanthropic status, too, has contributed to lack of internal control.

The expanding use of control devices in hospitals and a control mentality are being strengthened by growing consumer sophistication, government involvement in controlling sites in which it allocates monies, and rate control commissions, as well as growing professional sophistication of physicians, nurses, and others involved in the hospital enterprise. Consumer, governmental, and professional intervention in effective operation of the enterprise is intensified by the astronomical growth and complexity of modern society, its knowledge, and its institutions. This growth and complexity obscure observations that were once more apparent and demand that control of the enterprise be as clear, simple, and pertinent as possible, so that control devices will be effective in assessing essentials and able to penetrate the complexity surrounding modern hospitals and nursing.

Control, then, is the sum of the findings of the means in use to determine whether the goal is being achieved. It includes the disposition of such findings by consequent changes or corrections. Evaluation is an indispensable ingredient of control, because it is the means of collecting data or findings. Control is an indispensable ingredient of accountability, the cornerstone of management.

Newman[1] speaks of three ingredients of control: placing standards at strategic spots, checking and reporting on performance, and making consequent corrections. Stevens[2] corroborates the essentiality of these three ingredients. The heart of the control process consists of known, appropriate standards observable in the workers and the quality of their performance or finished work, which either verify or isolate portions that require correction.

Donabedian[3] identified three ways of looking at evaluation for control purposes: (1) structure, or the management process and devices that govern the operation and practice of the enterprise, (2) process, or the way in which the operation is unfolded, set in motion, and completed, and (3) outcome, that is, the state or condition of that to which the work was directed, as for example patients after they have received our ministrations and services. These form the bases for continuing efforts toward controlling.

Structure as the means of controlling the enterprise is the oldest and most widely used. We shall look at its components in use as we consider the relationship of control to other parts of the administrative process.

Process as a base of control has been in fairly wide use also; wherever we have been evaluating nursing care while it is in progress, by comparison with standards, procedures, or policies, we have been employing this device.

Outcome as a base for evaluating remains the most obscure for nursing practice, because it requires a view of the finished product in order to demonstrate the effectiveness of the care given. Our finished product is patients at discharge. We must explore and examine our expectations of their state at that point sufficiently to know specifically what the outcomes for patients are. Work to date has turned up few elements of the discharged patient's status to give us concrete data on which to judge. The common elements so far have been the state of locomotion as ambulatory, lack of fever, freedom from pain (which is often irrelevant because the trend to early discharge makes the presence of discomfort, if not actual pain, likely at discharge), and the degree of knowledge possessed by patients. Because we are still flagrantly defective in discharge planning, including instruction, this aspect of outcome almost universally needs correction. Admitting our lack of meaningful outcome criteria for evaluation and control is not to rule out the use of this base, but to point out the intensive work it yet requires. Also in regard to outcome as a base, there exist the fear and acknowledgement that patients may get better in spite of, not because of, our ministrations, sometimes leaving a potentially large margin for error to be excluded in appraisal based on outcome.

Taylor[4] describes the use of outcome status during the time the patient was cared for as opposed to time of discharge. It seems to be a corollary to the process audit whereby specific nursing care is evaluated, but it insists on outcome as the goal of the appraisal. She illustrates her point with reference to indwelling catheter care in which good condition of the urine determines the quality of the care, rather than a review and check of the necessary steps in the care to achieve this satisfactory state of urine after the indwelling catheter procedure. Her position regarding these outcomes is the assumption that because the goal has been achieved, either a problem did not occur or nursing assessment and intervention were appropriate.

Hagen[5] supports the need for pursuance of an outcome base for evaluating and controlling practice by pointing out that in education there continues to be reliance on structure and process, to the exclusion of outcome, even though it is known that there is not a high relationship between structure and process and outcome evaluation. She cautions against repeating the mistakes of education.

TERMINOLOGY

The controlling function embraces many aspects, both old and new. Confusion in terminology frequently accompanies proliferation of ideas and devices about a subject, and controlling is no exception. Peer review, quality assurance or control, and nursing audit are among terms used commonly and often interchangeably. Precision in terminology helps clarify this part of the administrative process as the control function receives increasing attention.

Peer review is the evaluation of a worker by peers in the scalar process, as opposed to evaluation by a superior. When applied to nursing care in general, it refers to evaluation of that nursing care by nurses, not by physicians, hospital administrators, or the public. For example, PSRO—the federal legislation requiring physicians to monitor medical care and bed utilization—applies to physicians only. That it should be extended to include nursing and other kinds of health care may be desirable, but it is not part of the legislation at this point. In mid-1974 a contract was awarded to the American Nurses' Association by the Health Services Administration of the department of Health, Education, and Welfare, to develop criteria for measurement of the quality of nursing care and to find ways in which nurses can participate in PSRO.[6] So in fact peer review can describe any and all particular programs that monitor the quality of nursing care so long as nurses are doing the evaluating and controlling of such programs.

Likewise, quality assurance or control refers to all programs or activities designed to evaluate and control the quality of the nursing care being given in a particular institution. The nursing audit is a form of quality assurance for nursing that embraces all such evaluating activities. A program involving regular, systematized, and routinized inspections of the nursing care of a particular patient, though called quality assurance, is only a part of it. The danger lies in the use of generic terms for a particular application of controlling, because they are not sufficiently definitive.

NEED FOR STANDARDS

Standards are the most important element of control, because without them there can be only diffuse or partial observation and correction. As noted, there is growing attention to standards of nursing care in directing the work of the enterprise. They are no less important in controlling; indeed, they serve the same purpose—clarity.

In Chapter 2 we remarked on the growth of standards for clinical entities deriving from nursing audit systems where the instructions to data retrievers and reviewers became standards for charting and in turn standards for performance. The outline below is an example of this growing body of clinical entity standards for patients with cerebrovascular accidents.

LONG BEACH COMMUNITY HOSPITAL
NURSING AUDIT CRITERIA*
Patients with a diagnosis of
cerebrovascular accident (C.V.A.)

Nursing observations should be documented relative to:
1. Level of consciousness
    a. Reaction to stimuli, verbal or painful
2. Pupillary state

*From Benedikter, H.: The nursing audit—a necessity; how shall it be done? New York, © 1973, National League for Nursing, pp.7-8.

3. Movement
    a. Description of paralysis or limitation
    b. Therapy given (range of motion)—use of foot boards, etc.
    c. Tolerance of activity
4. Mental state and supportive or protective measures including restraints
5. Speech
    a. If aphasia present, describe
    b. Ability to communicate by speech or writing
6. Incontinence and bowel function
7. Skin
    a. Color and condition
    b. Description of edema, if present
    c. Description of pressure areas and treatment
    d. Preventative measures
        (1) Positioning
        (2) Skin care
        (3) Use of protective devices, heel protectors, decubicare pad, etc.
8. Oral hygiene
9. Nourishment
    a. Type and amount taken; tolerance
    b. Ability to swallow
10. Respiration
    a. Description of distress, if present, and how relieved (O_2, suctioning, medication)
11. Pulse
    a. Quality and rate
12. Pain
    a. Type and location
    b. How relieved
13. Progression of signs and symptoms

There are three areas that might be added to the outline: psychological response of the patient (and family) to the condition; the patient's response to physical and occupational therapy, if and as they are brought into the medical regimen; and the discharge plan, including specific instructions to the patient and family, as well as a referral site if used.

Another example of audit criteria data as directional guidelines, in addition to their primary audit purpose, applies to the care of patients with cerebrovascular accidents (see Fig. 11). It demonstrates outcome standards in terms of discharge status and the possible complications, with anticipated critical management, that might develop. These data could be converted to more specific guidelines or even suffice as they are for standards of care for that type of clinical condition. Psychological responses would need to be added to the list of possible additional complications (for example, depression).

The above illustrations of standards represent current effort to expand the use of standards and the possibility for such use or conversion to standards when they arise secondarily, that is, out of the audit procedure. This secondary aspect may provide more precision as well as stimulus to standard setting, because in meeting the needs of the audit procedure an important standard-generating system is found. In short, by preparing directional and auditing criteria simultaneously, each one is likely to enrich the other.

In addition to current efforts to establish clinical standards, there are existing ones available: procedure and policy manuals and written nursing instructions found in most nursing services, as well as textbooks and journals, abound in standards in varying degrees of formulation. Not to be discounted as existing standards is the expertise of all practicing nurses.

Although discharge planning including instruction has been well known and within the range of comprehensive nursing for at least 20 years, as late as 1973 it was found necessary to pass a resolution at the ANA biennial convention to support this part of nursing practice. (The resolution also includes admission planning.) This action would seem to demonstrate our collective failure to establish and use standards more widely and particularly to activate this aspect of comprehensive care. The point here is not to note failure in a pejorative sense, but in a constructive way. Recognition of failure demonstrates the formidability of achieving what has not been accomplished in 20 years even though the knowledge was available, not to mention achieving implementation of new knowledge. We have failed to convert such knowledge to understandable, observable, measurable standards of nursing practice. The problem is one of getting a sufficient number of nurses internalizing comprehensive nursing care to make the significant difference in achieving such care generally.

RELATIONSHIP OF CONTROLLING TO OTHER PARTS OF THE ADMINISTRATIVE PROCESS

Controlling pervades all elements of the administrative process. We have noted the necessity of considering evaluation early in the formation of plans. One cannot control the enterprise if it is not clear at the outset what the goal is and the specific ways of implementing and achieving it. The control factor is further enhanced by the specificity of management by objectives, with its internal accounting system between superior and subordinate for the attainment of a specific piece of work in a specific period of time.

Organization of the enterprise builds control into the structure with the line function of accountability. Staff must have control of that for which they are accountable. They will not know whether the work is effective unless the accountability factor is fully operative. Clear-cut job descriptions make accountability, and hence control, easier to achieve, as does respect for the organizational principles of unity of command and span of supervision, because they both enhance personal accountability for maintenance and implementation of standards. Control is needed especially in decentralized organizations, where responsibility is more widely spread, in order to ensure the appropriate accountability.

Management by exception is an application of the control function. Where managers are apprised of only the exceptions, or those points at which the organization is not functioning appropriately, they can exercise control at those points.

Staffing has multiple control points. Clear-cut standards for recruitment, selection, placement, training, and evaluation of personnel provide built-in and ongoing control of staff achievement of the purpose of the nursing service. Contracts are controlling devices in that they are specific statements of conditions and procedures governing and binding both the employer and employee. Especially contributory to control are those contracts that guarantee professional performance committees through which all nurses participate in control of nursing practice.

Control is inherent in the growing efforts to quantify nursing care by patient classification, conservation of nurse time, statistical data collection, and the consequent interrelationships. Control is also found in the systemic view of staffing (see Fig. 5), where personnel in position and supported by interlocking parts engage with equipment, supplies, and the patients to move them to a state of optimum health.

Directing and controlling have the closest relationship: directing guides, counsels, coaches, and leads personnel in implementing standards of nursing care, while controlling determines the degree of success of the managers in such endeavors. The same standards are operable. If they are not, then there is need for review, restatement, or reinforcement of standards, assuming that they have been selected, prepared, and made known to the staff. An illustration of the strategic points for the introduction of standards can be found in the types of conditions chosen for formation and application of standards where the ten most common clinical entities in each of the clinical services are given precedence. Medical records departments have such data on hand.

Directing and controlling are paramount factors in supervision and are closely related to supervision. One cannot separate the direction and control exerted by any manager at any level from the supervisory process likewise engaged in by a manager. Directing, controlling, and supervising are not only collaborative and coordinating, but are essentially integrated into each other operatively.

Because nursing care plans are directional and controlling in the ministration of direct nursing care, the significant attention they receive as a controlling device by Nicholls[7] should be noted. She speaks of three parts of a controlling system at work in giving direct nursing care: standards found in the nursing care plan, feedback on the interaction of standards on patients' needs, and the consequent action necessary to keep standards serving patients' objectives and needs.

Coordination, reporting, and budgeting also have strong controlling ingredients.

Follett,[8] in considering the psychology of control, refers to the need to always view the total situation in order to see all the factors and their interrelationships. It is in the integration of the parts that she sees control emerge. She illustrates her position by pointing to the work of Elton Mayo, the anthropologist Malinowski, and the philosopher Whitehead. The interrelationships of control to other parts of the administrative process provide another illustration of her notion of the necessity to view the total situation and its interrelating parts if we are to control them. The plan for the implementation of an audit and standards of care system within the management by objectives structure (see Chapter 2) illustrates the use of consideration of the whole and interrelating parts in control. This plan combines two parallel considerations: the audit and standards of care in relationship to each other so that the whole standards for comprehensive nursing care and the proof of their use are mutually supportive, contributory, congruent, and cohesive.

Drucker [p. 496][9] says that controls cannot be objective, because the observer and the event in a social situation such as a business enterprise change each other. For him, the very act of observing alters the observer and the situation. The point is suggestive of Follett's total situation and relationships. It is an unsettling point of view, but one that is borne out by experience in a supervisory capacity. The fact is that the observer can and may change his or her perceptions while in the act of observing. For example, the more one observes carefully the parent-child relationship in the hospital situation, the more inclined one becomes to acknowledge the importance and therapeutic effect of such a relationship and in turn take steps to multiply opportunities for furthering the relationship.

CONTROLLING MECHANISMS
Accreditation procedures

There have long been licensure laws in each state that guarantee minimum standards of performance to the public and accrediting bodies that evaluate institutions on higher standards than do state licensing boards. Both provide controls for hospitals and their departments. The main agency for the evaluation of hospitals is the Joint Commission for Accreditation of Hospitals (JCAH), which was founded in 1951 with the collaboration of the American Medical Association, the American Hospital Association, the American College of Physicians, and the Canadian Medical Association. Its Board of Directors includes representatives from the American College of Surgeons, American College of Physicians, American Medical Association, and American Hospital Association. Conspicuously absent is the American Nurses' Association, though it is used consultatively in some aspects of the work. Schlicke[10] suggests the extension of representation on the governing board of the JCAH to the public, nursing and other health professions, and perhaps government. This accrediting body is voluntary: hospitals ask and pay a fee for inspection and certification if the inspection warrants it. Its consultative aspect is an important secondary contribution to hospitals. It accredits residential and extended-care facilities, nursing homes, and facilities for the mentally retarded and psychiatric care.

Criteria for evaluation of a nursing service during a hospital accreditation visit fall in two categories: examination of nursing care, which will be considered under audit procedures, and an appropriate administrative structure consisting of an organized staff; qualified director and assistants; sufficient number of RNs to give nursing care requiring specialized skills, to plan and evaluate nursing care, and to supervise the other personnel; proper distribution of staff, preplanned and periodically evaluated; a current written organizational plan; nursing service goals; cooperatively developed nursing care and administrative policies and procedures; nursing care plan for each patient; significant, accurate, and concise nursing records and reports; monthly staff meetings; formal programs of training and education; and professional reference material available.*

It is interesting to note that the first criterion, calling for an organized staff, may suggest that staff is responsible for its collective professional performance and seems compatible, if not identical, with the efforts of state nurses' associations to get professional performance committees established by their representation of nurses in contractual arrangements with individual hospitals.

Consultants

In addition to the consultant role of the JCAH, which contributes to the controlling function of hospitals, there are other consultants from different sources who are available and ready to assist. Perhaps the most common are the nonprofit organizations cooperating with or actually accountable to state hospital associations, Blue Cross organizations, and the like, where consultants serve hospitals and their departments in an advisory way, thus improving both the operation itself and the control of such operations, We noted the work of the Commission of Administrative Services (CASH) in hospitals at work in California and Battelle Northwest Systems Programs for Hospitals serving the northwestern states. There are also individual and private consultants of various kinds, as well as a growing body of commercial consultants who afford excellent counseling service preceding or accompanying use of their products by the institution.

Evaluation devices

In addition to accrediting agencies, there is an array of outside materials available to a nursing service, against which it can

---
*From Nursing Audit Workshop, Chicago, 1974, Joint Commission on Accreditation of Hospitals, pp. ST/12-ST/16.

measure its performance in its effort to control the organization or keep it operating in appropriate directions. Some of these devices are directed to the nursing care itself, to the nursing department, or to both in combination. Sometimes these devices are set up in such a way that the evaluation can be recorded in the device itself as the evaluation proceeds. Frequently they are accompanied by arithmetical weighting, which permits numerical scoring. They abound in potential strategic points for standard setting.

One device that provides an appraisal guide for the quality of the nursing care itself is the Quality Patient Care Scale [Wandelt and Ager[11]]. It is a companion piece to the Slater Nursing Competencies Rating Scale (see p. 121). This scale is set up similarly under the headings of psychosocial, individual, group, physical, general communication, and professional implications; and there are four to six example cues under each of 68 items in the Quality Patient Care Scale. For example, the cue indicating the quality of care and illustrating consideration of the patient as a family member consists of encouraging the family to take part in the patient's care. In the Slater Scale the cue to the competency of the individual nurse is encouragement of the family to engage in the patient's care. There is considerable reinforcement as the quality of care and the competency of nurses are observed. Moreover, the generous cue lists provide excellent examples from which a nursing staff can prepare larger numbers of cues with which to examine the quality of the care and also individual nursing competencies. There are guidelines for using the Quality Patient Care Scale. A 2-hour observation period is suggested for a patient or group of patients, whereas the Slater Competencies Rating Scale is used retroactively or by observation. The scales are not used simultaneously, because it is made clear to all staff that there is no identification of individual behaviors in the Quality Patient Care Scale.

An early appraisal guide for a nursing service [Mullane[12]] consists of eight criteria arranged in order of importance as viewed by experts in hospital and nursing service administration. They consist of organization, planning, appraisal of service, conservation of energy and material, reporting, staff, purpose, and budget. Each criterion except staff is broken down into six to ten items. Staff contains six parts, each of which contains four to nine items. The numerical accompaniment is simple, thus making use of the instrument easier.

Another appraisal guide for a nursing service[13] organizes the appraisal content around ten criteria in which the department of nursing service has definitive statements of philosophy and objectives; has an established plan of organization consistent with objectives and hospital organization; develops and implements written administrative policies, personnel policies, a program for provision of nursing care, a budget, and a system of records and reports; estimates and controls its equipment, supplies, and facilities; participates in in-service education; and maintains an appraisal system to evaluate achievement of objectives. Each criterion is elaborated in considerable detail, facilitating its use by self-appraisers.

Thomas[14] gives an exciting account of the involvement of a nursing service working in nine committees, each of which considered one of the above criteria. Besides healthy intercommunication among all levels of nursing personnel, there was investigation of such subjects as power-failure readiness, criteria for use of facilities by outside agencies, adequacy of facilities, equipment and supplies, line-staff application in units, the diversity found in application of procedures and policies, and the writing and review of policies. It is a firsthand account of a nursing staff "coming alive" in the process of this intensive analysis of its service in light of the nine criteria listed in the above guide.

Another self-evaluation guide[15] is set up around an interesting arrangement: realization of illness, patient appraisal, planned care (patient-oriented care and services and personnel); execution of care, restoration of health, extension of care, or terminal illness. There are copious entries under each broad title above that inform the staff of possible uses of this evaluation device. For example, under execution of care, preventive aspects, there are eleven such informative entries, such as whether the patient is made responsible and accountable for maximum self-help and whether he or she is helped to make proper selection when buying or renting equipment. Interspersed throughout the guide are administrative devices having direct bearing on nursing care, for instance, the topic of rounds. There are also less common administrative elements of nursing often regarded as outside nursing, such as financial charges that in fact do have at least an indirect bearing on nursing care, because financial matters though unspoken are often uppermost in the minds of patients. As with earlier evaluation devices, the organization of material as well as the items provide fresh insights into comprehensive nursing care.

An additional evaluating device is a framework developed into a master criteria list containing the following broad entries: the plan of nursing care is formulated, the physical needs of the patient are attended to, the nonphysical needs (psychological, emotional, mental, social, spiritual) of the patient are attended to, achievement of nursing care objectives is evaluated, unit procedures are followed for the protection of all patients, and the delivery of nursing care is facilitated by administrative and mangerial services. The latter two have strong administrative implications. There are 47 pages of excellent, detailed elaboration of these broad categories, affording any nursing staff a splendid device with which to gauge comprehensiveness and efficiency of nursing care [Jelinik and associates[16]].

The American Nurses' Association nursing practice standards, developed in the 1970s, offer an excellent evaluating system because they cover medical-surgical care, gerontological material, child health, psychiatric-mental health, and community health nursing practice.[17] Though these standards for nursing practice are new, both the American Nurses' Association and the National League for Nursing have been developing and revising such standards for some years.

Rounds

Rounds are probably the oldest controlling device in existence and a very important one. They have traditionally consisted of excursions into patient areas for the purpose of appraising the quality of nursing care being given, the performance of those providing such care, and the adequacy of supplies, equipment, and other supports in use. The directness and immediacy of rounds supply firsthand contact with the workers, cutting through administrative layers and providing the indispensable element of personal contact. This is a pertinent point for administrators in our complex health care institutions, where there is 24-hour responsibility.

Nursing rounds are a fundamental device because they permit and encourage the use of other devices whereby the one(s) making the rounds, fortified by such a formalized range of observations, uses them in the course of rounds; and they afford direct and immediate appraisal opportunities. Interception may occur if the person making rounds institutes possible corrective action, but at the observational level they are few.

Rounds are usually better when they are regularized but not scheduled precisely, allowing an opportunity to see areas at various times and in natural conditions. One presupposes that appropriate job descriptions and knowledge of them have been provided to the workers being observed. Donovan[18] notes the need for defined standards to provide a base for tangible observations and evidence. There should not be undue intrusion on the work being performed, though the one making rounds should talk to patients and personnel in order to achieve the purpose of the rounds. Corrective action, unless life threatening, should not be taken until the appropriate person can be apprised of findings that require investigation or correction. Sufficient structure is necessary to achieve the particular purpose of the rounds, but not so much that rigidity prevents agility in responding to directions and findings as they occur. Mental or written records are necessary in purposeful rounds. The manager may or may not be accompanied by the one responsible for the particular unit or department being visited, though that person should always be aware of rounds in progress and should be greeted, if not given a summary statement in general or particular terms. This is a form of courtesy to the person with jurisdictional responsibility for the area visited. Frequency is contingent on many variables. Grand rounds are more formal, less frequent, and inclusive of larger numbers of participants.

There is an inherent educational aspect to rounds, because there are usually occasions for the one making rounds to enter into the work being done at the site, such as helping a worker to turn or lift a patient. Such occasions are rich in opportunities to guide, direct, and counsel personnel in the actual conduct of the nursing care. They provide a partial role model too. Moreover, such opportunities bring manager and worker into collaboration, which contributes to the motivation of both in doing their respective parts in achieving nursing goals.

A long-standing variation of nursing rounds is that of visiting all patients (or more usually, selected critically ill patients or those with specific problems) in conjunction with the change of shift report. The patient is often naturally a part of such rounds. These are occasionally called interval or walking rounds. They seem, however, to be the traditional patient visits accompanying the change of shift report and responsibility. They reinforce the prime value of rounds: direct observation, in this case simultaneous direct observation of personnel from two adjacent shifts.

Physician-nurse rounds are another long-standing control device for seeing that the medical plan and regime are being satisfactorily implemented. The three-way meeting of the patient, physician, and nurse is indispensable to quality patient care, because it provides the opportunity for that coherence necessary to success in meeting patient needs. The need for this essential contact between physicians and nurses, whether inclusive of the patient and whether mobile or stationary, is pointed out by Mauksch,[19] who says that genuine continuity of care needs and demands open and deep communication between physicians and nurses. Sheps and Bachar,[20] in speaking of the interdependence of the physician and nurse, illustrate the point by use of a continuum: one end represents work that only a physician can perform, and the other end represents work that can be done by nurses' aides or volunteers, who possess no professional training. In the middle is that fluctuating body of work, mainly procedures and judgments, that can be performed by either the physician or nurse. Christman[21] observes the lost opportunities to remove risks to patients and to give excellent care because of misunderstandings arising from the incidental interaction and communication between physicians and nurses.

It is difficult to say why these rounds have fallen into disuse. The fast pace of the hospital, medicine, and nursing; the altering and ambivalent physician-nurse relationship; the habit of assuming operational or procedural needs as the only justification for nurse accompaniment; and the predominance of short- over long-range planning in medical and health care have probably all contributed to such disuse. Fragmentation, isolation, and working with only partial information have resulted from this disuse. There is no exchange so productive of good patient care as this three-way communication between patient, physician, and nurse, and we should work indefatigably to reinstate it. Moreover, it might reduce the growing need to interview patients, with its attendant repetitive and intrusive aspects, by synchronizing the getting and giving of information.

Interdepartmental rounds are another common type. These include regularly scheduled rounds to specific areas of the hospital by the hospital administrator and varying combinations of department heads, including those from personnel, finance, and purchasing. They have the advantage of all participants seeing the same situations or events simultaneously, so that observations and discussions have a common, pertinent, and objective base. Variations of interdepartmental rounds have managers other than the top ones make rounds with their interdepartmental counterparts for coordinating purposes. An interesting innovative addition to these traditional administrative rounds is that one of the persons making rounds eats an identical meal with a patient on a scheduled basis. Findings from such rounds are put in memorandum form, signed by the administrator, and sent to the appropriate department head, who then responds on the memo within a certain number of days. Because the memos are filed over a period of time, they may show patterns that require corrective action. These rounds have been extended to include evening and night shifts and outside areas and grounds. One can see the importance and extent of patient input in this system [Smith[22]].

Reports

Reports are related to direct observation of the work and the workers in order to control the quality of productivity of the enterprise. Change of shift, patient condition, untoward incident and accident, regular (weekly, monthly, annual, or progress), statistical (clinical analyses, nursing hours, opinion polls, regulatory or accrediting agency), and many other reports constitute ongoing control mechanisms for the enterprise. There are so many means of collecting data in our machine-oriented culture that we must exercise economy in this regard, not only for the well-being of the enterprise but of the manager. Drucker [p. 499][9] cautions on this point by asking what can be the smallest number of reports and statistics necessary to provide a reasonably dependable portrayal of the situation for controlling the enterprise.

As well as the internal reports, there is an external supply equally beneficial in appraising and controlling the quality of service in a given enterprise. These include the customary sources of pertinent data: professional associations and journals, related commercial or nonprofit organizations such as consultants, and suppliers. There are the reports of various commissions and committees at the local, state, and national levels, for example, the Report of the National Commission on Health Manpower. The recommendations of such an important and prestigious commission can well be used for informing and comparing the enterprise in efforts to control it. This Report advises attention to monitoring mechanisms of the quality of care being provided, which relates directly to control, and to gaps in communicating, coordinating, and controlling among both practitioners and institutions that affect costs, distribution, and quality of services. These recommendations are only now receiving considerable attention, though they were made in 1967.

Also related to external reports, and to an increasing degree to hospital practice, the provision of medical and hospital controls by PSRO and the Quality Assurance Program of the American Hospital Association may eventually extend to nursing and other aspects of patient care in hospitals. In convention in 1974, the American Nurses' Association passed a resolution supporting the inclusion of nursing in PSRO legislation. Likewise, the National League for Nursing praised the PSRO legislation and called for extension of quality review to all health care services.

We have noted a similar recommendation from the Academy of Nursing and the commissioned efforts of the American Nurses' Association to develop evaluation criteria and ways of participating in PSRO. Such resolutions, recommendations, and actions support nursing efforts to monitor and control its own practice and health care, of which nursing is a part.

Systematic routinized inspection programs

A fairly common practice has arisen in monitoring the care being given to hospitalized patients. The procedure is usually called a quality assurance program, though occasionally it is called a nursing audit procedure. These programs are precise combinations of rounds, supervision, and sometimes standards. Checklist forms for such a procedure follow a similar format covering various aspects of patient care, such as the cleanliness and storage of urinals, reflection of patient teaching and discharge planning in the nursing care plan, accessibility of fresh water, and safety of appliances and equipment, as well as various questions about patients' charts and the nursing unit. In some cases, all professional nurses engage in such patient inspections; in others, only selected nurses do the patient inspections. Frequently there is numerical scoring of the data.

Ramey[23] has developed a comprehensive checklist for making such patient care evaluations. It is divided into three sections: nursing process, administration, and in-service education. The nursing process consists of eleven questions under assessment and nine under planning; six sections under intervention, consisting of interpersonal, technical skills, environmental control, collaboration with other professionals, referrals, and record keeping, each containing five to twelve questions; and six questions under evaluation. Administration consists of six questions under objectives for the unit, nine under team nursing, and six under environmental control. In-service education consists of four questions under programs based on objectives, four under orientation plan for the unit, and five under utilization of reference material and resource persons. Though it has a common base with other such devices, Ramey's checklist is a sophisticated device for on-site evaluation of individual patients' care. It presupposes mastery by the staff of philosophy and objectives of nursing services, the nursing process, and comprehensive nursing care.

A variation of this device for evaluating nursing care is described by Pardee and associates.[24] It is confined essentially to patients and their charts and nursing care plans and may be used for an individual patient or all the patients in a unit. It consists of two to nine items each under sustenal, remedial, restorative, and preventive care. The results of such evaluations are used in many imaginative ways besides direct improvement of nursing care, such as for in-service education needs, determining effects of experimental change, providing evidence for staffing and budgetary changes, and strengthening of the nursing history.

Nursing audit

With the exception of supervision, which includes so many control components, there is no more compelling control device than the nursing audit. Essentially, a nursing audit is the examination of a patient's record to determine the degree to which nursing care was satisfactory according to prescribed standards and to collect data as a base for corrective action. The considerable attention it is receiving is merited. Extensive national work has been done and continues in this area by the National League for Nursing and the JCAH. The cause for the nursing audit may have been set back, however, by the failure of these two powerful organizations to collaborate in this endeavor. An excellent precedent for such collaboration exists in the long-standing joint educational efforts of the National League for Nursing and the American Hospital Association, of which approximately 10,000 nurse managers availed themselves. The American Hospital Association is a parent organization of the JCAH and holds seven of the twenty seats on its governing board. One can only speculate about impetus to potential collaboration if the American Nurses' Association were represented on this governing board. Perhaps an important coordinating and unifying opportunity was lost through failure to collaborate on a critical and timely project.

The great impetus currently given to the nursing audit has historical antecedence. The precision and refinement in current systems have evolved from the work of many in efforts to develop and use this important mechanism. The pioneer work of Esther Pfab in the Chicago area is quoted copiously by Deeken.[25] Her guide contains a list of 36 coded factors for use in the nursing audit. These coded factors facilitated the examination of charts and may well be the forerunner of auditing procedures in which data are retrieved by nonnurses from codified instructions. This guide also includes opinion polls of discharged patients as followup work on the chart audit, even to the use of such polls as a means of determining the effectiveness of the audit committee.

There has been some attempt to use the audit procedure on charts of current patients, with a view to upgrading the quality of care while the patient is in the hospital [Donovan[26] and Rubin and associates[27]]. The retrospective audit is, however, in greater conformance with the definitive view of the audit.

Essential characteristics. The Joint Commission on Accreditation of Hospitals describes six essential steps in a nursing audit program: (1) written standards of care against which to evaluate nursing care, (2) evidence that actual practice was measured against such standards, showing a percent conformance rate, (3) examination and analysis of findings, (4) evidence of corrective action being taken, (5) evidence of effectiveness of corrective action, and (6) appropriate reporting of the audit program.[10]

The three major audit programs have been developed by Phaneuf,[28] Benedikter,[29] and the JCAH.[10]

Phaneuf audit. The Phaneuf audit grows out of long experience and pioneering work with the nursing audit[30, 31] and is based on the functions of the nurse as described by Lesnick and Anderson.[32] One of these functions is dependent and six are independent. They consist of application and execution of physicians' legal orders; observation of symptoms and reaction; supervision of patient; supervision of others (except physicians) who contribute to the care of patients; reporting and recording; application and execution of nursing procedures and techniques; and promotion of physical and emotional health by direction and teaching. There are 50 items in these seven categories. For example, under supervision of patient there are seven such items, one of which is continuing assessment of patients' condition and capacity. There is provision for numerical scoring. This system is carried out by a representative professional nurse group, except for a cover sheet consisting of 22 items completed by a trained clerk. The Phaneuf system may be coordinated with the Slater Nursing Competencies Rating Scale for evaluating the performance of individual nurses and the Quality Patient Care Scale for evaluating the quality of nursing care. There are advantages to using a philosophically cohesive set of devices to measure quality of care, personnel performance on site, and retrospective nursing care.

Phaneuf sees some general nursing weaknesses arising from systematic auditing become easier to correct or improve because they have been illustrated so graphically. She mentions the need to completely carry out nursing responsibility before involving other departments or physicians. For example, the failure of physicians to tell nurses about their medical plans for patients was corrected when

NURSING I. OUTCOME AUDIT CRITERIA AND INSTRUCTIONS

AUDIT TOPIC: CEREBRAL VASCULAR ACCIDENTS
COMMITTEE: NURSING AUDIT
DATE: 11-5-73

	A. ELEMENTS	B. STD. 100% 0%	C. EXCEPTIONS	D. SPECIAL INSTRUCTIONS	
	HEALTH				
1	1. Skin in good condition	X	None	Discharge note re: skin condition, no	1
2				decubiti or reddened area noted.	2
3					3
4	**ACTIVITY** 2. Ability to ambulate	X	1. Intractable physical impairment on admission or ex-	Ambulation, ability to transfer to wheelchair	4
5			tention of CVA, cardiac or other secondary complication.	P.T. or Nurses Notes.	5
6	**KNOWLEDGE**		2. Transferred to Rehabilitation Skilled Nursing Facil.		6
7	3. Ability to perform activities of daily living	X	Same as above.	Documentation of skill in: feeding self,	7
8				bowel and bladder training, bath and dress,	8
9				orientation, ability to communicate.	9
10			**CRITICAL MANAGEMENT/REPORTING**		10
11	4. Extension of CVA	X	MD notified within 30 min. of degree of neuro. deficit.	Pupil non-reactive (PERLA change), flaccid	11
12				paralysis from spasticity. Change in level	12
13				of consciousness.	13
14	5. Pneumonia	X	1. Temp. > 101 reported to MD.	Progress notes for rales, chest X-ray con-	14
15			2. Ambulate within 1st 24 hours.	firms pneumonia.	15
16			3. Turn q. 2 hrs. until turning independently		16
17					17
18	6. Urinary tract infection	X	1. Urine sent to lab for C/S.	Nurses notes for urine color, or evidence	18
19			2. Report frequency, pain and Temp. > 101.	of frequency and pain. Lab report of WBC's	19
20				in urine, and/or bacteria	20
21					21
22	7. Pressure sores (decubitus)	X	1. Turned q. 2 hrs.	Decubiti are reddened and open areas. Use	22
23			2. Protective devices used.	of protective devices (sheep skin, flotation	23
24				pads, etc.).	24
25					25
26	8. Fecal Impaction	X	1. Remove impaction within 12 hours.	Records indicate BM q. 3 days.	26
27			2. BM checked daily for normal pattern.		27
28			3. Intake < 3000 cc/24 hrs.		28
29					29

Copyright 1973, Joint Commission on Accreditation of Hospitals
JCAH Retrospective Patient Care Audit Worksheet I/Nursing/Criteria

Fig. 11. Nursing audit procedure for patients with cerebrovascular accident. (Courtesy Joint Commission on Accreditation of Hospitals, Chicago.)

nurses communicated their nursing assessments to physicians—a conciliatory way to solve the problem. Other weaknesses of which she speaks include absence of a nursing process structure (the carrying out of physicians' orders remains the most successful and complete part of nursing), absence of health histories, depersonalization of care, and need for greater attention to the clinical component of nursing.

She does see significant influences at work in audit programs, such as the emphasis being placed on the patient rather than the nurse and the requirement to make nursing judgments openly, on documented data, and by peers.

Benedikter audit. The Benedikter audit system is a process audit, that is, nursing as it was provided rather than an outcome audit, or condition of patient on discharge. It is strong on predetermined standards that must be generated internally by the staff rather than taken from other sources. Such internally generated standards are more easily internalized into general practice and have a strong directional aspect. Representative nursing committees carry out the audit procedure. The professional nurses assume the judgmental responsibility for seeing that the prescribed standards are met; the licensed practical (vocational) nurses evaluate medication administration and whether all of the physicians' orders were carried out; and the nurses' aide and ward clerk check the mechanical aspects of the chart. There are guidelines for executing these latter two responsibilities.

JCAH audit. The JCAH nursing audit procedure is essentially an outcome audit, though it provides for a process audit where it is indicated by a special problem area or weakness found in the course of the regular audit procedure. It features conservation of professional nurse time by having charts checked and retrieved by clerks (usually medical records department employees), on the basis of criteria worked up by nurses and organized on a form entitled Outcome Audit Criteria and Instructions (Fig. 11).

This form is essentially divided into two categories: outcome, or discharge status, including the headings of health, activity, and knowledge; and complications, including critical management of them. The nursing audit committee develops the description of the disease entity to be used by the data retrieval clerk within this framework. We noted the difficulties involved in using the outcome status, but it is useful in demonstrating an important and seemingly universal nursing weakness, patient instruction. The compilation of possible complications, with their critical management (and the discharge status to a lesser degree), requires an examination of nursing care and charting in the units. With moderate alteration and addition, such examination could constitute nursing care standards. The work of developing complications for large numbers of disease entities can be reduced by using what must be one of the oldest systems analyses, the systemic categorization of anatomy and physiology. The selection of complications in the management by objectives plan for introduction of a nursing audit system (see pp. 11-12) can take place within the framework lists compiled around this systemic categorization. In short, there is a finite number of complications and much potential for transference and overlap from clinical condition to clinical condition. The audit committee may select all or part of the discharge status and complications to be audited. A prescribed number of consecutive charts (not randomly selected) is used for the audit.

This system is very sophisticated and highly structured, though it lends itself to modification. It has the strength of being presented by the accrediting agency for hospital quality. The collateral efforts in other departments, such as medical records, is advantageous. Seldom has nursing had such knowledgeable collaboration with other departments.

• • •

Audit systems show the potential for measurability in nursing care. They demonstrate (as do other control mechanisms) the congruent, economical, and cyclical nature of the control process because, besides providing a measure, they demand greater consideration of that which they are measuring. This forced consideration generates refinement of the standards and of the nursing care they represent in a relational spiral directed to achieving the goals of the nursing department.

REFERENCES

1. Newman, W.: Administrative action, ed. 2, New York, 1963, Prentice-Hall, Inc., p. 420.
2. Stevens, B.: Analyses of trends in nursing care management, J. Nurs. Admin. 2(6):13, 1972.
3. Donabedian, A.: Some issues in evaluating the quality of nursing care, Journal of Public Health 59(10):18-33, 1969.
4. Taylor, J.: Measuring the outcomes of nursing care, Nurs. Clin. North Am 9(2):337-348, 1974.
5. Hagen, E.: Research on nurse staffing in hospitals, Washington, D.C., 1972, Public Health Service, U.S. Department of Health, Education, and Welfare, (NIH) 73-434, p. 133.
6. PSRO contract awarded to develop care criteria, The American Nurse 6(9);1, 1974.
7. Nicholls, M.: Quality control in patient care, Am. J. Nurs. 74(3):456-459, 1974.
8. Follett, M.: Dynamic administration. In Metcalf, H., and Urwick, L., editors: The collected papers of Mary Parker Follett, New York, 1940, Harper & Row, Publishers, pp. 187-194.
9. Drucker, P.: Management; tasks, responsibilities, practices, New York, 1974, Harper & Row, Publishers, pp. 496 and 499.
10. Schlicke, C.: American surgery's noblest experiment, Chicago, 1974, Nursing Audit Workshop, Joint Commission on Accreditation of Hospitals, pp. ST/10 and OV/23.
11. Wandelt, M., and Ager, J.: Quality patient care scale, Detroit, 1970, Wayne State University Press.
12. Mullane, M.: Self appraisal guide for hospital nursing services, Detroit, 1959, Michigan League for Nursing.
13. A self-evaluation guide for nursing services in hospital and related institutions, New York, 1967, National League for Nursing, code no. 20-1291.
14. Thomas, Sr. M.: Implementing the criteria for evaluating a hospital department of nursing, Nurs. Outlook 16(2):49-51, 1968.
15. Quest for quality; a self evaluation guide to patient care, New York, 1966, National League for Nursing, code no. 20-1212.
16. Jelinik, R., and associates: A methodology for monitoring quality of nursing care, Washington, D.C., 1974, Public Health Service, U.S. Department of Health, Education, and Welfare, (HRA) 74-25.
17. American Nurses' Association: Standards of nursing practice, The American Nurse 6(7):11-22, 1974.
18. Donovan, H.: Making rounds with a purpose, Nurs. Outlook 8:394, 1960.
19. Mauksch, H.: The organizational context of nursing practice. In Davis, F., editor: The nursing profession; five sociological essays, New York, 1966, John Wiley & Sons, Inc., p. 136.
20. Sheps, C., and Bachar, M.: Nursing and medicine; emerging patterns of practice, Am. J. Nurs. 64(9):108, 1964.
21. Christman, L.: Nurse-physician communications in the hospital, JAMA 194:151-156, 1965.
22. Smith, R.: Administrators make onsite tours, Hospitals 46:45-48, 1972.
23. Ramey, I.: Setting nursing standards and evaluating care, J. Nurs. Admin. 3(3):31-34, 1973.
24. Pardee, G., and associates: Patient care evaluation is every nurse's job, Am. J. Nurs. 71(10):1958-1960, 1971.
25. Deeken, Sr. M.: A guide for the nursing service audit, St. Louis, 1960, Catholic Hospital Association.
26. Donovan, H.: The personalized nursing audit, Supervisor Nurse 2(12):37-41, 1971.
27. Rubin, C., Rinaldi, L., and Dietz, R.: Nursing audit—nurses evaluating nursing, Am. J. Nurs. 72(5):916-921, 1972.
28. Phaneuf, M.: The nursing audit; profile for excellence, New York, 1972, Appleton-Century-Crofts, pp. 120-129.
29. Benedikter, H.: The nursing audit . . . a necessity; how shall it be done? New York, 1973, National League for Nursing, no. 20-1501.
30. Phaneuf, M.: The nursing audit—for evaluation of patient care, Nurs. Outlook 14(6):51-54, 1966.
31. Phaneuf, M.: The analysis of a nursing audit, Nurs. Outlook 16(1):57-60, 1968.
32. Lesnick, M., and Anderson, B.: Nursing practice and the law, ed. 2, Philadelphia, 1955, J. B. Lippincott Co., pp. 247-293.

CHAPTER 10

COORDINATING

The coordinating function of administration is essentially relational, serving to articulate and unite various parts so that nothing that contributes to the achievement of the goal is omitted. This function is facilitating, because it embraces all the other functions sufficiently to see that they are brought into play at the right time and right place so that appropriate resources are marshalled to achieve the purpose of the enterprise. The coordinating function is also synthesizing, because union of parts brings integration and harmony to the operation.

Coordination is a supportive function. In unifying activity and effort, it helps to preserve balance and function in the organization. It provides cues to the workers so that there will be harmony and deftness in articulating complemental and relative parts and coherence of the contribution of each member to the whole. Coordination is required in direct proportion to the size and complexity of the enterprise—the more far flung the contributing parts, the greater the need for coordination.

There is a communicating component to coordination: in order to unite, facilitate, and synthesize resources, information must be conveyed to, from, and among personnel. This implies a human relations component.

Georgopoulos and Mann[1] speak of four kinds of coordination: corrective, preventive, regulatory, and promotive. An example of corrective coordination is found in the introduction of a weekly patient assignment schedule to replace a daily one, in the interest of keeping workers with the same patients long enough to enhance and particularize their practice. Preventive coordination is seen where such a schedule would be introduced to ward off the short-term assignment in a rehabilitation institute. Regulatory coordination could be a policy of staffing one day heavier than others for the purpose of releasing personnel for in-service programs, committee work, and so forth. Promotive coordination is operative in scheduling a newly appointed patient representative to meet with unit staffs to review particular patient care, in order to reinforce the general presentation of the patient representative's work.

COORDINATION IN NURSING

Coordination has been a part of nursing for a long time, perhaps because of the omnipresence of nursing in health care institutions. The nursing staff has had to notify other departments that their services are required for particular patients and to see that such services are duly carried out. This coordinating function perhaps derives also from the seniority of the nurse, after the physician, on the health care team. While this coordinating function is not necessarily detrimental to nursing, it may serve to perpetuate the undefined nature of nursing.

Mauksch[2] has intensively explored the coordinating function of nursing. He speaks of the hospital's functions as providing bed and board, services subsidiary and supplementary to the cure process, and assistance in the diagnostic and therapeutic function under direction of the physician. He sees services accruing from the degree of illness, physical incapacitation, and emotional stress as overlying the diagnostic and therapeutic functions. The nurse's work embraces many of these functions, but not exclusively; others in the hospital participate in them in varying amounts and degrees. There must be coordination in each of the above categories, but it is quite inconstant, depending on the number and degree of responsibilities of other departments and services in the particular hospital.

It should be noted that there is considerable movement in the direction of departmental autonomy, as demonstrated in some instances by the assumption of almost complete responsibility for medication by the pharmacy, but with observation of effect and administration of fewer medications left to nursing.

It is also worth noting that the coordinating function may camouflage the erosion of nursing. A case in point is the work of the inhalation therapist. This work was formerly done exclusively by nursing, but is now done more expertly by the specialized group, apparently recruited out of the precise needs of thoracic specialists who apparently thought nursing was not meeting the needs of their patients. Here, too, there is residual work left to nursing, such as supervision of deep-breathing exercises and monitoring of therapy after it is instituted and instructions have been given by inhalation therapists. This residual work of the nurse becomes less therapeutic and assumes a more coordinating and extending nature. One wonders if the coordinating aspect should be curtailed or expanded, in view of the overriding question of the essential nature of nursing.

RELATIONSHIP TO OTHER ELEMENTS OF ADMINISTRATION
Planning

Because planning includes the goal determination of the enterprise for which long- and short-range plans are made, support of the coordinating function is required. Where plans are well understood and communicated, the contribution of the interrelating parts is expedited with less strain. For example, the introduction of the position of patient representative will be expedited considerably by unit-by-unit review of particular patients, with the patient representative and workers following the general presentation. This is coordinating action in which staff understanding of the new position is enhanced by particularized reviews by small groups or units. In a proposed plan for assessing existing nursing care for a given institution (see Chapter 5), a polling device was to be used to obtain information from the physicians, patients, their families, and communities. This activity constitutes coordination by bringing together responses from widely diversified groups.

The coordinating function is apparent in planning when nurses are involved early in hospital architectural development. Indeed, the coordination provided by such prime users results in appropriately balanced and integrated plans. Breger[3] gives an excellent account of such coordination.

There are questions arising from the coordinating function that deserve consideration, for example, whether business corporations have obligations to social purpose inherent in good personnel relations, as well as excellence of operation and profit. Siegel[4] found both pros and cons in interviewing top executives and economists, with responses ranging from the claim that profit is the sole purpose of the corporation and any money used for social purposes violates the corporation's imperative, to such social practices as placing employees on salary to teach in black colleges. However, because hospitals are not industrial corporations and are essentially nonprofit, the question and arguments do not fully apply. The social obligation of the hospital takes another form in the consideration of volunteerism as low-cost health care testing and such public service directed to its primary work of health care. Though such external coordination may be an academic question at the moment, it may in time have consequences for hospital decisions.

Organizing

The organization of the enterprise is the perfect example of coordination. Its skeletal structure provides the basic articulations of positions necessary to achieve the purpose of the enterprise and to generate the energy to set the organization in motion and tie the prescribed parts together systematically and economically. Coordination is seen in all phases of organizational operation. Delegation, accountability, and evaluation of achievement cannot exist without such interlocking activity—the team leader with the team members, the supervisor with the head nurses in a division, clinical specialists with the staffs they support, and so on.

Moreover, as complex organizations departmentalize there is the concomitant need for coordination. Specialized clinical areas, though having some separate or specialized objectives, must remain an integral part of the whole organizational structure in order to participate in meeting institutional goals and make certain that departmental and institutional objectives are in proper alignment and are compatible. An example of such coordination is the synchronization of staff in coronary care and often adjacent definitive, or secondary coronary care, units. These backup staffs, prepared and trained for such service, can be enlisted immediately from the adjacent units to relieve coronary care nurses when a patient in the coronary care unit or elsewhere in the hospital requires their special continuing services. Any subdivision of the organization and its work demands coordination in order to keep the subdivision a participating, articulating part of the whole.

This coordination that derives from departmentalization can be restrained or reduced by exploitation of the commonalities of departmentalization. The monumental work of Beland[5] and the definitive work of Abdellah and associates (see Chapter 3), provide a comprehensive, firm base for the exploration of commonalities. We must identify the core of care common to proliferating specialties, for example, in rehabilitation, alcoholic treatment, and dialysis units.

In staff relationships those who observe, study, and provide information are serving the coordinating function. Decisions made by line personnel are enriched by the work of staff personnel, who increase the knowledge of and the relationships involved in the projected decision. For example, the collection of pertinent articles and the preparation of abstracts of such articles by an in-service director or librarian would greatly facilitate the decision of where in the organization to place a newly employed clinical specialist.

The movement to flattened organizations contains a coordinating element, because its purpose—to reduce layers of accountable personnel—increases accessibility of superior to subordinates and thereby facilitates communication among related positions.

Important management theorists [Newman,[6] p. 405] point out a potential danger in the relationship of coordination to organization. The danger of deficiencies in organization when excessive coordinating devices are needed is signalled by an increase in devices such as use of added specific positions and committees. Examples of underutilization of coordination seem more prevalent in nursing, however, as shown in the introduction of a new service such as cardiac surgery when no one is charged with seeing to the articulation of all the parts (for example, the preparation of the general nursing units for their admittedly more remote but still necessary participation in the project). Overutilization of coordination occurs when there is overparticipation in review of a specific problem. For example, when a head nurse is charged with reviewing an untoward incident involving a patient in the unit on other than the day shift and other departments and a supervisor or an assistant director do a simultaneous review of the same incident, there is overcoordination, which shows a lack of understanding of accountability and line responsibility. This is not to say that the supervisor or assistant director could not contribute to the collection of data with the knowledge and consent of the head nurse, but only that a concurrent review is excessive. This can and does happen out of officiousness, ignorance, or lack of confidence in the head nurse and should be dealt with to eliminate overcoordination. In practice there often is collaborative but not concurrent effort in putting the review together.

We have been slow to acknowledge this sometimes oppressive coordination borne by the head nurse at the unit level, thereby deterring efforts to remedy the situation or render it bearable. Such remedies as extension of other departments to their logical limits and introduction of the ward clerk and ward manager might have come much earlier.

Stevens[7] acknowledges the coordinating burden of the head nurse when she says that the great number of encounters found in the head nurse position increases the frustration level of the position. However, she seems to perpetuate the thinking that has long kept head nurses outside the administrative pale by referring to them as filling "the juncture between administration and staff" and "meeting her (the head nurse's) responsibilities to patients, staff and administration." It is precisely this veiled separation of the head nurse from the administrative group that has perpetuated the overload of encounters; it makes this work something separate from the work of other managers, rather than a part of carrying forward the goals of the organization to which all management personnel are committed. If there were this uniform commitment to known, coherent goals, the great number of encounters would be reduced, given priority, or viewed constructively within the framework of the commonly held goals.

Relative to coordination, Drucker[8] points out overstaffed organizations where work rather than performance is produced and coordination abounds. This admonition is valuable as we add positions to the nursing service that vie with existing ones. The position of unit manager may be such a position. If this person is to be the superior or equal of the head nurse, he or she becomes the coordinator and works with other departments to see that the care plan is maintained and services and scheduling are kept efficient. This function is ordinarily carried out by the ward clerk, under direction of the head nurse.

Staffing

Pigors and Myers[9] see coordinating as part of their definition of management: "Organizational leadership . . . one of its central tasks is effective coordination and utilization of available human and nonhuman resources to achieve the objectives of the organization." One can see the pervasiveness of coordination in the enterprise in this definition, with its attendant effect on other functions of administration such as planning, organizing, controlling, or budgeting. All are brought into play in appropriate order and amount as the goals of the organization are achieved through utilized and coordinated resources of all kinds. Implied in such coordination is not only the articulation and welding together of positions, but the more formidable task of achieving such articulated group effort through the welding of individual personalities, making coordination both more necessary and difficult. The multiple facets of staffing the enterprise, which place competent personnel in the right mix in position to meet the nursing needs of the patient population, are intimately involved in the coordinating function.

A clear-cut illustration of coordination in the staffing function is found in the position of the liaison nurse developed at Rancho Los Amigos Hospital [David[10]]. These nurses demonstrate the coordination component in two ways: coordination of component parts of comprehensive continuous nursing care of which they are masters, and coordination of the articulating parts of patient care within the institution's and the community's vast array of services according to the individualized needs of particular patients. Such liaison nurses demonstrate knowledge and command of both internal and external resources from which they approve, select, or guide selection of those resources appropriate for a particular patient. Their special strength lies in being experts in both internal and external nursing care, or in melding the advantageous properties of the clinical specialist with those of the public health nurse in individualized ways.

Steen's[11] account of a liaison nurse practicing in a general hospital in which 57% of admissions were for treatment of chronic diseases essentially follows the above description of the liaison nurse in wide-ranging nursing coordination, with the added dimension of ombudsman whereby the liaison nurse represents the patient or family where difficulty is encountered in reaching and obtaining the services of other agencies. It might be said that this is policing the coordination of the patient's care, a not uncommon occurrence in patient needs beset by the complexities and intricacies of our social welfare system.

Directing

The close relationship of directing to supervision is served by the coordinating element of administration.

Inherent in the supervisory process is the need to keep all the work in progress under scrutiny so that the person, committee, or whoever charged with the responsibility carries it out, continues to do so, gives an accounting periodically, or reports a quiescent period while collateral effort is made. This part of the supervisory process may be called coordinating, or following through, because it consists of persistent effort to see that all parts are working toward the goal.

In a mobile age and profession such as ours, in which turnover is high, this aspect of supervision becomes doubly important. If it is not done conscientiously and knowledgeably, fledgling projects or activities begun by another may die, not from inappropriateness but from lack of follow-through by a successor in seeing that the project is nurtured to maturity.

The supervisory process gives and maintains direction—day to day, week to week, month to month, and year to year. This direction is essential to bring continuity to bear on people, their projects, and their work. This direction is coordination of a linear nature, as compared with the lateral nature described earlier: it monitors the work of others while it is in the process of being achieved or carried forward. The supervisory work involved in the installation of a problem-oriented medical record system, for example, requires that the day-to-day progress be checked, personnel counseled and helped to master the techniques, data reviewed with workers, and the system reworked where necessary until all staff are performing appropriately.

Supervision as described by the American Society of Personnel Administration in *Employer's Labor Relations Guidebook*[12] corroborates the thinking of Follett and Newman about coordination. Their notion of voluntary coordination deriving from good organization and communication lines is paralleled in this source by advice to supervisors to give clear and uniform job assignments, adequate training and recognition for achievement, and instructions that allow for verbal exchange and questions in the interest of well-informed workers.

Controlling

The numerous controlling devices in use in nursing services are coordinating devices in the sense that they bring together such multifaceted mechanisms as audit systems involving all levels and departments of nursing in cooperation with medical records departments, medical staffs, other departments, patients, and sometimes the public; as rounds often involving multicategory participation for varied reasons; or as guidelines or standards from different sources, including those prepared on site, with which nursing staffs compare their practice and refine their working conditions. The more articulations involved in the coordination of these evaluating or controlling devices, the more comprehensive they will be. Such articulations, when thought of as possibilities from which to select the most appropriate, versatile, or effective systems with which to evaluate the work of the enterprise, are valuable coordinating devices. Similarly, written reports, manuals, records, minutes, and such, help coordinate the many parts of the enterprise and contribute to control by keeping all the parts in sight.

The most ultramodern coordinating device is probably the computer, by which data storage and retrieval make possible unlimited coordinating material for unlimited purposes. There is already one hospital, Canyon General Hospital in Anaheim, California, that has no written medical record; the patient record is completely computerized.

We have noted the existence of computerized nursing care plans drawing on standards of care for specific disease conditions, combined with the individualized data on the patient. All changes in medical or nursing orders are stored, coordinated, and printed out for daily use by the nursing staff. Other departments receive printouts, too, so that the large job of coordinating all the patient contacts with other departments by nursing is obviated [Cornell and Carrick[13]].

However, a statistical study[14] carried out in the late 1960s showed that nursing services have made only limited use of computers. Administrative and financial functions, followed by medical records and inventory control departments, were the greatest users of computers in hospitals.

Barker[15] did a masterful review of computers in which she specifically addressed nurses and pointed to the fact that the 1970s are the years of computer use. She pointed to the need for nurses to become involved seriously and thoroughly so that the benefits of computer systems can be used by nursing to purify, strengthen, and enrich nursing care. She described successful efforts of Charlotte (N.C.) Memorial Hospital to incorporate computer service into nursing service. Work at this hospital is also clearly described by Smith.[16] These accounts point out the imperatives of getting nursing involvement in computer work, assignment to one nurse of the responsibility for incorporation and extension of such work in the nursing enterprise so that it can be given the concentrated attention it requires, and use of existing excellent nursing computer centers to expedite the work nationally. Charlotte Memorial Hospital or Barker could become the agent for expansion of computerized nursing service nationally in the way Rancho Los Amigos Hospital was the agent for expansion of rehabilitation nursing and the University of Wisconsin Extension was the model and agent for continuing education in nursing. These imperatives are impregnated with coordination, because their need arises precisely from looseness and dissipating isolated or diffuse efforts. We must build collectively on existing strength. Holding such building together is an important aspect of coordinating.

Barker eloquently lays out for us the direction we should take:

When the traditional nursing Kardex has been eliminated; when the medicine card is no longer necessary; when patient charging is no longer the time-consuming chore resulting in much useless information; when nursing care plans, tailored to meet individual patient needs, are automatically generated; when staffing and personnel assignment are generated, matching skills of personnel and needs of patients; when errors are reduced by legible printing, periodic reminders for safety checks on incompatible drugs and treatments; when the profession's clerical work load is reduced and more time is available for direct nursing care; when necessary information as to bed availability, treatment procedures, disease processes is instantly available; when inservice education can proceed to meet individual needs at the learner's rate; when students can be scheduled to coordinate their needs to experiences available; when learning is more palatable and requires a logical thinking process in evaluating and choosing alternatives; when alterations in nursing practice are based on study of actual nursing actions and results; when charges for professional nursing can be calculated; when the quality of nursing care can be objectively measured; then let the nurse be able to say it was a cooperative effort between the nurse as the user of the computer and the data processor who has the technical knowledge to make it possible. She can then stand proud of her own creative accomplishments in streamlining the nursing information system."*

Brown and associates[17] describes a computerized health information service in use in the care of a 9,000-member Indian tribe, which provides comprehensive current information at any time on any member. One can imagine the boon to the health worker of such an instrument in rendering high-quality care in a widespread geographic area.

COORDINATION WITHIN COORDINATION

Follett's[18] concepts of responsibility as cumulative and authority as residing in several locations to describe the ways in which responsibility and leadership are extended through the organization in order to take advantage of the strengths and contributions of all workers demonstrate coordination within coordination. She notes the need to transact, whereby various departments confer and keep in touch so that their responsibilities will be mutually supportive in achieving the ultimate goal. She thinks that this coordination of cross-functioning was deterred by lack of appreciation for coordination, the hierarchical nature of organizations, and the tendency to use such coordination only to eliminate existing difficulties. She links this need for transacting to acknowledgement of accumulating responsibility and authority as residing in several locations. It is in the early stages of planning, organizing, and staffing for parts as well as the whole that one provides for this cross-functioning, or sharing of information and ideas laterally, so that the results will be satisfactorily coordinated. The final responsibility is thus shared with those directly involved or concerned peripherally, laterally or transactionally, on a continuing basis and early enough for the participation to be fruitful rather than corrective.

Inherent in Follett's ideas are the concepts of consultative management (every employee a manager) and participatory democracy or management. Underlying them all is the obligation to not only permit but encourage employee input in the planning, organizing, and staffing for both personal enrichment and that of the enterprise. In Follett's context, there is enrichment in practice and procedure by the exchanging, contributing, and uniting aspects of coordination.

In this matter of early coordination Gill[19] speaks of the process of lateral coordination by which managers at each level are given the opportunity to address ideas before they are adopted, not so consensus will be achieved but that the act of contributing in the formative stages will improve the ideas and enrich and engage the contributor. Again, there are undertones of consultative management and respect for people, which support and verify the interpenetration of various concepts with such common elements as consultative activity and illumine the relationships that generate lucidity and clarity, not only in the parts but in the whole. The underlay provides for interweaving that strengthens clarification, understanding, and commitment to the concept it is supporting.

Related to these concepts of cross-functioning and lateral coordination is Newman's[6] idea of voluntary coordination [pp. 410-411]. Voluntary coordination consists of informal lateral conferences. It grows from good relationships based on good organization and communication lines, visible and compelling objectives, and congruous plans. Teamwork and similar coordinated activity grow from such specifics, as seen where classical team nurs-

---

*From Barker, M.: The era of the computer and its impact on nursing, Supervisor Nurse **2**(8):36, 1971.

ing is practiced. If one specific is missing, the goal and its achievement are altered negatively. All efforts to maintain these specifics should be nurtured because they often lie in informal, gracious occasions adjacent to the formal organization.

COMMITTEES

The committee, a structural device of great importance, has multiple coordinating aspects. It embraces all of the elements of administration in various combinations and for various purposes. The built-in coordinating mechanism is the formal arrangement of selected people to deliberate and make decisions about selected topics for presentation to the person or group that convened the committee.

Because the specificity of committees is so wide ranging, the coordinating factor involves the various parts of administration to a considerable degree. The executive committee, which assists a manager in decision making, is long-standing and potentially powerful. The power is contingent, however, on the degree to which the manager functions consultatively. The decision of this committee may touch on all aspects of the enterprise. Standing committees, of which the executive committee is one, vary, but frequently in a nursing service they include procedure, administrative policy, budget, personnel, and in-service education committees. Temporary, or ad hoc, committees are established to do a particular piece of work and are terminated at the conclusion of the work. Committees can be action oriented, advisory, or both. The procedure committee is an example of both because its work in preparing and keeping procedures up to date is frequently put into effect with formal approval by another person or body. This dual role of the committee in acting and advising is a common one and helps to see that the work of the committee is utilized. There is always the potential danger that such work will be filed and forgotten, either accidentally or deliberately, in which case the committee work has been "busy work."

There are advantages and disadvantages to the use of committees. Among the advantages is the value of working out plans or decisions both on a one-to-one basis and collectively. Committee work should produce growth upon growth of the plan as well as of the members themselves. Corporate thinking should produce richer results, especially when the membership of the committee is representative of all levels, departments, and shifts. The committee allows for input of differing points of view and from wider perspectives. It permits distribution of the work load, such as in data collection and review of the literature. It should produce better decisions because of its representational nature, though this is not guaranteed: autocracy is possible in group as well as individual activity, for as many reasons as there are types of personalities.

The disadvantages derive essentially from the diffused authority that makes it easy for each member to avoid or shift responsibility. This permits floating and lack of commitments, which render the work of the committee less effective. The chairperson can and should be held accountable if drift sets in. He or she is answerable to someone or to a group for the mission of the committee and in turn has the responsibility to demand performance on the part of the committee members.

Committees cost money. Payroll considerations must be made for the time of the participants. Thus, it behooves all concerned (those authorizing committees, the chairpersons, and members) to use the time advantageously.

Randall[20] has some remarkable points to make about committee effectiveness. Besides an agenda circulated in advance, any necessary staff papers to the point and summarized, and a chairperson so in control of the position that he or she states issues in his or her own words, Randall suggests having a proponent of the issue or idea explain it and then solicit opinions, first from those opposing the issue or idea, followed by opinions from all others, so that no one can avoid the responsibility of placing thoughts and opinions on record. This latter point of insisting on individual responsibility for the deliberations keeps individual accountability operative in carrying forward committee work.

There is a point of view that committee activity involves people in the objectives and issues of the enterprise. In such institutions, every professional nurse serves on a committee. This ensures and encourages involvement of personnel in the enterprise, provided the committees are strong and functioning properly. This idea of having each nurse a member of a committee is akin to the in-service project where each nurse belongs to a seminar group, with ongoing commitment to studying specific problems and needs of the enterprise.

A form of committee, though not labeled as such, is described by Gill[21] as "a strong central staff . . . a small versatile staff of nurses working together for the good of nursing as a whole [which] can learn and apply a host of specialized skills." If executive committees were more representative, they could sometimes approximate such a group. The planning, perspectives, and priorities committees of the national nursing associations also provide a comparable model for Gill's kind of group.

The professional performance or nursing practice committees that are being instituted, usually at the request of state nurses' associations in their representation of nurses for contractual purposes, have strong coordinating implications in that they apparently aspire to obtain input of the nursing staff in deliberations and decisions affecting nursing care in the particular institution. This proposal seems to point to a deficiency in the deliberative and consultative function ordinarily carried out in the committee structure of the enterprise, but probably also to the absence or inhibited nature of the formal staff organization of the enterprise.

Committees, then, serve a vast coordinating, interpenetrative service in the enterprise, uniting and weaving various parts, projects, and interests in the all-embracing effort to achieve the goals.

INTRADEPARTMENTAL COORDINATION

As the coordinating function in its secondary, or embracing, role supports planning, organizing, staffing, directing, and controlling in the nursing enterprise, its interpenetrative nature is apparent. Its cohesive nature is similarly demonstrated, and its contribution to coherence in the management function of the nursing enterprise is shown. Such activities and deliberations sustain the intradepartmental contribution to coordination.

INTERDEPARTMENTAL COORDINATION

There is little doubt that composite patient care in our health care institutions has been seriously deterred by absence of interdepartmental coordination. There is also little doubt that our collective failure to coordinate our efforts toward achievement of patient care goals can be attributed to the lateness of administrative thought and practice in reaching us in the health care field. The monolithic and isolated view of the hospital, which has been permitted to predominate, has in no small measure been both a cause and effect of our failure to incorporate such management theory and its coordinating component. Currently there are growing and successful management development programs in colleges. Though there is a universal need for management training among hospital personnel, they have not made use of these programs. Energetic coordination is necessary to bring hospital management personnel into these programs. Coordination will surely be one of the vehicles by which we meet patient needs collectively and competently and has much to offer in accelerating achievement of this objective, making all hospital workers mutually supportive and in touch with resources wherever they are.

We have noted the growing interweaving of the work of the personnel and nursing departments. When the staffing function is coordinated in terms of recruitment and other facets, it will be more efficient and fruitful. Likewise, where in-service education is coordinated, it is strengthened and streamlined. In the budgeting process, time and energy-consuming lone efforts are rendered more efficient and effective and certainly less frustrating when departments work collaboratively under the guidance and direction of the person in charge of the whole budget operation.

Closer to the actual work situation and in operation longer than either personnel departments or budget directors are the housekeeping, laundry, pharmacy, and other operational departments. At a recent workshop for hospital managerial personnel, the duty list for a worker in housekeeping was projected on a screen. It was a revelation to the nurses there, who were apprised of the comprehensive range of this worker's duties. It reinforced the importance of this work in quality patient care and its direct contribution to freeing nurses to nurse, rather than the former concern for if not the actual performance of some of these duties.

At the same meeting a dietitian was heard to say how disturbing and destructive it is when nurses' aides exclaim, as they remove the cover from a plate of food, "What in the world is this?" It gave nurses pause to think about how easily the work of other departments can be undermined. Similarly, a hospital administrator was heard to ask a nurse what will be left for nursing to do as jobs are stripped away from it. While it may have been intended as a provocative question, it also constituted a meaningful one to which nurses would do well to address themselves, alone and in concert with colleagues in other fields. Health care work is rife with such actual and potential questions. Coordination is the means of explaining and tempering attitudes and work in the light of such questions.

Interdepartmental meetings are the chief means of bringing about greater appreciation for and contribution to the work of others, or harmonizing the collective efforts of all to the goals of the institution. If the goals are kept paramount in such deliberations, the probability of keeping such deliberations to the point, well thought out, and fruitful is greater. Where projected changes are subjected to interdepartmental scrutiny in such meetings, they stand only to be justified, improved, or postponed until such time as the necessary changes or conditioning of those concerned occurs.

There are variations of interdepartmental meetings to which nursing is or should be a part. These meetings are often interdepartmental only to the degree that a department is granted attendance privileges. Medical staff meetings, including meetings of clinical specialty groups, are examples of such meetings. There is growing nurse representation at them, as there should be, so long as nursing carries such heavy responsibility for the implementation of medical care plans for patients.

Meetings of the board of directors that include only hospital administration would be enriched by representation from hospital departments on a regular basis. (In some contractual negotiations, nurses are asking for such representation.) It could be argued that the hospital administrator represents the hospital departments at board meetings, but the coordinative function would be better served by departmental representation, as it is in medical staff meetings, and for a parallel reason, namely, that nursing assumes considerable responsibility for implementing the board's plans and policies.

As there are interdepartmental meetings to facilitate and coordinate departmental efforts toward goal achievement, so there are interdepartmental meetings to facilitate and coordinate patients' goal achievement. This fine effort is found most commonly in rehabilitation institutes. These interdepartmental meetings devoted to patient care usually take one of two forms, which run concurrently. At one session the total staff will deliberate about a group of patients under their care; at an alternate session, there will be in-depth deliberation about one particular patient. The effort is directed to maximizing and synthesizing the respective contributions of the interdisciplinary participants to patient care.

Probably the most crucial of all interdepartmental relationships in carrying forward the goals of the institution is that between medical and nursing staffs. There are so many areas of concern and current issues that would yield to the combined wisdom of the two professions that one can only lament the separation while diligently working to increase the communication and coordination.

Though there are a few viable attempts at coordination of these two groups, such as representation at medical staff meetings and the beginnings of physician-nurse conference groups, under the impetus of the National Commission for the Study of Nursing and Nurse Education, they are infinitesimal when viewed against the enormity of the need.

In the mutual problems engendered by extension of nursing into medicine, pediatric nurse practitioners (perhaps the first of nursing's extensions into medicine) and their certification merit attention. Because the American Academy of Pediatrics withdrew from collaboration with the American Nurses' Association in the certification of these pediatric practitioners, the National Joint Practice Commission of the American Medical Association and the American Nurses' Association (in existence because of the influence of the National Commission for the Study of Nursing and Nurse Education) took the position that certification within a profession should be the responsibility of that profession—a decision in favor of nurse autonomy.[22] The National Joint Practice Commission went on to say that by keeping state nursing and medical practice acts general and flexible, role changes when they occur can be made official by joint statements. It is interesting to note that this Commission, in existence only since 1971, has studied interdisciplinary education and health care for the aged and those in rural areas, three fertile fields for physician-nurse coordination.

Happily there are continuing efforts to strengthen and expand these fragile beginnings. There is growing evidence of interdepartmental collaboration and coordination. There are the beginnings of joint meetings in which all hospital members consider the total contribution to goal achievement, share ideas with each other, and reap the benefits of joint study of management or subjects common to all departments. The inclusion of nurses and nursing in medical specialties such as associations of thoracic surgeons has given rise to closer coordination and also to the clinical strengthening of these nurses.

The literature is also showing signs of coordination. When professions share each others' journals, there is likely to be improved coordination. There is more material dealing with coordination problems in general and physician-nurse coordination in particular. Aradine and Pridham[23] suggest that physician-nurse collaboration be directed to learning how to collaborate in work, maintaining such collaborative relationship, providing the services of patient care, and formulating policy about such services. Their work suggests that we have not done enough definitive work on the problem but have left it in an amorphous state.

Another example of interdepartmental coordination comes from the increased utilization and sophistication of medical records departments where charts of discharged patients are finalized more expeditiously than when the charts remain in units, awaiting completion of incomplete portions before finalization. The unit staff, especially the ward clerk, is spared this coordinating job of completing charts and assembling incomplete parts. Maintenance of charts is the responsibility of the medical records department, which has the tools and sanctions necessary to keep all charts complete, filled, and ready for re-use, study, and so forth. Completion of the nursing portion and correct order remain the unit responsibility. Thus burdensome and unnecessary coordination in the units is removed as a result of strengthening another department.

In addition to formal efforts at interdepartmental coordination, there is the aspect of lateral coordination, where informal groups and contacts are more purposeful and directed. One might well ask whether we have capitalized on the good and fruitful relationships found at the operational level, that is, in the unit, the operating room, or a particular clinic. Conversely, has a harmful relationship been examined or explored in order to be corrected? Goodwill, good working relationships, and communication often characterize such coordination. Are the participants able and willing to intrude consideration of the more remote aspects of professional coordination and collaboration in such relationships? It might be very productive if done deliberately.

EXTRAINSTITUTIONAL COORDINATION

If coordination falls short of the goal within the hospital, it falls more so in its relationship with the outside—the community in general and particular parts such as other health care institutions, related services, and social action. The hospital has always had a separatist character, perhaps because of the uniqueness of its contribution and the fact that people have no choice but to use its expertise and services when their health demands it. For whatever reasons, there is an aloneness about the hospital and other health care centers.

There has been a growing effort in the last decade to close the gap and bring the health care institution into the mainstream of community life, as seen in the flourishing Womens' Auxiliary Movement, the growing use of the hospital emergency department in lieu of a visit to the physician's office, the growing volunteerism of hospitals and staffs in health promotion, such as clinics for testing for glaucoma and measuring blood pressure, the opening effect of such vast governmental programs as Medicare-Medicaid, the participation of the hospital in civil defense planning, and the American Red Cross blood bank program. The external analysis and environmental scanning found in hospital planning and the presence of hospital personnel amid health and welfare planning groups offer additional evidence that the hospital is indeed breaking out of its solitary position.

Despite these and other efforts in progress, much remains to be done in coordinating the contribution of the hospital to the needs and desires of the community. Such coordination begins with the institutions themselves. They must collaborate, cooperate, and coordinate in the interest of better and more economical services. Should every hospital aspire to a complete range of services; or should specialized and expensive services be distributed among hospitals, such as pediatrics to one and obstetrics to another, or rehabilitation to one and oncology to another? The proliferation of hospital beds attests to the empire building of individual hospitals at the expense of the taxpayer and consumer. Though comprehensive health planning bodies have come into being in an effort to conserve health services, and state regulatory agencies and utilization review committees are at work on such conservation, these bodies apparently need more powerful mechanisms to curb this unwarranted expansion in hospital beds, which would in effect force the cooperation of hospitals that has been missing during these many years of Hill-Burton hospital financing. A study showing the presence of 60,000 unneeded hospital beds, which cost $1 billion annually to sustain, gives concrete testimony to this chronic condition [Cohn[24]]. It is estimated that an empty bed costs from two thirds to three fourths as much as an occupied, revenue-producing bed. Joining forces, not competition, is the way to reduce overbedding and bring coherence into the system.

Comprehensive health planning groups recommend and state regulatory bodies require and force consideration of merger, consolidation, collaboration, or some form of active cooperation by hospitals, rather than the long-standing practice of individual, independent expansion and growth. Absence of accountability from hospitals themselves, as well as state, regional, and national hospital associations, governmental regulatory agencies, and third-party payers such as Blue Cross has permitted this costly failure to collaborate, cooperate, and coordinate, despite continuous outcry from the public about exorbitantly high rates.

A pertinent illustration of community agency coordination is contained in the following account. A study of a tri-county health department by a county health and welfare planning council, at the request of the medical director, produced the recommendation that an administrator be hired to free the medical officer from administrative duties to allow time for more professional work. The recommendation was adopted and the loaned executive who set up the position became the permanent administrator in charge of budget, funding, personnel administration, public relations, program development, and evaluation.[25] In addition to coordination, this account demonstrates conservation of professional time.

Coordination is at work in communities, in response to phenomenally high accident and injury rates, where hospital emergency departments, ambulance services, and state patrol, police, and fire departments work together to get expert care to patients quickly and efficiently. An illustration of such unifying work is found in Illinois, under the aegis of the State Public Health Department, where a network of local, areawide, and regional trauma centers serves the population expertly and comprehensively. Trauma coordinators employed by the State Public Health Department and stationed in each trauma center coordinate the work of these trauma centers and act as liaison for the various types of workers involved in the program.

The attention given to coronary heart disease in all aspects of community life (coronary care units in hospitals and widespread educational efforts of organizations such as the American Heart Association) is providing a valuable means of coordination between community and hospital. The tremendous work of the American Heart Association in education and research has in large measure given rise to the vast network of services for heart care wherever they are found. The coordinating work of local and state heart associations encourages emergency departments to provide full cardiac service and in some cases to be certified as such by the particular unit of the heart association when specific criteria are met. This coordination spreads internally from the emergency department, because it is often coronary care personnel who train or examine employees and even professionals (such as physicians) in emergency coronary care, using the guidelines and instructions of the American Heart Association. Coordination becomes a network of synchronized care from wherever the stricken patient is found to the coronary care unit, by way of an emergency or specially equipped ambulance, with support from police or fire departments. There is no reason to think that there will not be expansion of these coordinated efforts in the interest of potential patients with other types of disease conditions having an emergency component (for example, diabetes).

In this kind of coordinated care the circle is completed by agencies such as the American Heart Association, which does so much work directed to education and prevention that ultimately one would find reduction in the need for the emergency coronary services. The systems approach supports such circular coordination in that discrete programs of the Association are synchronized to provide comprehensiveness of its total program. Another integrated and articulating part is the work the Association does in preparing nurses and other health personnel for this work and strengthening the expertise of those already so engaged. There are more obscure coordinating possibilities in the community whose findings and services could enrich or supplement the patient care given by hospitals.

Under the aegis of groups such as the Black Panthers, there are people's clinics for the poor, usually in black areas, organized to provide first-level care and staffed by volunteers. These may be coupled with health study groups that analyze the health care situation and possibilities for such deprived populations. Donovan[26] raises the question of whether we have the courage, openness, and security as professional nurses, individually or in professional organizations, to meet with such groups on their terms in the interest of the health needs of such a deprived population. The same question could be asked of an institution, its nursing service, or individual nurses within that service. To what degree would they be willing to meet with such groups or extend their services into such grass-roots health facilities, in the interest of coordinating health services for such populations? Corroboration for the need to explore and act upon reasons for nonuse of traditional services by the poor, even in modern neighborhood health centers, is found in Perkin's work.[27] She sees education and outreach as necessary to ensure utilization. Outreach to the extent that it reaches right into people's own efforts in a learning as well as teaching way is seen by Donovan as the way to ensure utilization. This is really coordination of people's own efforts with traditional services, whereas Perkins suggests direct contact with persons and families. The presence and number of such grass-roots efforts is a determinant: where they do not exist,
they cannot be used. Searching them out may be a preliminary step.

Another type of coordinating community service is the volunteer research group. These are often found among youth groups and are quite sophisticated in their operations. Their model and inspiration may be Ralph Nader and his research organization. One such group is the Oregon Student Public Interest Research Group. Among its various inquiries it has included a study of nursing homes, and findings were neither alarming nor heartening.[28] Other findings pointed out the need for education and training of staff and speedier remedial work on violations found by state inspectors (a 56% correction rate was found at the time of the next inspection). One can see the implications here for hospitals, which often drain off nonprofessional staff from nursing homes by offering higher salaries, and for community health and welfare organizations and the educational community, which can help in upgrading the quality of the staff in nursing homes. The sense of continuity between hospitals and nursing homes, which has improved patient care, could carry over into other aspects of operation where coordination exists, generating constructive action and cooperation.

• • •

Coordination is a marvelous device for bringing an organization to fruition in achieving its purpose, because it keeps releasing collateral aspects of functions, activities, and relationships that, if recognized and used, can regenerate and strengthen other functions, activities, and relationships while they all contribute to purpose achievement.

REFERENCES
1. Georgopoulos, B., and Mann, F.: The community general hospital, New York, 1962, Macmillan, Inc., p. 277.
2. Mauksch, H.: The nurse; coordinator of patient care. In Skipper, J., and Leonard, R., editors: Social interaction and patient care, Philadelphia, 1965, J. B. Lippincott Co., pp. 251-265.

3. Breger, W.: Nurse participation in nursing unit design for health care facilities, J. Nurs. Admin. **4**(1):52-57, 1974.
4. Siegel, B.: Minding the corporate conscience, United Airlines Mainliner **18**(8):32-34, 1974.
5. Beland, I.: Clinical nursing, ed. 2, New York, 1970, Macmillan, Inc.
6. Newman, W.: Administrative action, ed. 2, New York, 1963, Prentice-Hall, Inc., pp. 405 and 410-411.
7. Stevens, B.: The head nurse as manager, J. Nurs. Admin. **4**(1):36-40, 1974.
8. Drucker, P.: Management tasks, responsibilities, practices, New York, 1974, Harper & Row, Publishers, p. 549.
9. Pigors, P., and Myers, C.: Personnel administration, ed. 7, New York, 1973, McGraw-Hill Book Co., p. 6.
10. David, J.: Liaison nurse, Am. J. Nurs. **69**(10):2142-2145, 1969.
11. Steen, J.: Liaison nurse, Am. J. Nurs. **13**(12):2102-2104, 1973.
12. Employer's Labor Relations Guidebook (revised), Indianapolis, 1970, Indiana State Chamber of Commerce, p. 28.
13. Cornell, S., and Carrick, A.: Computerized schedules and care plans, Nurs. Outlook **21**(12):781-784, 1973.
14. National Center for Health Services Research and Development: The use of computers in hospitals (no. PH110-233), November 1970, pp. 12-15.
15. Barker, M.: The era of the computer and its impact on nursing, Supervisor Nurse **2**(8):26-36, 1971.
16. Smith, E.: The computer and nursing practice, Supervisor Nurse **5**(9):55-62, 1974.
17. Brown, V., Mason, W., and Kaczmarski, M.: A computerized health information service, Nurs. Outlook **19**(3):158-161, 1971.
18. Follett, M.: Dynamic administration. In Metcalf, H., and Urick, L., editors: The collected papers of Mary Parker Follett, New York, 1940, Harper & Row Publishers, pp. 154-160.
19. Gill, W.: The process of lateral coordination, Supervisor Nurse **3**(1):10-14, 1972.
20. Randall, C.: The folklore of management, Boston, 1961, Little, Brown and Co., pp. 35-38.
21. Gill, W.: The concept of the strong centralized staff, Supervisor Nurse **3**(2):16, 1972.
22. National Joint Practice Commission supports intra-professional certification, The American Nurse **6**(3):1, 1974.
23. Aradine, C., and Pridham, K.: Model for collaboration, Nurs. Outlook **21**(10):655-657, 1973.
24. Cohn, V.: New report claims U.S. has 60,000 unneeded hospital beds, Portland, Ore., The Oregonian, September 13, 1974, p. 8.
25. Health agency seeks position, Vancouver, Wash., The Columbian, April 28, 1972.
26. Donovan, H.: Can we work with the Black Panthers? Nurs. Outlook **18**(5):34-35, 1970.
27. Perkins, Sr. M.: Does availability of health services ensure their use? Nurs. Outlook **22**(8):496-498, 1974.
28. Nacheman, A.: Report sees nursing homes not bad as pictured, Vancouver, Wash., The Columbian, June 24, 1974, p. 32.

CHAPTER 11
REPORTING

The ongoing responsibility of nursing services demands a reporting structure appropriate for transmission of important information necessary to carry on the nursing care of groups of patients, as well as the maintenance of records for reporting our ministration to and observations of patients individually. Reporting and recording have been intimately involved with both nursing care itself and the entire administrative process in achievement of the goals of nursing.

Reporting consists of written and verbal communications between and among persons associated with the nursing enterprise. Recording consists of preserving such communications, either in writing or by various electronic media. Reporting and recording are specific kinds of communication. While they partake of many aspects of general communication, carrying or providing information is the primary ingredient. Documentation may be used interchangeably with recording and reporting, though it suggests a stronger authenticating, substantiating, or corroborating component. More frequent use of the term document in all affairs of the nursing enterprise can only enhance the reporting and recording structures by providing the more stringent requirements inherent in the term. The more we strengthen our reporting and recording structures the better will be our nursing care and administration.

RELATIONSHIP TO THE ADMINISTRATIVE PROCESS

Reporting is related to all other parts of the administrative process. It is a secondary function because it supports planning, organizing, staffing, directing, and controlling; it is interwoven with them all.

Plans can neither be formulated nor implemented without integrated reporting: collection of data, consideration of alternatives, and decision making are dependent on some kind of reporting interactions.

Likewise, an organization cannot function unless there is provision for planned intercommunication both up and down the hierarchy and laterally among and within the work groups at department, floor, or unit levels. Getting reports from those most intimately connected with the work remains a goal that is far from realized. Flexibility is in order, however, because the idea of a report may intimidate those whose contribution is most needed. Simply hearing from and listening to workers closest to the operation may be more comfortable and productive for some people.

Staffing the nursing enterprise involves large and growing amounts of reporting and recording, and personnel departments may be second only to medical records departments in the amassing of records. The institution and its employees must be protected as they engage in the work of the enterprise. Such protection requires much recording or committing to writing in order to be effective and to guarantee the appropriateness and efficiency of the operation. Day-to-day supervision requires countless reports and recording as one goes about ordering means to ends in goal achievement. We have noted the need for written standards for the nursing care to be given and job descriptions for the workers. Both standards and descriptions are basic records for the benefit of the patients and of those providing the care.

The growing number of articulations of personnel departments with outside agencies, such as in contractual arrangements with professional organizations or unions or with parts of the community in which the hospital exists, mandates copious record keeping to provide the necessary verification and evidence needed for satisfactory encounters with these outside organizations.

Controlling is dependent on reports and records to a high degree where the enterprise is complex, as indeed it is in the case of nursing. The Joint Commission on Accreditation of Hospitals lists "significant, accurate, and concise nursing records and reports" among its evaluation criteria. Reporting and recording are integral parts of all control systems or devices, from the budgetary program for the institution to checking off the return demonstration of a new employee.

SOME GENERAL ATTRIBUTES OF REPORTING AND RECORDING

Accuracy is crucial to users of reports or records. Accuracy must derive from honesty, precision, and clarity. The reporting-recording effort must address the issue or information being reported or recorded directly and pointedly, with sufficient detail to elaborate it properly but not so much that clarity and precision are jeopardized. Accuracy depends in some degree on the clear thinking of the reporter or recorder: the more knowledgeable, experienced, sensitive, and insightful he or she is, the greater the probability of accuracy in reports and records.

Objectivity is likewise related to accuracy in reporting and recording. Strict adherence to the matter under consideration, accompanied by identification of contributory, tangential, or parallel considerations, is essential if correctness is to prevail. The freedom and ease with which the content of reporting and recording can be checked contributes to accuracy and is tantamount to openness. For example, the assembled data (such as cost-of-living index, prevailing rates in the locality and region, and comparable rates within the institution) presented freely to the workers for examination and checking, ensures more accuracy than closely held information. Opportunity for such checking also encourages healthy openness rather than troubled secretiveness.

Timeliness and promptness generate better reports and records: up-to-date data at the right time contribute much to smooth managerial functioning. For example, a statistical description of the increase in bedsores and grievances to demonstrate the effect of consistently lowered nursing hours on both nursing care and staff shows the importance of timeliness and promptness. Such a report also demonstrates the importance of factual data, balance, and relationships in addressing problems by skillful reporting, as well as showing many other good managerial practices and their relationships in a broader context.

Need for good writing techniques

The problems of written reports, records, and communications in general often arise from failure to develop appropriate mechanical and technical skills. We are cautioned in two companion sources about these dangers in communicating with large numbers of people.[1,2] The implications are the same for related reporting devices. Writers in management are advised to use simple words and sentences, to avoid the passive voice in favor of pronouns and strong verbs, to take care with use of connotation (emotional undertones) and denotation (dictionary meaning) of words, to avoid repetition, and to think the communication through in advance. One perhaps should qualify emotional in regard to connotation. Connotation is always contextual, that is, embedded in surrounding words, the times, and the place. The context, then, may or may not generate the emotional undertones. Additional safeguards for effective writing are trying it out on one or two persons in advance, so that weaknesses and discrepancies can be found and removed, there is a time lapse between preparation and finalization, and it can be reviewed from a fresh vantage point.

Williamson[3] identifies the parts of a report that, if used and synchronized, ensure a well-organized, logical presentation. These parts consist of the title, an abstract for quick review of the problem, introduction, body, and conclusions and recommendations. Such structure is valuable to the communicator because it exerts discipline that forces rework and refinement of thought and allows for better understanding by the one receiving the communication.

Need for appropriate circulation and storage

Good circulation of reports and appropriate provision for storage are crucial to good management practices. Unless the right people see the right material, there is weakening of the organizational fiber and consequently of goal achievement. Moreover, one should be cognizant of whether the material is evaluated and used (we are a nation of report filers rather than users).

In general, the wider the circulation the better, even of confidential material, in the interest of well-informed workers. That which contributes to understanding contributes to goal achievement. There is the excuse that "they won't read it anyway"; yet there are always enough discerning, interested people sprinkled among the many nonreaders to justify the practice of wide distribution laterally at all levels. Their interest makes them valuable in achieving goals. Moreover, the use of highlighting or abstracting techniques, which reduce the time necessary to read such material, greatly enhances wider utilization. Some organizations provide speedreading courses to their management personnel to increase the coverage and utilization of large amounts of material.

Standard routing devices are useful in that they keep the circulation system under control, reduce the need for multiple filings, and respect individualization. An accompaniment to the usual routing system is the assignment for coverage of various sources to particular individuals so that there is surety that all sources are monitored and that pertinent general or individual information is noted and routed accordingly. Our reproduction systems are so efficient and fast that the actual materials or pertinent parts can be provided each person following such monitoring. Such routing is really a part of librarianship and can be integrated into the hospital library, which assumes responsibility for it. The practice of providing small, regular amounts of time to workers for perusal of such material supports the individual's use of it. Facilitating utilization of information in all ways possible demands one's own commitment to the worth of using and disseminating information. Efficient ways to do so will follow such commitment.

Reports and records are primary supports for a well-informed and understanding work force, who are the achievers of the goals of the enterprise. Storage and retrieval are essential secondary supports and require as much attention as does dissemination. Indeed, continuous access to these materials must be provided if dissemination is to be projected into the future as well as meet immediate needs. Easy and uniform retrieval is at the heart of the storage systems and devices. Systematization of such materials is important; the simpler the process, the easier utilization will be. Unwieldy procedures militate against easy accessibility and utilization. For example, the use of substations or satellite locations decentralizes the operation and increases accessibility; however, decentralized materials are more difficult to control. The decision to decentralize requires that the relative merits of easy accessibility and control be weighed carefully.

There is the collateral need to keep materials up to date to ensure high usability.

We have noted the provision for revision and currency in procedure and policy manuals so that subsequent statements can be incorporated into or supercede earlier ones. The need for maintaining historical and unbroken sequences also requires ongoing vigilance, and filing arrangements must be made responsive to easy retrieval and utilization.

INTERNAL NURSING SERVICE REPORTS AND RECORDS
Change of shift reports

The change of shift report is the oldest report in the nursing service; indeed, its longevity attests to its importance in carrying forward the goals of the enterprise. Though it has undergone many changes over the years, it remains essentially a transmission instrument for the care of patients from one set of workers to another, using a written report, the nursing care plan as contained in a card file, and patients' charts. It provides the staff the opportunity to learn salient points about patients that have occurred during the preceding hours.

The change of shift report has both critics and supporters. The critics hold that the time thus spent is not justified, that much extraneous material and irrelevant matters creep in, that workers need hear only about specific patients to whom they are assigned, that team conferences can reduce the time thus spent, and that patient needs are unmet during reporting times.

Supporters contend that it is the most important part of the day, because the greatest number of workers can be assembled for direct information enhanced by collateral questions and issues and checking on pertinent information relating to nursing care of patients under their collective care. They also contend that it is vitally important to have well-informed workers so that the nursing care they give will be more deliberate and purposeful. They see a teaching potential inherent in the change of shift reports. Moreover, these supporters think that it is so crucial that every effort should be made by managers at other levels, such as supervisors and assistant directors, to be present also.

As timesaving efforts increase, tape recorders are being used with more frequency and effectiveness. The overriding limitation of such devices, however, is their elimination of two-way exchange. Where such exchange between collaborating persons is deemed important, the tape recorder is of little use except for subsequent reporting of the same material. However, our current state of staff instability justifies electronic retention of material for repetitive communication purposes. Our growing sophistication in increasingly complex nursing care requires the most careful attention to the transmission of essential and supportive information in carrying forward the goals of the nursing department in their most particularized way —the actual nursing care of individual patients. The change of shift report constitutes the best means to date to achieve such particularized attention to so many patients and workers.

Perhaps the most important factor in favor of the change of shift report is that it survives. If survival demonstrates worth, then efforts to make these reports more productive are justified.

A corollary to the change of shift report on units is the change of shift reports in nursing offices or departments where size dictates them. Wherever responsibility rests, personnel must be provided the requisite information and tools to carry out the responsibility. The base for such reports rests on written summary reports from constituent units rather than patient care plans in card files in the units.

There are many formats for such overall reporting. For the most part, they consist of outline forms to provide essential information such as discharges, transfers, and admissions; immediate pre- and postoperative patients; critical patients; those receiving important procedures such as blood transfusions, those with complicating factors such as decubitus ulcers, isolation, neurotic states, or untoward incidents; and VIPs. An excellent example of a comprehensive report format also provides pertinent staffing information such as numbers of patients in each of five classifications, the number of private duty nurses, and the number of patients to be fed [Warstler[4]]. The magnitude of the responsibility continues to be best served by such comprehensive, summarized reports. Evening- and night-shift managers require the same formalized base for carrying forward the goals of the nursing department as do personnel at the unit level.

General periodic reports

Less well established than change of shift reports is the periodic report on the state of a unit, department, or service. For the most part, where they are in effect they have started at the top: the nursing service director discharges accountability by preparing a written annual report for the hospital administrator. The process should and does fan out from there: the nursing service director requires similar accountability in the form of a written report from the department heads or supervisors, who in turn require them from head nurses. Such reports consist of progress toward achievement of objectives, demonstrated by factual and statistical material; impediments to such progress, which are also elaborated in factual if not statistical ways; the status of projects under way; and the aspirations and plans for the future that result from previous or freshly introduced material. Such periodic reviews keep managers in the habit of evaluating more deliberately and continuously. This practice has a generalized effect in that it focuses the whole operation and its parts more sharply. Interdepartmental factors should be included because they show the importance of such relationships in achieving institutionwide objectives. For example, introduction of new services or specialities, increased outreach into the community, or similar factors should be reflected in these reports.

Such reporting devices down through the organization should be accomplished more than once a year in order to subdue the complexities that abound in institutions. Managers who must submit quarterly achievement reports will do so more thoroughly and efficiently because of inherent continuity and proximity factors. Such reports demand judgments from us that were hitherto often unknown, ignored, or left diffuse. Coherence and cohesiveness are well served by having all levels engaged similarly in performing this part of their accountability responsibilities.

There are specialized reports that attend and serve these generalized reports. The growing collection of data surrounding the staffing function, such as numerical patient classification, summary of nursing hours, and distribution and kinds of workers, is frequently compiled in reportorial fashion. The introduction of new methods such as a retrospective chart audit system or a revised personnel evaluation system requires reports and records. The compilation of such reports provides data to be examined in the same way in which untoward-incident reports can be examined for trends, exceptions, and so forth. Minutes of committee meetings are reportorial material too.

HOSPITAL ANNUAL REPORT

The hospital annual report is perhaps not so important as is its counterpart in industry, where there are stockholders and various publics to whom it is addressed, because hospitals for the most part are nonprofit institutions. However, they too have various publics besides the boards of directors. The employee population, contributors, and consumers have considerable interest in such information, if national protests to rising prices are any indication.

Because nursing comprises such a high percentage of hospital personnel and budget, there should perhaps be more input from nursing than is usually the case.

An insightful commentary [Detman[5]] on annual reports in the industrial sector speaks to the need for candor, less pomposity, and less effort toward public relations. There is at least some applicability to hospital annual reports in this commentary.

An example that seems to offset these deficiencies, namely the absence of nursing input, the need for candor, and a more personal touch, is shown in the Annual Report of Long Beach (California) Community Hospital 1972-73, entitled "The Truth of It Is. . . ." This report takes an actual patient through hospitalization and shows the components of care involved and the percentage of cost accruing to each component. Nursing takes its place with other departments in a satisfying breakdown and review. It is informative, comprehensive, and clearly stated.

EXTERNAL NURSING SERVICE REPORTS AND RECORDS
Regulatory or accrediting agency reports

Because the hospital, and correspondingly the nursing service, is increasingly subject to the influence of outside agencies, attention must be paid to reports and records that emanate from these sources. The multitudinous reports required and provided by the Joint Commission on Accreditation of Hospitals are a case in point. Managers must stay in touch with such materials and reports, not only in order to comply with the requirements but also to use beneficially the ideas and suggestions contained therein. Reportage is also a part of such regulatory bodies as state health departments, Medicare-Medicaid legislation involving as it does third-party payers, Social Security Administration personnel, and so forth. Keeping order, pertinence, and continuty in such reportage is imperative if the complexities and difficulties are to be surmounted.

Other pertinent reports

An ever-widening array of reporting devices is at the disposal of nurse managers and contribute in varying degrees to the effectiveness with which they preside over the multitudinous activities of a nursing department. The goal of the nursing service is better served by the degree to which nurse managers can enlist other managers to use these devices. We have mentioned library resources that abound in reports and records of great significance to nursing service administrators. For example, several nursing journals carry regular columns on the legal aspects of nursing. There are independent services to which one may subscribe, such as *The Citation* of the American Medical Association and the Regan Report on Nursing Law.

There is also a growing number of reports of commissions, councils, and other deliberating bodies, which nurse managers must attend to if they are to keep abreast of outside contributions to their work. The Report of the National Advisory Commission on Health Manpower is an example. Much can be gained from such contemporary sources in managing the nursing enterprise. All such reports and data are not uniformly advantageous or useful, but nurses have the obligation to check them out in order to find what is or is not useful to their circumstances.

THE CHART

The chart is the document par excellence of the health care institution, because it is the repository of all data pertaining to a patient's hospitalization(s). All findings, results of examinations and tests, observations, details of what was done to and for patients, and their responses to these therapies and ministrations are contained in the chart. It also carries enabling records such as consents for treatment, surgery, autopsy, acknowledgements of informed consent as they come into practice, and so forth. It is not only a cumulative and comprehensive record, but a potential legal document in the case of possible litigation regarding any part of a patient's care and welfare while he or she is hospitalized. It is also privileged information, denied even to the patient, though this denial is being challenged as patients' rights are being increasingly asserted.

There have been innumerable efforts to streamline, refine, and update this instrument in all health care services. Triplicate physicians' order forms, permitting carbon copies to be sent directly to departments for processing, were a big step in refinement of the chart. Separate sheets for recording medications and treatments or serial findings such as blood pressure, prothrombin times, and neurological signs have been developed. Frequently these serial recording arrangements have been called flow charts, to indicate the progress of a single item over a period of time. It is well to remember that though the term flow chart is new the concept is not, for that is precisely what a graphic sheet for vital signs consists of. The Commission for Administrative Services in Hospitals (CASH) has demonstrated some of these improvements in the chart.[6]

As nursing refines its practice, a nursing history is being more widely used, related to if not stemming from the assessment part of the nursing process from which plans, implementation, and evaluation of nursing care proceed. The nursing history has an antecedent in the traditional admission note, which included objective and subjective symptoms and findings as well as any use of prosthetics, though it did not note the habits of daily living such as dietary preferences and sleep and elimination patterns.

There is a need to correlate the nursing history with the medical history so that the patient is not subjected to repetitive questioning. The medical history is being taken more frequently by various assistants, principally physician's assistants and nurse practitioners as they become available.

There is a fairly common complaint that nurses' notes are lacking in quality and precision; they seem to suffer by comparison with the charting done by European nurses. Walker and Selmanoff[7] have found corroborating evidence in an extensive study of nurses' notes taken in a university hospital. They found the notes unimportant in the communication among nursing personnel as well as between nursing and medical personnel. Though there was some evidence that there were more entries by medical than surgical units, entries in both remained low. They found infrequent inaccuracies, but omission of much pertinent data. The authors state that the chart is seldom being used as an answer to the growing problem of communicating descriptive patient information. Though this research was done in 1964, there is little evidence that the quality of nursing notes has changed. The complaints continue. If this is so, why? Have our observational skills degenerated? Do we not know enough about the etiology of disease to make appropriate observations? Is our effort to build nursing in a comprehensive direction deflecting us from our traditional prowess in observing patients in their essential relationship to the disease condition and therapeutic plan? It is paradoxical that in our earlier vocational days these patient records were of better quality than they are now, if current inadequacy is as widespread as is claimed.

PROBLEM-ORIENTED MEDICAL RECORD

An alternative to traditional charting, with its fragmented source orientation in which categorically parallel records are kept, is the problem-oriented medical record founded by Dr. Lawrence Weed.[8] It is claimed to be scientific, logical, analytical, and consistent. There are four essential parts: the data base, the problem list, plan for each problem by number and title, and progress notes. These four parts are supported by the SOAP process (an acronym for *s*ubjective findings [patient complaints], *o*bjective findings [those made by personnel], *a*nalysis [subjective and objective findings in relationship to each other], and *p*lanning [action contingent on analysis]), and flow or parameter sheets.

The data base is the sum total of the information known about the patient. It must be defined because it will vary according to the patient population and the hospital and its practices [Woody and Mallison[9]]. It consists essentially of the history, physical examination, laboratory and x-ray findings, and a patient profile that is a psychosocial overview of the patient. The data base can be as sophisticated as resources allow, as for example computer testing and history taking [Cononi and Siler[10]], use of trained aides for specific testing, use of professional nurses skilled in primary care, and physicians' assistants.

The complete problem list embraces psychosocial problems as well as those related to the primary and secondary disease conditions. All personnel chart in the same place so that all entries are easily found. This brings greater interprofessional activity and thought to the patient's care.

The SOAP process as a technique for dealing with problems gives the necessary structure, if one becomes habituated to it, that provides stability and uniformity in both considering and recording a problem.

Flow or parameter sheets replace many repetitive entries in nursing notes. The graphic sheet is an illustration of a flow sheet, as is any arrangement for recording periodic observations or findings for both ease of recording and ease of visualizing the data.

Feinstein,[11] in a critique of the problem-oriented system, says that good medical records have always been problem oriented and proposes rather that this system is problem structured. He likes the totality found in the patient profile and admires the effort in the direction of patient education. However, he finds illusory the claim to continuity of patient care, claiming that medical specialization is too pervasive to be overcome by a recording system. He goes on to say that the fragmentation that is lamented in source charting remains present in the problem-oriented chart too. He also points out the time involved in record keeping in this system and questions its justification. Apparently much supervision is required to introduce this system.

If problem-oriented charting can bring cogent nursing data (interspersed with that of others) back to the chart, it would be justified. One can only wonder what equally concerted effort to revitalize traditional nurse charting would produce. It seems somehow fallacious to compare an admittedly devitalized method with a new and vibrant one. One thing is clear: nurses' notes need strengthening, as does the nursing care from which they flow. Concerted probing and effort are required because the quality of the record will be no better than the quality of the care given.

REFERENCES

1. Do your memos and reports sound artificial? Hospital Supervision 7(17):1-2, 1974.
2. Brock, L.: Do your memos confuse or communicate? Supervisory Management 19(9):18-21, 1974.
3. Williamson, J.: Prescription for report writing; leadership on the job, New York, 1957, American Management Association, pp. 82-84.
4. Warstler, M.: Some management techniques for nursing service administrators, J. Nurs. Admin. 2(6):29-30, 1972.
5. Detman, A.: Will anyone read your annual report? United Air Lines Mainliner 18(3):25-27, 1974.
6. Nursing service—improved nursing notes procedure, Santa Ana, Calif., 1964, Commission for Administrative Services in Hospitals.
7. Walker, V., and Selmanoff, E.: A study of the nature and uses of nurses' notes, Nurs. Res. 13(2):113-121, 1964.
8. Weed, L. L.: The problem-oriented record as a basic tool, Chicago, 1970, Year Book Medical Publishers, Inc.
9. Woody, M., and Mallison, M.: The problem-oriented system for patient-centered care, Am. J. Nurs. 73(7):1170, 1973.
10. Cononi, G., and Siler, M.: Automated multiphasic health testing in a hospital setting, J. Nurs. Admin. 2(6):70-80, 1972.
11. Feinstein, A.: The problems of the problem-oriented medical record, Nurs. Digest 1(9):36-44, 1973.

CHAPTER 12
BUDGETING

The relatively recent use of budgeting in nursing services and the hospital industry parallels the newness of formal administration and application of its concepts in hospital and nursing operations. The nonprofit nature of the hospital and the uniqueness of its services have tended to permit the continuance of nonbusinesslike practices long since denied the general business community.

There is a concerted growing effort to bring standard business practices and procedures into the hospital, supported by expanding, sophisticated consumerism that demands fiscal accountability by hospitals for soaring costs. This effort is culminating in state legislative action in the form of state hospital commissions to review hospital rate increases and develop uniform accounting systems.[1] Inclusion of productivity as well as rate review is sometimes sought by such commissions. Impetus is also being given to budgeting and accounting by the federal government through its Medicare program, more stringent controls on hospital building and renovation, and comprehensive health planning programs.

Economic theory that categorizes and examines industries contributes to the fiscal responsibility of the hospital. Knowledge of tertiary industries that include services of all kinds can throw important light on hospitals as economic units in this classification, because we are part of the larger national economy. The more we know of economic theory, the more constructively we can operate within the sphere of its applications and contribute to it.

Inside influences also foster the increase of sound business practices in financial management. There are growing numbers of prepared personnel found in all categories in the hospital enterprise and evidence of improved practices deriving from increasingly competent managers.

Items and issues that have lain dormant and obscure are being exteriorized and examined by budget procedures. The cost of nursing care is a good example. Because the payroll is such a large portion of both the hospital and nursing budgets, there is considerable effort being made to free nurses of long-standing accretions to their work so that they can practice well-delineated nursing care. The compilation and study of nursing hours, patient classification for time determination of nursing care, and all such efforts contribute to the elaboration of nursing costs.

There is growing recognition that nursing must be considered an independent service rather than immersed in room-and-board charges. Kovener[2] speaks of the need to make routine nursing charges explicit so that nursing is reimbursable, as are services of other professionals. By so doing, the consumer is made aware of a concrete nursing component of hospital care. Nursing care certainly generates as well as consumes income; it needs to be reckoned specifically and entered as such on both sides of the ledger. Germain[3] reiterated this need when she predicted that we will eventually get to the point of charging specific amounts for specific components of nursing care. Keller[4] addresses the submergence of nursing in general hospital costs with the expectation that nursing practice will become more visible and accountable in the hospital as a result of the work of nurses in independent, private practice outside the hospital.

Patient classification systems and nursing hours, numerically determined for staffing purposes, should be convertible to a reimbursement scale on their categorical bases. An alternate method would be a base rate for routine services such as bathing, bed making, observation of temperature-pulse-respiration, supervision, and coordination, to which would be added specific charges for care of incontinent patients, frequent observation, and all treatments, medications, and services on an itemized individualized basis. Fee for service may be closer than we think. Definitive, itemized nursing care would do much to refine the nursing care itself and its reflection in the budgeting process.

THE BUDGET

The budget is a concrete, precise picture of the total operation of an enterprise in monetary terms. It is comprehensive and shows interdepartmental relationships. It underpins and melds all elements of the administrative process and the parts of the hospital enterprise. Budgeting is really management by objectives on a large scale. Morever, it shows the value system and priorities to which the enterprise commits itself.

Public opinion has been most expressive in relation to these hospital value systems and priorities. There is a consistent flow of factual data in the popular press that addresses itself to such values and priorities, and much of these data have strong budgetary implications.

Kelly[5] states that only about 40% of pediatric beds in the country are used, that only 3% of hospitals equipped to do open-heart surgery use such facilities more than four times weekly, and that cardiac-monitoring units are excessive in number. On the positive side, the account notes institutions where values and priorities reflect budgetary concern: Long Beach Hospital in California has rooms at $20 a day for such procedures as minor surgery; Albany Medical Center in New York uses its operating rooms and laboratory services 24 hours a day, 7 days a week; and Baptist Memorial Hospital in Memphis utilizes minimal care units, though such units are perhaps not uncommon.

Keeping abreast of this flow of factual data is not only immensely informative, budgetarily and otherwise, but also provides formalized consumer input. It should give professionals pause to realize the extent to which they are dependent on the popular press for such information.

There are essentially two kinds of budgets. Operating, or planning, budgets are most commonly used and involve the nursing department. Financial budgets show projections, origin, and disposition of funds and working capital and are used primarily by the hospital administrator and his fiscal staff. Even in this area the knowledgeable director of nursing can provide input and contribute to long-range plans and policies. The more fiscally competent the nurse managers are, the more their influence will be felt in overall hospital policy. Competence in operating budgets, however, usually precedes input into hospital financial budgets and is given higher priority.

Effective budgeting requires an organizational structure that provides clear-cut authority and responsibility, an accounting system that provides appropriate and current data, interested and supportive top and middle management, and a budgeting system appropriate for the particular needs of the enterprise.[6]

There is usually one administrative officer, often the controller, who assumes overall responsibility for the budget by setting the schedule, providing the forms, guiding and advising department heads, assembling and finalizing the budget, monitoring its progress during the fiscal year to identify variances (departures from the operating budget) when they occur, and seeing to the examination, correction, or compensation of these variances, in concert with the appropriate department head.

EXECUTION OF THE BUDGET

The budget falls into two large parts: broad, philosophical, goal-oriented deliberation; and conversion of such deliberations to concrete, systematized, numerical data that result in the final budget. Final approval of the budget is usually made by those ultimately responsible, the governing board. There can and should be projections beyond one fiscal year for continuity of plans and operations and amortization of very costly items.

Prior deliberations are made by department heads, who together review the objectives and their achievement, long-range plans, new directions in service, personnel, plant, equipment, and so forth. These deliberations facilitate organizational equilibrium and encourage the cooperation and give-and-take necessary for good interdepartmental working in terms of integration, correlation, and parallel functioning. For example, the move to a complete unit-dose system of medication, in which the pharmacy assumes almost all responsibility for medication, requires that nursing and pharmacy adjust personnel requirements accordingly. Likewise, a shift from the nursing in-service program to hospital-wide service requires budgetary adjustment and synchronization. The clearer the view of the precise nature of nursing and the nursing department, the more one can contribute to such interdepartmental deliberations and protect the interests of nursing in this arena.

Interdepartmental deliberations require comparable intradepartmental deliberations for the same assessment of objectives, long-range plans, and new directions in service, personnel, plant, equipment, and so forth. For example, strengthening one clinical service or specialty by additional personnel, increased preparation of present personnel, or new equipment may require maintenance of the status quo or retrenchment in other clinical services.

Such considerations should reach down to the unit level for both input and collaboration. Involvement of all levels is important, so that the planning and controlling of the operation are in a sense shared by the workers (Myer's concept). Likewise, the Scanlon plan, in which there is not only participation of workers in planning and controlling but also financial remuneration on a share basis, flourishes where there is staff involvement in such deliberations. Budgets, because of their generalized yet specified components, are important vehicles for any participatory incentive plan.

PERSONNEL PORTION OF THE BUDGET

From broad deliberations one moves to the concrete: the actual numbers of various categories of nursing personnel necessary to meet the nursing needs of the projected patient population. Unless the budget is for a new institution or service, the last year's figures provide a base for examination and proposed alteration. The current staffing pattern also will yield the necessary base for a projected budget. Usually, each department is given a list or print-out of all personnel assigned to it, with the necessary computed figures for reckoning holiday, vacation, and sick time; and necessary explanation of terms (for example, full-time equivalent that facilitates reckoning of part-time personnel). One must know how many unfilled positions there are and how they are covered currently. Personnel policies have a profound effect on the budget, influenced as they are by third-party input, prevailing conditions in the locality and region, and their own internal sophistication. For example, the number of days allowed annually for educational and personal use alters the budget.

Wage and salary administration plays an important part in budgeting for the personnel needs of the institution. Are there comparative analyses and justification for salary ranges among department heads, for the responsibility factor between unit managers and head nurses, or between nursing and dietary or physiotherapy aides, and for the tension factor between critical care, operating room, and general medical-surgical nursing personnel? Is compensated lateral progression provided in an effort to keep nurses as staff nurses?

The general nursing payroll has separate categories other than clinical and administrative, such as the staff of the in-service department. A survey of in-service programs in 814 hospitals and nursing homes found a wide range in budgets, from under $10,000 to over $100,000, with an average of $38,400. Sixty percent of those reporting operate with their own budget.[7] Another category is research and development, an important and growing endeavor in hospitals. There is an estimate that 3% to 5% of income should be allocated to it. The nursing department should know in actual and budgetary terms what proportion of its own or other staff or consultant time is devoted to such activity.

There are budgeted items in direct support of the payroll part of the budget, such as advertising used in recruitment, convention and conference fees, meals and transportation for personnel attending professional meetings, parking facilities, consultant services, and recreation.

EQUIPMENT AND INVENTORY MAINTENANCE

Equipment takes a large section of the budget. Budgeted items consist of projected new, replacement, or additional pieces of equipment, amortization of those already procured but not completely paid for, and charges for service to existing equipment. (This latter item might alternatively be included in the engineering budget.) When such items exceed a predetermined figure, they are given individual consideration. This section of the budget is increasingly important and expensive as equipment grows in sophistication and quantity, paralleling technological advances. Less expensive improvisations should not be overlooked in budgetary control.

Because smaller equipment and supplies (treatment trays, thermometers, syringes, and needles) are increasingly centralized, the budget for central supply becomes substantial, though centralization enhances budgetary control. The phenomenal increase in disposable equipment and supplies also greatly affects the budget and makes close scrutiny necessary to determine the economy of disposables over nondisposables in budgetary considerations. Centralization facilitates such scrutiny.

Precise and specific inventories are valuable adjuncts to the budget. If checked routinely and periodically, they show utilization and replacement figures from which future needs can be ascertained. When compared with figures that reflect changing conditions such as new procedures, expanding services, and tightened administrative practice, inventory figures provide a stable base from which to estimate additions and subtractions where necessary. Efficient and spacious storage methods greatly assist in inventory maintenance.

Simple record keeping for inventories provides better accuracy and conservation of time. The nursing service that maintains stocked supply shelves in each unit, with replacement service twice daily, illustrates a simplified recording system. As an item is used, an attached gummed sticker is placed in a card file, which shows charges made and facilitates replacement, for inventory maintenance.

Stationery supplies are another substantial part of the supply budget.

FINANCIAL INCENTIVES

There are isolated beginnings of efforts, which have immediate and continuing budgetary implications, to use financial incentives to increase productivity and conserve materials. Two concerted efforts are the employee financial incentive programs of Memorial Hospital Medical Center of Long Beach, California, and Baptist Hospital in Pensacola, Florida [Jehring[8]].

The plan in Long Beach consists of a fund to which employees contribute regularly. Annual savings to the hospital that result from improved use of labor and supplies over the preceding year are contributed to the fund and are held in trust for employees until they leave the hospital's employ. The accounting procedure and formula are very precise and sophisticated. The program originated in 1961, and by 1969 the amounts contributed by the hospital and employee savings exceeded $3 million, of which over $240,000 was paid to employees.

The Baptist Hospital program operates departmentally and consists of monthly cash bonuses for each member of a department where productivity exceeds preestablished norms. The productivity figures include man-hours and supplies. The procedure was carefully designed and executed and is precise and sophisticated.

A third possible financial incentive [Sand and Berni[9]] describes an experimental attempt to show whether a financial incentive would improve the quality of nursing care specifically. The goal was to increase patient socialization and activities in the nursing home setting. Criteria for goal achievement were posted, explained, and reinforced through discussion. The observation method was used. It was a terminal project of three weeks, and aides and patients received a total of $122.00.

The above plans provide concrete examples of arithmetical evaluations and estimations of the work performed and supplies conserved in hospitals and nursing homes, demonstrating not only the possibility but the benefits of such efforts in increasing or perfecting employee output. They reinforce the use of budgeting, cost accounting, and cost containment in reducing hospital costs or getting increased or improved service for the same cost. Such plans also strengthen the measurement component of all services, including nursing. They increase the involvement of personnel in the operation of the enterprise in a meaningful way.

An older incentive device is merit pay for exceptional performance, but it is sometimes confused with periodic automatic pay increases for satisfactory performance. It is unpopular because it smacks of elitism and of a time when there were no uniform and systematized salary schedules. There still may be a place for monetary compensation for those performing beyond the call of duty or for exceptionally high-quality performance; for example, bonuses may be given. Such incentives can properly be raised in budgetary considerations.

ECONOMIC WASTE

Bluestone[10] speaks of two kinds of economic waste in health care institutions. She labels as concrete waste that which derives from the poor use of supplies and equipment, lost or stolen equipment, or careless use of electricity. By contrast, "fluff waste" derives from poor organization and improper use of facilities for patients. Such waste is carried over into the budget. There must be constant vigilance in reducing waste. She offers some pithy advice: do not assume that quality nursing care is tied exclusively to finances, for to do so may be illusory; and know enough about fiscal matters so that the activities of others, including fiscal officers, can be monitored and contribute to planning for use of available resources.

ADVANTAGES OF BUDGETING

As long ago as 1957, Young[11] promoted the nursing service budget as a means to cost control, better and more careful planning, a guide for operation, departmental and self-evaluation, source of information and hospital policy review, and financial accounting for the nursing service department. It is equally applicable today. A National League for Nursing survey [Aydelotte[12]] showed that only nursing services in hospitals with 300 or more beds (at least 50% of respondents) submitted and administered annual budgets for personnel, supplies, equipment, and other expenses. Nursing services of 200-299 beds submitted budgets for personnel only. The same survey[12] showed unfilled budgeted positions, ranging from 3.8% to 8.5% [p. 40]. The greatest number of unfilled budgeted positions were in the RN classification [pp. 41-42].

Fiscal expertise and competence are the order of the coming day. The budget is the major vehicle for fiscal activity and involvement.

REFERENCES

1. Hospital agency created, Vancouver, Wash., The Columbian, March 27, 1973.
2. Kovener, R.: The twenty-five-cent aspirin, Nurs. Forum **6**(4):399-402, 1967.
3. Germain, L.: Determining the cost of nursing care; myth or reality? National League for Nursing News **21**(6):13, 1973.
4. Keller, N.: Letters, J. Nurs. Admin. **4**(4):8, 1974.
5. Kelly, J.: Our $125-a-day hospitals; where does all that money go? Family Weekly, September 29, 1974, pp. 4-6.
6. Managing the budget function; studies in business policies, National Industrial Conference Board, Inc., no. 131, 1970.
7. Profile of a training director, Nurs. Outlook **22**(6):393, 1974.
8. Jehring, J.: Motivational problems in the modern hospital, J. Nurs. Admin. **2**(6):39-41, 1972.
9. Sand, P., and Berni, R.: An incentive contract for nursing home aides, Am. J. Nurs. **74**(3):475-477, 1974.
10. Bluestone, N.: One course Sue Barton never took; health care economics, J. Nurs. Admin. **3**(6):24-28, 1973.
11. Young, E.: The nursing service budget #22, New York, 1957, National League for Nursing, pp. 14-15.
12. Aydelotte, M.: Survey of hospital nursing services, New York, 1968, National League for Nursing, p. 40.

PART III

ADJUNCTS TO NURSING SERVICE ADMINISTRATION

CHAPTER 13
IN-SERVICE EDUCATION

In the last two decades, there have been great strides in in-service education. Directors of in-service education are now present almost universally in nursing services. Though it is the most commonly recommended corrective agent for problems and faults plaguing nursing services, it must be remembered that in-service education has limits and is not a panacea for all ills. General education, of which in-service is part, is the hope for helping all people to develop their job potential and to become knowledgeable citizens, family members, friends, and co-workers.

In-service education is the vehicle by which goals and the multiple articulated means available to achieve them can be explored. It can be used to consider and solve problems; institute and advance new learning; elicit, analyze, and systematize individual ideas for group, individual, or institutional betterment; develop the idea of the hospital as another community agency; and struggle to understand ourselves, others, and the inherent relationships.

CONTINUING EDUCATION AND IN-SERVICE EDUCATION

Continuing education consists of all opportunities and facilities for personal and professional growth outside of formal education programs that lead to degrees or certification (though it should be remembered that degrees and certification have eventually been achieved through continuing education).

In-service education is the part of continuing education that is carried on within the work environment and provided by the employing organization to enhance workers' knowledge, skills, and attitudes so that they may continually improve the quality of service or care they provide to patients. Staff development is a term sometimes used interchangeably with in-service education, though it is broader in that it includes educational experiences extraneous to, though possibly supported by, the institution. Responsibility for continuing education resides with the individual, who either uses the opportunities available or not, whereas responsibility for in-service education rests with the enterprises in which the workers are employed.

In both continuing and in-service education, workers should help formulate the opportunities, because participatory planning is necessary to ensure that the needs and operational input of the workers are present. Apropos of this essential participation of the learner, Knowles[1] suggests involving them in the teaching too, which leads to cooperative pursuit of learning and self-diagnosis as participants evaluate what they have learned and where related needs will direct them. The needs and characteristics of adulthood, essentially the making of choices constituting self-direction, with direct and indirect consequences, abound in continuing education. They should be recognized and respected. Ortega y Gasset[2] points out that need, rather than desire, is the requisite to learning. In-service education benefits from the theory and knowledge of adult education, as does continuing education of which it is a part.

Drucker[3] notes that, though the huge structure of formal education militates against the centrality of continuing education, our economic structure supports such centrality. Because costs of education are so high, students are forced to acquire their learning in stages over long periods of time, thus providing the shift to continuing education within the regular academic structure. At least one college (Marylhurst) has made such a conversion from an academic liberal arts college to an education center dedicated to lifelong learning [McDermott[4]].

INVOLVEMENT OF PROFESSIONAL ORGANIZATIONS

Continuing education is so important a vehicle for professional and personal growth that the American Nurses' Association has a special section for people engaged in directing continuing education and is deliberating at all levels on whether continuing education should be tied to continuation or renewal of licensure. Enthusiasts of mandatory continuing education tied to licensure think this will hasten the day when there is clear-cut progress in the nursing care of patients. Those opposed to mandatory licensure deplore its rigidity and think that nurses have availed themselves of educational opportunities and will continue to do so. They see the problem as one of providing more and better opportunities to all nurses wherever they are and providing some structure for evaluation of effectiveness, as well as overall structure where none exists. Moreover, it is thought that duress to involve the nurse in continuing educational opportunities hinders rather than encourages growth.

In 1972 the American Nurses' Association voted to endorse voluntary continuing education. It has accepted the program developed by the National Task Force on the Continuing Education Unit of the National University Extension Association. Continuing education unit (CEU) is defined as 10 contact hours of participation in an organized continuing education experience under conscientious sponsorship, capable direction, and qualified instruction.[5]

The National League for Nursing has issued a statement (February 1974) with guidelines for the development of continuing education programs in nursing that support the ANA position.

Five states (California, Colorado, New Hampshire, New Mexico, and South Dakota) provide for evidence of continuing education in their nurse practice acts. In 1973 twelve states were considering bills to make continuing education a requirement for relicensure.[6] Additionally, nurses are collecting certificates of attendance, keeping records of their educational activities, and thinking about and participating more in such offerings.

These are the beginnings of national and state formalized structures that will account for better-evaluated offerings more systematically proffered and formulated. Wisconsin could serve as a model because of the efforts of Signe Cooper and her colleagues in a state where continuing education is deemed important and systematic continuing education for nurses has been offered for a long time. The state has consistently employed innovative as well as standard techniques and methods.

It is not accidental that Mrs. Cooper was the director of a project to explore continuing education needs and possibilities in five north central states (Michigan, Minnesota, Montana, North Dakota, and Wisconsin). A report by Cooper and Byrns[7] points out that the lack of planning in continuing education in nursing has resulted in "scattered, fragmented, inadequately planned and poorly conducted continuing education offerings" in which there is uneven geographic and subject coverage, accompanied by poor use of educational resources. It recommends a broad program to get the greatest involvement at all points, by means respectful of conservation of faculty and systematized offerings coordinated centrally in order to structure the present randomness. It speaks to the need for guidance and help in assessing individual needs and recommends special attention to the following:

a. Geriatric nursing
b. Application of new technologies to nursing practice
c. Principles of mental health applied to all areas of nursing practice
d. Principles of rehabilitation and teaching of patients (including positive health teaching)
e. Nursing care in emergency and ambulatory care settings
f. Patient assessment*

The findings of this landmark report by a national expert in continuing education, based in a state that excels in continuing education and grounded in personal contact with large numbers of affected nurses, has not only regional and national implications but is of value for in-service programs for nurses everywhere who are searching for internal and external enrichment of their programs.

PLACE OF IN-SERVICE EDUCATION IN THE ENTERPRISE

The nursing in-service education staff must know how they will articulate their work with similar work within the hospital as a whole, so that there will be economy of resources and effort. An example of such articulation is the historical development of orientation programs, which often began in nursing departments. Subsequently, budding personnel departments and payroll offices were asked to provide information, usually about paychecks and related matters. As personnel departments grew, they assumed some responsibility for at least that part of orientation dealing specifically with their work. In some cases the personnel department took over the responsibility for general orientation, while departmental orientation continued to be conducted by personnel in each department. This transition from nursing responsibility to shared responsibility to delegated departmental responsibility illustrates appropriate division of work and respects all departments. For the most part, however, nursing departments pioneered in-service education in hospitals. It often happens that the in-service function in nursing serves as the model or actually moves into hospitalwide in-service education, which also accounts for the number of nurses who carry out this function for the hospital.

In-service coordinators or directors are staff persons, responsible for the overall direction of in-service education and accountable to the director of nursing. They cannot command, but must work out content, participation, and so forth, with line personnel. Line personnel (and indeed all personnel) are represented by an advisory committee responsible for advising and assisting the in-service director and assistants.

Personnel departments may assume or be delegated responsibility for ongoing programs in which nurses and other workers participate. These may deal with safety, disaster, the role of the hospital as a community agency, regional planning, accreditation, new services, and incorporation of mental health concepts, to mention only a few possibilities. There is a need, too, for such institutionwide programs to increase interdepartmental appreciation and understanding. An interesting account of an ongoing management program using in-house staff working with a training director illustrates this sharing and its good effects on interdepartmental relations [Goldenberg[8]]. Day-long sessions in off-site workshops for hospital supervisory personnel, conducted by various groups, are effective and give evidence of interdepartmental collaborative growth.

An advisory committee, representative of all levels of workers so that the views and opinions of all can be channeled into deliberations, is important. Nursing and hospital in-service programs can operate independently but collaboratively, but the trend is toward hospitalwide programs.

The in-service staff and advisory committee will be concerned about providing diversified educational opportunities geared to self-directing adults, to meet the

---
*From Cooper, S., and Byrns, H.: A plan for continuing education in nursing in five north central states, Madison, Wis., 1973, Department of Nursing, University of Wisconsin Extension, p. 1.

appraised needs of these adults in an organized, imaginative, and educational way. More important, it will foster a learning climate that will nurture self-development, improve the readiness factor of the workers, and set the stage for openness. In such a learning climate, ideas are encouraged and thought exciting; people are urged to question and try other ways; change is not obsessive, but subjected to scrutiny of the new and old to avoid the "bandwagon" pitfall; people feel a part of the health team not only locally but abroad; reading is encouraged and promoted by easily accessible wide-ranging materials; seizing the moment to see, hear, and explore is commonplace; and field trips and use of library services are standard operating procedure.

Inherent in a good learning climate is a sense of sharing, a kind of collegiality in which all are participants. These factors underlie the motivation of workers to learn. A climate of this kind is difficult to achieve, because the pressure of work militates against it. There is also the societal disdain for the intellectual life, shown by the dilution of the academic side of general education, the growing number of nonreaders, and the national decline in I.Q. test scores.

DETERMINING WORKER NEEDS

Determining needs for in-service education is an essential and ongoing job. It is difficult, because diagnosis of needs of self or the enterprise is related to self- and enterprise awareness and requires breadth and depth of vision and perception and a clear view of goals of the institution and societal factors, among other factors. There are essentially two kinds of needs: felt needs and those proposed by individuals, which range from impromptu thinking to carefully thought out needs. Improving the quality or method of determining felt needs is an educational activity in itself. If personnel are asked about such needs by questionnaire, group meeting, or interview, the collected findings need group review to mesh, distill, elaborate, explore, or otherwise clarify these needs of individuals. Group review of findings is an exercise in analytic thinking, not only for the staff and advisory committee but for all personnel. Moreover, such review may be a means of reconciling felt needs with observed needs, or those needs seen by others such as management personnel in nursing, clinical specialists, and outside observers (professionals, lay people, and consumers). With adroit leadership, the partially recognized or stated and random or isolated felt need may be brought into partnership with other needs and thus channeled into a more comprehensive set of needs. Caution must be exercised to ensure that such deliberations embrace both kinds of needs so that they do not end up as observed needs only; this would be prejudged manipulation, a violation of the staff's right to contribute.

Improved communication is a felt need often expressed by nurses. It requires group exploration and analysis to discover what people think it means, what it actually means, how the lack is manifested, and what the bad effects are, before learning opportunities can be formulated to correct the diffuse notion of communication.

This kind of intermediate stage, that is, between collection of findings and plans for meeting them, is an excellent place to introduce ground rules for the general conduct of the in-service program. For example, methods of problem solving can be used for reduction of gross data (the collected findings of felt and observed needs) to a synthesized, structured list. An interesting correlation exists between problems and needs. Problems are things done improperly, incompletely, or not at all. Needs are things that must be understood and resolved in order to eliminate problems.[9] Application of problem solving at this point might produce not only the desired list but a collateral benefit in terms of suggested improvements in standard procedures and policies in the organization. Such an exercise illustrates the complemental nature of in-service education and administrative-clinical practices. Distinguishing between the two is essential because it allows more precise and effective use of each. Discussion at this intermediate stage might point out the need to review the reporting structure in operation—an administrative function—as well as the need to explore general communication theory or patient-personnel communication—an in-service function.

Another useful ground rule is the application of the platonic dialectic structure to tighten and give form to all deliberations. It consists essentially of movement from names to definition to examples to understanding and, if used consistently, circumscribes the discussion, deliberation, or argument in such a way that clarity prevails. It helps to keep relationships discernible, thus reducing diffusion. It also keeps tangential thinking in its place: not suppressed, but tabled for future use.

A related ground rule is what Schwab[10] calls habits of mind, or response to other people's points of view; response to their problems and how they are expounded, rather than to conclusions; and response to others' problems, first in their terms, then in related terms, and finally by suggestions and collaborative pursuance of related problems.

Decisions about the in-service program and its priorities can be made only after determination of felt needs; reconciliation of them with observed needs insofar as possible; weighing of the composite list against the literature, the experiences of others, the current major health concerns, or the position of the enterprise in its pursuit of excellence; and review of the problems involved.

Medearis and Popiel propose a significant list of questions for determining training needs, aimed at systematically studying personnel performance:

1. How well does the patient understand what's happening to him?
2. How well coordinated is the patient's care?
3. Is each employee adequately prepared to perform his functions?
4. Does he understand the nursing care standards?
5. Are there any such standards defined in nursing service and within specific units?
6. How well prepared are team leaders to handle the interpersonal relations of their team?
7. What resources are not being utilized?
8. How are nurses prepared for supervisory and acting positions?
9. How does in-service education relate to these problems?*

Knowles speaks about the steps involved in the diagnosis of learning needs:

1. Identifying a model of desired competencies.
2. Assessing our present level of achievement of these competencies.
3. Identifying the gaps between where we are now and where we want to be. These gaps are our needs as learners, and the concrete experiencing of such gaps by the learner is the best functional definition of motivation to learn.†

It is easy to see similarities in the thinking of Medearis and Popiel and Knowles: both defined standards and modes of desired competencies are elaborated clear views of comprehensive nursing care and appropriate administrative behavior. There are also strong similarities to Cooper's list of needs, in which five are concerned with the concept of comprehensive nursing care and two with administration.

In 1956 Donovan[11] suggested such a beginning point for in-service education, that is, a concerted effort to study and implement comprehensive nursing care and appropriate administrative behavior at the precise point along a continuum where the nursing service is at the time.

If such standards, models, and suggestions are centered for attention and seen in relation to summarized, synthesized felt-observed needs and to the current state of the enterprise—all clearly coordinated and integrated—a realistic starting or restarting point in in-service education has been reached. The more visible and understood the many relationships in-

---

*From Medearis, N., and Popiel, E.: Guidelines for organizing inservice education, J. Nurs. Admin. 1(4):30, 1971.
†From Knowles, M.: Gearing adult education for the seventies, Journal of Continuing Education in Nursing 1(1):11-16, 1970.

volved, the firmer the base and the clearer the objectives, priorities, and articulating parts of a comprehensive in-service program.

CENTRALIZATION AND DECENTRALIZATION

Cooper and Hornback [p. 181][12] note the need for both centralized and decentralized programs, operating simultaneously, so that in addition to the servicewide centralized program under the direction of the in-service staff, there will be ongoing unit(s) programs serving those particular staffs. They view these decentralized efforts as means of maintaining spontaneity, interest, and enthusiasm.

Berni and Fordyce[13] recommend that formal classes be arranged that are easily accessible to the ward. They suggest a revolving continuing education schedule that would be helpful to new nurses and provide review for others. Programs should be periodically updated "in order to positively reinforce the experienced nurse's continued participation." Reinforcement is central to behavior modification and in-service education: improving nursing skills is related to if not consonant with modifying behavior by appropriate reinforcements.

Decentralized programs encourage more general participation because of the closeness of staff relationships and physical proximity. Additionally, the small-group experiences of decentralized activities afford practice opportunity for participation in group deliberations. Another advantage of the decentralized program accrues to the evening and night staffs, because with some assistance they can plan and execute programs for themselves independent of other shifts and of the in-service staff.

All decentralized programs should be reported centrally so that the total record can be maintained. Moreover, those involved in decentralized programs should have access to centralized personnel for help in getting equipment and materials, as well as for purposes of coordination.

ELEMENTS OF IN-SERVICE PROGRAMS
Personnel

A staff must be available to aid the in-service director in carrying out the goals of the department. Personnel for in-service programs come both from within the institution (members with special abilities, interests, or expertise; units willing to present patient conferences for the entire staff; persons from other departments and reports of meetings attended) and from without the institution (resource people from the community, educational personnel, community workers such as health and welfare planning groups, and health and social agency staff members; and from outside the community, such as personnel from state regulatory agencies and those who may be in the area temporarily). In addition to moral support of the nursing service director, the hospital administrator, and the nursing staff, there must be financial resources to cover salaries, secretarial help, equipment, library, and outside assistance. Sharing of expenses between institutions for outside personnel to arrange or conduct in-service programs, either within or outside the institution, is becoming more frequent.

Scheduling

Scheduling of all facets of the in-service program is necessary to keep order in the use of faculty, facilities, equipment, and so forth. Coordination with those in charge of staffing permits the necessary planning to release as many people as possible to attend programs and sufficient backup personnel so that staff will be unharried while they participate. Such scheduling should be widely distributed so that it is well known to staff in advance.

Opportunities for in-service education must be evenly distributed and during on-duty or repaid time. Predictions of slack periods (such as during summer or holiday times) may provide opportunity for scheduling in-service programs. Thought and effort must be given to scheduling programs so that they are readily available to personnel on all shifts. This is especially important for the evening- and night-shift personnel; for far too long in-service programs have been offered during the day shift, which required personnel from other shifts to attend during their off-duty time. Repeating programs for the evening and night shifts is possible more often than we realize, for example, at quiet times such as during visiting hours and at midnight when the night work is well under way, or around 11 PM when both evening and night shifts can be accommodated. Tape recorders, though useful, are not the whole answer for repetition of programs, because personnel on these late shifts deserve the same attention as those on the day shift. We should presume willingness and generosity in asking in-service educators to repeat programs personally. Another group that has been deprived of in-service opportunities is the part-time staff. They too deserve the benefits that will help them to improve their practice. Inclusion of part-time staff is also conducive to cohesiveness.

Types of in-service education

In-service education is usually divided into four parts: orientation, on-the-job training, ongoing education, and executive development. New and growing parts are patient education and incidental teaching.

Orientation. Orientation consists of experiences designed to help the new worker become proficient as soon as possible. It provides for verbal presentation of information; physical tours; time to examine descriptive material, reports, and procedure and policy manuals; and introduction of personnel to the work of the enterprise in general and to the department and the unit in particular. A sufficient length of time should be allotted for absorption of all that is presented. Orientation is usually accompanied by a checklist to ensure completeness. It may be individualized to meet specific worker needs that are not provided for in the general program.

On-the-job training. On-the-job training is a miniature and simplified nursing arts program, including supervised clinical practice, that provides auxiliary workers such as nurses' aides, nursing assistants, and orderlies with the knowledge and skills necessary to do their jobs. Some junior colleges and high schools provide such training, not for the needs of hospitals and nursing homes primarily, but to move marginally employable persons into service positions. Because it is often more economical and efficient to prepare personnel centrally, training may be purchased for new employees by hospitals or nursing homes in lieu of providing their own training programs. There are even large institutions that provide no on-the-job training for auxiliary workers, because they are able to find sufficient numbers of personnel who have been trained in community colleges or elsewhere [Sauer[14]]. Additionally, neighboring institutions are beginning to combine training programs.

There is a lamentable inequity in auxiliary training: nursing home managers complain about bearing the cost of training workers, only to have them move on to hospitals for higher wages. Perhaps there should be some kind of compensation to the training institution or promise of certain length of service after training.

Because there is difficulty in finding nurses who are experienced in such specialties as coronary or intensive care and emergency units, a specialized in-service program of orientation and on-the-job training must be devised to prepare personnel to meet these particular needs. It must be systematized, and staff must be freed to assume responsibility for such training in the special units so that prospective workers will be able to master the necessary skills.

Centralization of such special training is useful and efficient where it can be provided at regional coronary care training centers, demonstration emergency departments, and so forth. The institution must be reimbursed for or donate such instructional staff for this kind of training purpose. Such centralized programs resemble postgraduate courses.

Refresher programs for inactive nurses fall within on-the-job training. Originally, individual hospitals organized and offered these as a means of recruitment, though nurses were not compelled to stay with the particular hospital. Gradually there was a tendency to centralize these programs too, often under the aegis of a state or local chapter of the National League for Nursing or educational institutions. In this regard, one of the recommendations of the University of Wisconsin Extension report,[7] directed to agencies providing nursing service, is noteworthy. It suggests that these agencies offer the use of their educational resources to both inactive nurses in the community and those employed in other institutions. Because many nurses would be interested in availing themselves of the library resources and program offerings of the hospital or public health center near them, these resources could be an important part of the community outreach program of a hospital and would lead to greater involvement of these nurses in the affairs and concerns of nursing, even if they do not return to active work, and would keep the reentry door open.

There are interesting additions to help the inactive nurse remain in touch professionally. A statewide telephone network provides such a service in Wisconsin, including the Nursing Dial Access from which the nurse may hear a 3- to 9-minute discourse from 100 or more nursing tapes and 500 medical tapes, free of charge from any telephone in Wisconsin or for the price of a long-distance call from nurses outside the state [pp. 173 and 204-205].[12]

Refresher courses for inactive nurses are a good example of flexibility in the use of resources. The initial effort is made by a hospital and in turn moves to an educational institution or organization for wider applicability and possible enrichment from more broad and versatile experiences.

Ongoing education. Ongoing education is the most unstructured part of a total in-service program. There is an ever-widening list of means of presentation, but essentially it is attuned to the adult learner who can discriminate among the possibilities on the basis of discerning freedom of choice. Ongoing education programs should consist of parts that contribute to a whole, such as improved clinical performance or management (the essentials of overall goals). Relationships must be kept visible and operating, in order to avoid the pitfalls of randomness, isolation, and dead ends. The more closely these programs relate to current experience, the better the progression for growth.

The study of alcoholism is a case in point. There is tremendous effort in all parts of the community, for example, churches, industry, the media, and financial aid from various sources to bring about improvement in identifying and treating alcoholics and in supporting and using their families therapeutically. Little attention is paid to alcoholism in institutional in-service programs (excepting psychiatric), because these patients are seen in general hospitals only briefly. However, the American Hospital Association has prepared a multimedia program for its member hospitals that is designed for both professional and community use to educate personnel to deal with alcoholism, because many patients admitted to general hospitals have a secondary medical condition attributable to alcoholism.[15]

Several interesting questions arise here. How skilled are we in identifying secondary diagnoses and aiding the physician in this pursuit? What is the range of possibilities in secondary diagnoses? Can they be classified? How obvious, subtle, or obscure are they? What are the ways in which they can be identified? How many have societal implications or are public health related?

In-service education and nursing care of alcoholic patients require that cohesiveness be maintained, relationships be seen, the vast array of contributing parts be kept orderly and productive, and the central goal be preserved while being subjected to multifaceted scrutiny. This is no easy job and requires a sophisticated in-service management program for staffs of member hospitals. Use of materials such as the AHA program is an example of how timely audiovisual matter can fill some in-service program needs or be the medium for extensive enrichment of staff and service to patients by introspection, exploration, collaboration, extension, and integration. The skill of the in-service staff and its advisory committee will determine the degree of effectiveness of such a program. Moreover, such a project can be secured and made more productive if it is accompanied by an institutionwide search for patients with a secondary diagnosis of alcoholism or any other disease.

Universal topics can be developed similarly. The fascination of a 14-year-old girl with the stages of sleep and consequent eye movements (material gleaned from a nursing journal for her science project) reminded one nurse of both the mystery and familiarity of sleep. There is considerable and growing literature to be used in evaluating and analyzing sleep as it applies to the sick under our care or in maintaining the health of others. The assault of the internal and external environment on people's rest and sleep, the thoughtlessness of intrusions on it, the lack of planning to protect it, the possible range of medication schedules, the effect of nursing ministrations or lack of them, and the routinized scheduling of health care facilities all provide fascinating questions about sleep and rest that must be raised, expanded, and considered. Judging from patients' opinions, we are quite remiss and thoughtless about encouraging and protecting this vital part of their lives while they are under our care. There is certainly considerable range in the probing of sleep for an in-service project. It could have immediate application for nursing care and provide ongoing improvement in understanding and refinement of that care.

In the early days of in-service education, diseases and new drugs were frequent topics of physicians' lectures. Some said these choices stemmed from the gross limitation of nurses. These topics are still discussed, because we have found that the more clinically competent nurses are, the more they know about the clinical condition and are able to keep abreast of medication today. However, the expansion of the nursing component of patient care has made such topics adjuncts to or frameworks for nursing care, rather than the sole or major consideration they once were.

Demonstration of new equipment, nursing or patient care conferences, and programs to prepare for the introduction of a new service or specialty are among the many practices and possibilities for ongoing in-service education.

Executive development. All efforts of an ongoing program to develop management skills is a first step in executive development. There are growing opportunities for nurse managers to take part in executive training provided to hospital managers from all departments. Participation in the group services and deliberations of consulting organizations (for example, CASH and Battelle Northwest) retained by the hospital to assist in improving management and use of in-house staff, including a training director, are now available to nurse managers.

Another medium for executive development is discussion built on selected readings. One such program uses *Supervisory Management,* a journal of the American Management Association, and its companion *Hospital Supervision,* published by AMACOM, a division of the American Management Association, as bases for discussion as well as for personal use of the managers. A minimum structure directs the reading and its application. There are also individual selected experiences for promising personnel as understudies in the organization.

Odiorne [pp. 344-347][16] describes a training plan in behavioral and specific terms for increasing the delegation factor

for supervisors:
1. Description of the supervisors—supervisors as successful engineers and technicians raised to the supervisory level
2. Evidence of this need to increase the delegation factor—supervisors doing the work themselves, little coaching or instructing actions observed, and reports omitted, delayed, or done at home
3. Desired outcomes—supervisors doing less than 10% of the work of subordinates; supervising, directing, and coaching; preparing reports during the workday
4. Results to be shown—productivity increase, turnover reduced by 20%, work of subordinates increased, release of supervisory time by 50%, reports in on time, and improved decision making and reporting time by 20%
5. Results to be demonstrated by ratio delay studies (random sampling technique)—frequency rate of late reports, including those delayed at the supervisory level

Patient education. The newest component of in-service education is patient teaching, one of the weakest parts of the practice of comprehensive nursing care. By centralizing it under the direction of the in-service staff, material and format can be assembled and used in either an individualized or collective way, with considerable increase in effectiveness and economy. Such centralization derives from the growing demand to meet the needs of patients for information and knowledge regarding their health and its variations, accompanied by the growing openness of health personnel toward the public and their increasing attention to health.

The Patients' Bill of Rights (see Chapter 4) has no less than half of its parts devoted to the patient's right to know. This further supports the imperative to strengthen patient teaching in all its aspects, essentially clinical but administrative too where items such as bills and fees are involved.

An exciting form of patient teaching is that conducted by Rutgers Medical School in collaboration with two community hospitals.[17] A 1-week period included the following impressive list of offerings: a class for diabetic patients, a series of classes for expectant parents, and nightly preoperative instruction (1 hour for 5 days) via closed circuit television. In addition, hospital staff spent 12 hours teaching high school students about venereal disease, drug abuse, and sickle cell anemia and gave first aid instruction to squads of lifeguards at other points in the community. Two classes were held for the professional staff, dealing with the obstetrics and teen-agers' units. One patient received 1 hour of preoperative and 4 hours of postoperative instruction in colostomy care.

This linkage of patient teaching with the in-service education department has unlimited possibilities for formalizing this fragile component of nursing care. It could eventually be reimbursable, because it makes an explicit, quantifiable contribution to patient care.

Incidental teaching. Because incidental teaching is often impromptu, it is difficult to record and include within the overall program. However, since it is on a one-to-one, -three, or -four basis and is built around a particular patient, procedure, or occurrence, it can contribute substantially to the growth of personnel. Incidental teaching will be richer where personnel are interested enough to see that such opportunities are identified, used, and counted.

OUTSIDE LEARNING EXPERIENCES

Learning experiences beyond the institution, payed for by the institution, are important additions to the inservice program. One point of view contends that such learning opportunities and offerings may be more beneficial than inhouse in-service programs. Because they are offered centrally, they can accommodate all hospitals in an area and therefore are economical, efficient, and provide interinstitutional colleague exchanges, especially if the hospitals are clustered around an academic institution with its many resources. Community colleges, with their strong community-need orientation, are excellent arenas for outside learning experiences, particularly if they have a school of nursing. Supervision and management courses are frequent offerings in such institutions. Yet hospital personnel have been slow to avail themselves of such resources, which frequently are instigated, advised, partially staffed, and used by the business community. Clinical offerings become more and more common. Centralized out-of-house in-service offerings are an intensification and more closely related use of the traditional offerings of such institutions. Scheduling may present problems, but there are increasingly innovative ways of managing it.

Modular instruction units or packages containing readings and audiovisual material, enabling learners to move at their own speed, are adaptable to such centralized in-service education because they allow the flexibility and repetition necessary for busy institutions in releasing and scheduling personnel.

Coordinated opportunities are related to centralized learning opportunities for economy and strengthening of in-service programs. Evans [18] describes such coordinating activities in a large metropolitan area. An audiovisual committee of the in-service and staff-development instructors' group surveys materials and equipment for cooperative use. This group also provides low-cost workshops on a wide variety of fascinating and timely subjects for staff nurses in the area. The collaborative action of in-service directors effectively meeting the collective needs of their constituents is a fine achievement and can serve as a model for collaboration in other localities as well.

Other resources that might be classified as staff development include reduced tuition plans for employees; workshops, institutes, and educational offerings of professional and related organizations at local, state, and national levels; and field trips. Correspondence courses offered by universities are currently in favor and provide excellent opportunities for administrative and clinical self-development of managers.

Because the institution provides such experiences, care should be taken that they result in better nursing care or management. There should be ample opportunity for personnel not only to report to the staff what was learned, but to implement changes that are applicable and can be incorporated. Often acquisition of permanent gains is dependent on further action in the home site or unit situation. Such actions as review of all or selected parts of the content, selection of priority elements or those parts immediately useful, discussion with colleagues, immediate reinforcement of learning by review and discussion and integral or related reading, and immediate action including a plan to bring about specific individual or group attitudinal and performance changes deriving from the learning experiences can contribute to permanent gains. There should be a rotation system, so that all have an opportunity to learn from such experiences. It so often happens that these privileges befall the upper echelons only.

METHODS OF IN-SERVICE EDUCATION

Methods of in-service education grow steadily as the marvels of technology become more available. Audiovisual equipment is continually becoming more diverse and sophisticated [Price[19]]. There is an abundant and growing library of materials to be used with such devices; the American Journal of Nursing Company has an excellent comprehensive listing, and any issue of the quarterly *In-Service Training and Education* is a veritable treasure house of materials.

There are the traditional methods of lecture with discussion and seminars with material assembled and presented by one or more participants, followed by group response and discussion. The nominal group process is a way of structuring group discussion so that more uniform input is secured. Participants are assigned to small groups in which they discusss that part of the total to which they are assigned, followed by listing of ideas addressed to the particular assignment. This is done one at a time and in turn; then each is discussed. This is followed by selecting and listing the key ideas, from which a priority listing is made. Finally, these lists from each small group are presented to the whole group.

Library facilities are invaluable, mainly for independent study and preparation for group work. Ward libraries have always been useful because they are easily accessible. Nursing libraries in hospitals or agencies and hospital libraries that provide nursing materials are becoming more common. Public libraries will increase their permanent collection as requested, and they also provide a wide service through interlibrary loan. The literature is invaluable as a base for group sessions, providing food for deliberation and allowing for the collective wisdom of the group to materialize. Whole issues of journals devoted to a single topic, such as care of the aged and death, lend themselves to such institutional deliberations. National health organizations and the U.S. Government Printing Office provide up-to-date inexpensive clinical information. There is a growing number of journals for patients with diabetes, emphysema, or other conditions, which would be valuable for nursing personnel. Anthologies are valuable for such deliberative beginnings, because they provide opportunities for choices within the direction of a format. Another form of literature that can provide a base for ongoing in-service programs is the growing amount of programmed material for all media. The American Journal of Nursing Company provides an interesting collection of these programmed instructions.[20]

Case studies are yet another valuable base with which to launch in-service programs (see Appendix B). This method encourages growth in attitudes as well as clinical or management skills. The give and take of case-study discussions provides different insights and views as the whole group concentrates on a particular situation.

Pigors and Pigors[21] describe the steps of case analysis as studying the case or incident in advance, finding and organizing the information for facts and underlying considerations, formulating an issue in preparation for decision and action, making decisions and deliberating about them, and then thinking again of the case as a whole for what has been learned. Further work by Pigors, Pigors, and Tribou[22] and Mooth and Ritvo[23] provide excellent background and material for this kind of experience.

Odiorne's [p. vii][16] list of questions to be used for examining cases includes some additional points. He cautions against mixing facts with hunches or biases and suggests setting a priority for identified problems, selecting optional solutions for consideration, considering them in relation to objectives, and developing specific plans for selected solutions. This advice is applicable in any case or incident material.

An excellent compact program [United Hospital Fund of New York][24] for human relations and communication skills was designed for in-service instruction in nursing homes, but is equally applicable to other health care institutions. It is accompanied by a concise, cheerful, and meaty planning guide.

In-service programs can provide an excellent medium for discussion and solution of problems with which nursing staffs are confronted. Division of staff into study groups that meet regularly can make an impressive dent in existing problems, weaknesses, or confusion. Topics, which should be chosen by each group, can deal with visiting hours, optimal conservation of time, intake and output methods, admission notes or interviews, and so forth. Moreover, these choices that grow out of the actual work experience of nurses make study groups reality centered and immediate. It is also advisable that the literature be reviewed to see what ideas and solutions can be gleaned from others.

In an effort to effect change as a result of the learner's experience, some programs are scheduled to allow a time lapse before the final meeting. This permits the learner to assimilate the content of the learning experience, apply it to the work situation, and later share results in a final session of the learning experience. It also applies the pressure we all need to assimilate content and apply it to our work in order to meet the deadline of reporting honestly at the final session. When staff implement what is learned in study groups, this method of in-service education contributes directly to the improvement of the nursing service.

EVALUATION OF IN-SERVICE EDUCATION

Evaluation of in-service education is increasingly important, because it is becoming more expensive and is reflected in patient costs. If it does not serve its purpose—the improvement of the performance of workers so that patient care is improved—it is wasteful.

A small study Skipper and King[25] of a federally funded continuing education program involving 796 participants in 14 separate disciplines showed that nurses feel that continuing education helps their individual practice but not the work situation. This demonstrates the isolation of learning and the inability of the institution to incorporate individual learning into institutional practice. Such incorporation will require step-by-step analysis of learning and integration in the home site by all collaborators in the nursing care. Verbal reports of such learning are not enough if behavior is to be changed by the learning experiences, not only for learners but for their colleagues too.

The Tyler[26] rationale of evaluation is a good base for all concerned with in-service or any other type of education. It proposes that the objectives or outcomes desired from the learning experience be clearly stated, understood, and articulated step by step, so that the degree of consequent learning experience can be evaluated precisely. It is a coherent, logical system, because it demands of the teacher (or whoever is in charge of the learning experiences) such a clear, realistic view of what is to be achieved and the means of achieving it that the learner's acquisition of new or improved performance, knowledge, or attitude will be easily apparent to both teacher and learner.

Specificity is the hallmark of the Tyler rationale. In order to evaluate achievement of an objective, everyone must be thoroughly familiar with it, be able to speak about it easily and in different ways, and see relationships in it if they are to know clearly whether the learning experiences are appropriate and the objective achieved. Moreover, if relationships were more discernible, the fragmentation so often noted could be altered in the direction of integration and coordination. To aid in attaining specificity, review of optimal care of patients with a particular disease entity common to the institution might help because it concentrates the range of comprehensive nursing possibilities on a particular group of patients. Nursing care studies would be valuable in helping the staff to move from the abstract to the concrete in such deliberations. Immersion in broad concepts of nursing definition and their application or nonapplication to current specific care in the institution over a sufficient period of time is necessary to familiarize staff with the possibilities available.

One can see here the need for complete collaboration of the in-service staff and line personnel. The objective must have unified support if it is to have any chance of being achieved, and it must receive reinforcement at every opportunity.

The questionnaire is the most common evaluation device. It is set up in various ways, all designed to elicit the greatest range of responses. It is intended to measure participants' reactions to the offerings for the benefit of the providers, as well as the participants' personal acquisition of knowledge, skills, or attitudes. It is in this latter case that there is considerable lack of certainty about what was in fact acquired from the learning experience. It can range from rather superficial stimulation to deeply rooted acquisitions.

An overall evaluation questionnaire

Rate Your In-Service Education*

( ) Teachers have the major say in determining what their in-service program is to be.

( ) A system for assessing in-service needs of all professional staff is in use.

( ) In-service education is an integral part of program improvement and takes place before any curriculum changes begin.

( ) It is intrinsically satisfying to participants.

( ) Each teacher has the opportunity to learn how to do his job better.

( ) Teachers have the chance to learn from colleagues in the same school or district.

( ) They also have the opportunity to visit schools and teachers in other areas.

( ) The school board sees in-service education as an imperative.

( ) There is opportunity to prepare for career advancement if a teacher wishes.

( ) Administrators have in-service education, too.

( ) The program offers more alternatives than just college courses or workshops.

( ) The resources of nearby teacher education institutions are utilized in planning and implementing in-service programs.

( ) The community understands and supports the need for in-service education.

( ) The school district bears the cost of in-service education for all staff.

( ) There are tangible rewards for in-service growth.

If you have checked every item, LET US HEAR FROM YOU IMMEDIATELY. The professional world should know about you!

If you were able to check only three or four, the students in your community are probably being shortchanged. Your association needs to get busy.

Margaret Knispel, professional associate,
Instruction and Professional Development, NEA.

---

*Also known as staff development, professional development, continuing education, on-the-job training.

Fig. 12. Evaluation form. (From Graves, W.: Rate your in-service education, Today's Education **63**(2):43, 1974.)

from general education that has relevance for nursing points out some essential elements of in-service education: its crucial relationship to practice (curriculum); its need for all personnel, including top levels; its use of available resources, including collegial relationships; and the necessity of its being recognized, systematized, and supported (Fig. 12).

The checklist is also useful where the learning can be itemized, such as in orientation programs that allow for demonstrations and return demonstrations where appropriate.

Written tests are valuable, especially where concrete factual information is involved.

• • •

In-service education is an essential ingredient of the work situation because staff must be given opportunities to learn how to perform optimally. Because it is expensive, all effort must be made applicable and integrated into individual and institutional practice. It must be measurable, specific, and concrete to avoid waste of time, talent, and energy.

REFERENCES

1. Knowles, M.: Andragogy, not pedagogy! Adult Leadership **16**(10):350-352, 1968.
2. Ortega y Gasset, J.: Some lessons in metaphysics, New York, 1969, W. W. Norton & Co., Inc., p. 18.
3. Drucker, P.: What education needs, Continuing Comment (Claremont College Special Academic Programs and Office for Continuing Education), Spring 1973.
4. McDermott, J.: Maryhurst sets lifetime learning goal, Portland, Ore., The Oregonian, June 24, 1974, p. 6.
5. Standards for continuing education in nursing, Kansas City, 1974, American Nurses' Association, p. 9.
6. Thirty-two of 40 states support voluntary C.E. programs, The American Nurse **6**(2):8, 1974.
7. Cooper, S., and Byrns, H.: A plan for continuing education in nursing in five north central states, Madison, Wis., 1973, University of Wisconsin Extension, Department of Nursing, p. 4.
8. Goldenberg, T.: An economical approach to management development, Supervisor Nurse **4**(11):29-37, 1973.
9. United States Civil Service Commission: Training the supervisor, Washington, D.C., 1956, U.S. Government Printing Office, p. 18.
10. Schwab, J.: Backtalk from abroad, University of Chicago Magazine, March-April 1974, p. 12.
11. Donovan, H.: Inservice programs and their evaluation, Nurs. Outlook **4**(11):633-635, 1956.
12. Cooper, S., and Hornback, M.: Continuing nursing education, New York, McGraw-Hill Book Co., pp. 173, 181, and 204-205.
13. Berni, R., and Fordyce, W.: Behavior modification and the nursing process, St. Louis, 1973, The C. V. Mosby Co., pp. 90-91.
14. Sauer, J.: Cost containment—and quality assurance, too. Part I. Hospitals **46**:78-93, 1972.
15. News . . . AHA develops audiovisual program on alcoholism, Nurs. Outlook **22**(4):218, 1974.
16. Odiorne, G.: Personnel administration by objectives, Homewood, Ill., 1971, Richard D. Irwin, Inc., pp. vii and 344-347.
17. The patient education explosion, In-service Training and Education **2**(5):25, 1973.
18. Evans, V.: Continuing education in a metropolitan area, Supervisor Nurse **5**(3):25-29, 1974.
19. Price, A.: The effective use of the multimedia approach to staff development. In Popiel, E., editor: Nursing and the process of continuing education, St. Louis, 1973, The C. V. Mosby Co., pp. 118-127.
20. Catalog, New York, 1974, American Journal of Nursing Co., Educational Services Division, pp. 4-5.
21. Pigors, P., and Pigors, F.: The incident process; a method of inquiring, Nurs. Outlook **14**(10):48, 1966.
22. Pigors, P., Pigors, F., and Tribou, M.: Professional nursing practice cases and issues, New York, 1967, McGraw-Hill Book Co.
23. Mooth, A., and Ritvo, M.: Developing the supervisory skills of the nurse, New York, 1966, Macmillan, Inc.
24. Getting it all together; teaching human relationships and communication skills in nursing homes, New York, 1972, United Hospital Fund of New York.
25. Skipper, J., and King, J.: Continuing education; feedback from the grass roots, Nurs. Outlook **22**(4):252-253, 1974.
26. Tyler, R. W.: Basic principles of curriculum and instruction, Chicago, 1950, University of Chicago Press.

CHAPTER 14
PERSONNEL POLICIES AND CONTRACTS

HISTORY AND TRENDS

Employment agreement is the formal title for arrangements that result in a contract. Though contracts are commonplace in the business world, they are far from common in the health care field. Indeed, their presence at all may be due in greater part to the efforts of outside agencies such as professional associations and unions than to good personnel practice.

Because hospitals are rooted in service, there has been the long-standing notion that one embraces this kind of work for humanitarian reasons. Service is thought to be its own reward, an attitude that stems substantially from the religious origins of health care institutions. Such attitudes have had an inhibiting influence on the entry of the hospital to the modern personnel scene found in industry and other service enterprises such as government.

Long-standing attitudes are difficult to change. Philanthropists and business leaders, who often comprise hospital governing boards, have tolerated inadequate salaries and inferior working conditions in the name of the lofty goal of caring for the sick. It is only recently that wider societal representation is seen on such governing boards. It is hoped that this movement will facilitate appreciation of the need for adequate and equitable compensation and working conditions.

Galbraith[1] speaks succinctly about this fallacious philosophy of service to others being its own reward and resulting in salaries not commensurate either with the job performed or with comparable jobs in the economy. He calls it the "convenient social virtue." Though he sees this phenomenon of partial pecuniary reward as mainly affecting women in general, he speaks of "nurses, custodial personnel and other hospital staff . . . other tasks for the public good—those commonly characterized as charitable works—are also greatly reduced in cost by the convenient social virtue."

In hospitals and nursing there has been an air of secrecy about matters of money, including salaries. Nurses were cautioned not to discuss salary with colleagues, because it was unprofessional. When one dared to be so unprofessional, surprising discrepancies were discovered. Salary schedules arrived late on the hospital scene. Indeed, there are still nurses who think it is unprofessional to secure increased salary and other benefits in an aggressive way such as that employed by the American Nurses' Association and its affiliates.

In support of the "unprofessional" aspect of collective bargaining, Erickson[2] offers cogent arguments that center around the notions of the power struggle and adversary system that are involved. She sees the movement to professional practice issues, after usual items such as salary are secured in bargaining, as a mistake, because they become rigid, reduce professional judgment, and cannot be interpreted appropriately by nonnurses who represent nurses in negotiations. She sees inconsistency between bargaining collectively and the individual responsibility expressed in the 1968 ANA Code of Ethics.

She reports that provision for professional performance committees included in some contracts in California, which provide for discussion with hospital administrators of patient care and professional issues, are not supported by nurses. However, it has been reported that the professional performance committee will remain in a recent contract in California, over opposition of hospital management.[3]

Grand[4] sees an ideological dilemma in the collective bargaining program of nurses. She says that in order to counteract the self-seeking motives of securing higher salaries, contrary to the prevailing Nightingale philosophy of service before economic self-improvement, nurses are obliged to relate better salaries to higher quality nursing care. However, when a nurses' strike in which this relationship between quality of care and salaries had been pointed out, it was found that quality of nursing care was not in fact an issue.

The militancy of nurses' associations and unions has had the greatest effect on salaries and contractual arrangements; yet there is a long way to go before nursing personnel receive compensation appropriate to the degree of compensation and job security found in other fields. The hourly rate for a staff nurse in the highest column for tenure and shift in a northwestern metropolitan hospital in early 1974 was $5.12 an hour, while a journeyman plumber in the same area received $7.68 an hour. This is an interesting comparison when one weighs the educational and experiential differences.

There is still considerable apathy on the part of personnel who stand to gain from protective contractual arrangements. They seem not to appreciate the time, effort, and money expended to get the privilege —or right—of a contract for less fortunate colleagues, nor to appreciate the business soundness of a contract even where working conditions and salaries are good. Such apathy is slowly giving way to involvement in issues arising in the work situation. The Physicians' National House Staff Association (PNHA) is reported to be actively involved in organizing house staffs, in the interest of patient care as well as salaries and working conditions, despite potential opposition from hospital administration.[5]

There has always been opposition to efforts to increase salary and improve working conditions. The history of unionism, as well as that of the American Nurses' Association, is filled with struggle against those in control of the purse strings. This struggle, including reprisals, has been documented over the years in the *American Journal of Nursing*. Efforts in the area of economic security have required courageous, determined, and psychologically strong people to carry them forward. Ugly things have happened to some of these people, from harassment in a wide range of overt and covert ways to dismissal or prejudiced terminal evaluations. Fear is a natural concomitant to such devices and a deterrent to obtaining contracts.

Metzger and Pointer[6] attribute low wage scale in hospitals to:

1. The attempt of hospitals to hire otherwise unemployable at low wages
2. The bimodal skill mix
3. The relatively large amounts of payment in kind
4. The predominance of women
5. The lack of union organization in health care facilities [p. 12].

Somers (in Metzger and Pointer[6]) points out the crucial situation existing in today's hospitals, as regards the move into the mainstream of modern personnel and labor relations practice:

> It seems almost incredible that 35 years after the great labor upheavals of the Thirties, the adoption of the Wagner and Taft-Hartley Acts . . . , and the acceptance of unions as integral parts of American society, one of the largest and most vital industries in the nation should be condemned to relive all the turmoil, the trials and efforts of that period [p. xxii].

EFFORTS OF PROFESSIONAL ASSOCIATIONS AND UNIONS
Professional nurses

"Economic protection has always been a goal of organized nursing [p. 34]."[6] In a historical sketch, Metzger and Pointer show this goal of economic protection dating from 1897, when the Nurses' Associated Alumnae of the United States and Canada was organized. The professional association was thought to be the best means of protecting economic security. In 1946 the American Nurses' Association officially began its Economic Security Program; response by the state associations was moderate. These authors attribute a greatly stepped-up program in 1960 for contractual arrangements for nurses to the work of Barbara Schutt, through the pages of the *American Journal of Nursing* of which she was editor. Mass resignation and picketing in the mid-1960s and removal of the no-strike policy by the American Nurses' Association in 1968 provided acceleration to the programs of the ANA and its state affiliates [p. 35-37].[6] The greatest success in contract negotiations has been on the West Coast and in industrial states of the east and midwest. Approximately one third of the ANA membership is now covered by a contract negotiated by state nurses' associations.[7]

A trend to areawide negotiation is natural, especially in large cities where there are hospital councils. The Washington State Nurses' Association, for example, which represents nurses in twenty hospitals, entered agreement with the Seattle Area Hospital Council, which embraces these hospitals (pp. 221-223). One can readily see the economy of time and effort in such areawide negotiations and contracts.

The recent passage of amendments to the National Labor Relations Act (Taft-Hartley) to extend coverage to employees of nonprofit hospitals is a welcome boost to the Economic and General Welfare Commission of the American Nurses' Association, because it will provide the same protection to those nurses engaged in contract procurement as is enjoyed now by other groups seeking contracts.

Licensed practical nurses

Licensed practical nurses are energetically seeking contractual arrangements with hospitals. Although unions have approached and enlisted professional nurses, their impetus to unionize LPNs has been much stronger, probably because these nurses constitute the middle position in the hierarchy between professional nurses and nurses' aides, attendants, and orderlies. However, practical nurses have usually followed the professional pattern for achieving contractual arrangements covering salaries and working conditions, that is, through their professional organizations.

Hepner and associates [pp. 332-337][8] have excerpted much material of the National Federation of Licensed Practiced Nurses, Inc., which provides guidelines for contract procurement by way of the state association (as in the case of professional nurses) to handle the actual negotiation. A sample employment contract for licensed practical nurses is included in their work.

The Vancouver Memorial Hospital employment agreement[9] identifies the legal authority in the state for such an agreement, spells out management's rights specifically, contains an equal employment opportunity clause, adds personal birthdays to holidays, declares employer provision for hospital and medical insurance for full-time employees, cites coverage by either state workmen's compensation or a substantially equivalent plan, includes a conference committee of both licensed practical nurses and management for discussion of the agreement, and includes both the feminine and masculine genders in the document. These inclusions illustrate the growing sophistication of LPNs and the spelling out of contracts. It is interesting to note the specific timely societal influences, for example, the equal employment opportunity clause and the statement of gender.

Unions

The vast number of nonprofessional workers in nursing and other hospital departments, coupled with the slowness of hospitals to incorporate modern personnel policies and practices, has provided a fertile field for union activity. The National Labor-Management Act of 1947 (Taft-Hartley) had an inhibiting influence on union activity in nonprofit hospitals, though eleven jurisdictions at least partially protected and regulated the organizational and contract negotiation activity of employees of voluntary hospitals. Therefore, prior to the amendments in 1974 to the Taft-Hartley Act, voluntary nonprofit hospitals in 39 states were not required to recognize or bargain collectively with their employees. Voluntary institutions constitute the largest single sector of the hospital industry. They account for 48% of the total number of health care facilities, 66% of admissions, and 54% of total payroll expense. One can appreciate the extent of the deprivation to workers prior to recent amendments.

The goal of the hospital, namely, the care of the sick, has provided another deterrent to union activity in that such activity implied an attack on this humanitarian institution for which there would be little public support. Despite the traditional antipathy of hospital management to union activity, there are hospitals that have had long-standing labor contracts and where a reciprocally respectful attitude has generally prevailed. Kaiser-Permanente Health Group hospitals are in this category.

Despite deterrents to unionism in hospitals, there has been widespread activity to gain improved wages and working conditions for nonprofessional workers, a large number of whom work in the nursing department. A substantial and growing number of hospital employees are covered by union contracts. Service Employees International Union is the largest one serving these employees.

The main difference between the union contract and one negotiated by a professional association (such as a state nurses' association) is that the union maintains a sustained and strong role during the term of the contract, whereas the professional association does not. Provision of bulletin board space for official notices and meeting space for local unit meetings (with or without association representation) and later stages of the grievance procedure constitute the ongoing activity of the association, whereas the union's continuing involvement is extensive.

All new employees are affected by a union, because they must either join it or pay a fee to the union equal to the dues, presumably for services provided by the union. Union personnel may visit the hospital periodically, and the union appoints employees as shop stewards to represent it on the premises. Job descriptions of all positions governed by the contract are provided to the union. There is probably more detail and spelling out of articles in a union contract.

NEGOTIATING PROCEDURE

Hepner and associates [pp. 320-327][8] include copious excerpts from manuals and materials of the American Nurses' Association to describe the process of informing and guiding the membership in the method of procuring contracts through collective bargaining.

The operation starts essentially with local units in hospitals, which investigate needs and mobilize nurses to participate in contract procurement. At one time, a simple majority (including nurses who are not members of the ANA) could give their bargaining rights to the state association. The percentage of nurses requesting representation has steadily increased, and membership in the American Nurses' Association is now required. The state association representative then makes the contact with the hospital administration. Together, the state representative and officers and members of the local unit carry on negotiations with the hospital administration until a contract is signed by both parties on behalf of nurses in the institution.

The American Nurses' Association and the state nurses' associations have enlisted the aid of legal and industrial relations consultants, because there is considerable expertise required in the process of contract procurement. Familiarity with labor relations in general as background for the specifics of hospital negotiations is useful. Such a brief concentrated description is contained in *Employer's Labor Relations Guidebook* (1970) of the Indiana Chamber of Commerce. It includes a glossary and information used by unions.

Baer[10] has provided an excellent compendium of 101 elaborated guidelines for supervisors in the conduct of labor relations. For example, the supervisor is advised not to settle grievances on the basis of what is fair (guideline #42). On cursory examination this advice seems at odds with proper conduct, but in the labor relations context it is the agreement itself that determines fairness or unfairness. The agreement cannot be tampered with or modified during its extant course. Additionally, the supervisor is advised to use grievance settlements to strengthen relationships with employees (guideline #43). The key to this strengthening lies in being able and willing to admit error when circumstances warrant such admission.

Position of the director of nursing and nursing managers

The director of nursing is a member of hospital management and does not participate in the affairs of the local unit.

> Preferably, the director of nursing should participate in negotiations as a full partner of the management team. . . . [As such she] is management's "expert resource" on matters involving the nursing service. . . . While there is likely to be substantial agreement on the goals of the nursing service there can be equally substantial differences over how to implement goals and the ordering of priorities [between the director and the representatives of the local unit].[11]

Interdependence is in order, because the director of nursing belongs on both sides as a member of management and as a professional nurse, with something to say to both.

There is a growing national debate about the place of the director of nursing in contract negotiations. Three articles originally published in The Journal of the New York State Nurses' Association, along with an editorial in the June 1974 issue of *Supervisor Nurse*, do much to illumine the problems inherent in the nursing service director's position regarding contract negotiations.[12-14] One points up the myth of the "two hat" idea, which essentially promotes the do-nothing or stay-uninvolved philosophy, thus supporting the historic hospital position of rejection of collective bargaining and contractual arrangements. This article calls for strong, expert nursing representation at the bargaining table in the person of the director of nursing. The second article acknowledges the benefits of collective bargaining in the personnel function where policies are spelled out, documentation is maintained, and openness is encouraged and promoted.

The third point of view supports collective bargaining for economic purposes, but rejects its intrusion into the professional practice area on the grounds that the authority and responsibility for the quality of nursing care in a given institution rests with the director of nursing service, according to the American Nurses' Association Standards of Nursing Service (1973). This is a startling position in that it contradicts the thrust of the ANA Economic Security Program, which aims not only to strengthen the economic position of nurses but their clinical practice as well. It also seems in opposition to such well-established administrative concepts as participatory and consultative management whereby workers are involved in goal determination and achievement. Application of these concepts does not replace ultimate top administrative responsibility and decision for such goal determination and achievement, nor does it reduce the accountability of such persons. The application does, however, enrich that determination and achievement in important ways. Such enrichment is found internally through staff organization and a climate of openness and externally through the thoughtful efforts of local units, state nurses' associations, patient opinion polls, and the data-procuring and deliberative resources of health and community organizations.

Associate and assistant directors, as well as supervisors, are not members of local units, because they are clearly management personnel. They could, however, choose to be represented by state nurses' associations for contractual purposes, though the Taft-Hartley amendment requiring hospitals to negotiate with them would not obtain. If the management function were better understood and more fully operative, associate and assistant directors and supervisors would be standing by directors of nursing while they assert the rights of nurses to organize under the aegis of state nurses' associations. The director of nursing alone should not bear the intimidation of withdrawing from the ANA because of its collective bargaining effort currently exerted by hospital administrators. All management nursing personnel should bear the brunt, because they are collectively carrying forward the goals of the nursing enterprise.

Head nurses are usually members of the local unit, further demonstrating the unfortunate alienation and separation of this group from the levels of administration to which they properly belong.

Directors of nursing should have their own contracts, as should all nurse administrators.

In a comprehensive review of the state of collective bargaining Schutt concludes:

For . . . nurses—and potentially for the profession itself—there is a new sense of power, fed by a new awareness of rights, sense of conviction, and feelings of worth. The power is in more than their determination to change things; it is in the knowledge that together they can do it.[15]

Bowman and Culpepper[16] corroborate the idea that the time has come for nurses to study and use power constructively, for their own good and the good of the patients they serve; to move from a subordinate to a superordinate position in their own affairs and their relationship to others in the health care field; and to take action rather than react to the actions of others.

STRIKES AGAINST HOSPITALS

Both the American Nurses' Association and the National Association for Practical Nurse Education and Service, Inc., have guidelines for conduct during a dispute or strike of other groups in the hospital. Both recommend that neutrality of registered and licensed practical nurses be maintained. No longer do they do the work of the disputing group, or any other, unless a clear and present danger exists. They should recommend and assist with reduction in the census in the interest of patient safety; cooperate and work in support of other groups to further mutually favorable conditions of employment and work; and acknowledge the right of all employees to organize, choose their own representative, and determine their own goals.[17] Considerable difficulties have arisen over the right to organize and be represented, as well as over the conditions of negotiation. This has been the precise point of the effort to get the Taft-Hartley Act so amended.

This policy of neutrality and performing only one's legitimate duties has not been easy, because nurses have traditionally and generously done whatever needed to be done. This indeed is what they did in early strikes before the situation was thought through and a policy was established.

EXAMPLE OF A SPECIFIC CONTRACT

Because by far the majority of practicing nurses, including nurse managers at all levels, do not have or have access to a contract, it is useful to review some of the major components of a sound contract. The Employment Agreement by and between Seattle Area Hospital Council and Washington State Nurses' Association,[18] effective through June 30, 1976, is an excellent example because it displays considerable expertise, sophistication, specificity, and precision. It also represents areawide coverage (twenty hospitals), which gives it stability and strength through the uniformity it provides to a geographic area. This contract is composed of a preamble that speaks to improved nursing practice through appropriate standards of employment. The preamble is followed by twenty articles.

Article 1 recognizes that the Washington State Nurses' Association represents all registered nurses up to and including head nurses.

Article 2 describes arrangements for payroll deductions of dues for mandatory American Nurses' Association membership during the life of the contract.

Article 3 gives definition of nurse classification, including resident nurse who is a recent graduate or who has recently returned to active practice; general duty nurse who is immediately responsible for nursing care or has recently completed a refresher course; head nurse; assistant head nurse; charge nurse; full-time nurse who works 40 hours in 1 week, 80 hours in 2 weeks, or 70 hours in a 10-hour day over a 2-week period; part-time nurse who works less than 40 hours a week; per diem nurse who works less than 16 hours per week or 32 hours in a 2-week period; and temporarily licensed nurse. A month consists of 173.3 hours, and a year is 2,080 hours.

Article 4 deals with hours of work and overtime. There is provision here for monthly work schedules posted by the twentieth day of the preceding month. Full-time nurses shall have at least one weekend off in three, and there shall be effort to allow two out of four weekends off. When nurses must work on a third weekend, they will be compensated at time and a half the regular rate.

Article 5 describes employment practices, such as annual laboratory tests; provision for a probationary period; regulations regarding termination, discharge, layoff, and recall; access to one's personnel file; and orientation and in-service education. There is provision for a nursing practice committee, which shall meet at least quarterly, composed of staff nurses of whom half are to be elected by their peers and half selected by the nursing management. This committee will work with the nursing audit committee. Also included are provisions for bulletin board space, distribution of contract, meeting space, discussion and review of each hospital's retirement program, proximate parking for on-call nurses, voluntary withdrawal on low-census days, orientation for float nurses, and compensation for time spent on hospital-determined committees.

Article 6 provides for salaries, ranging from starting salary of $768 per month to $1,103 after 5 years of service, effective May 1, 1975; provision for cost-of-living adjustment; specific placement of newly hired nurses in the salary schedule; and maintenance of specific service premiums antedating July 1, 1969, and still extant.

Article 7 describes premium pay conditions, including shift differential, standby, callback, temporary assignment to a higher position, and reporting for work but leaving because of low census.

Article 8 incorporates specifications for vacation.

Article 9 pertains to holidays, of which there are eight.

Article 10 delineates sick leave for oneself and bereavement leave.

Article 11 provides for medical, surgical, and hospital insurance and workmen's and unemployment compensation.

Article 12 covers leaves of absence for maternity, military duty, educational and professional meetings, health reasons, jury duty, personal leave, and re-entry after leave.

Article 13 provides for a conference committee of three representatives of management, one of whom is the director of nursing, and three nurse representatives, for purposes of communication about personnel and other mutual problems. This committee will meet at least quarterly.

Article 14 spells out the grievance procedure in steps beginning with the nurse and her immediate supervisor, followed by the nurse, the local unit chairperson and the director of nursing, and the administrator and the state nurses' association representative, and finally leading to arbitration.

Article 15 provides for retention of any benefits already held that are more favorable than those included in the agreement.

Article 16 states management's responsibilities to the public for the orderly and efficient operation and management of the hospital, maintenance of standards, assignment and direction of employees, determination of materials and equipment, staffing needs and facilities, and selection, hiring, promotion, transfer, discipline, demotion, discharge, recall, and overtime of employees, within the provision of the agreement.

Article 17 assures uninterrupted patient care during the term of the agreement.

Article 18 states that each party is free to propose appropriate topics during negotiation and waives similar rights during the term of the agreement unless by subsequent mutual agreement.

Article 19 provides that anything in the agreement found to be contrary to law will be renegotiated immediately.

Article 20 gives the effective dates of the agreement.

There is an interesting addendum that provides guidelines for performance evaluation, which calls for a framework of written policies, job descriptions, and well-informed evaluators who frequently observe and provide day-to-day guidance.

Performance evaluations shall be provided at completion of 90 days, annually, and prior to termination. They are always to be discussed and signed at prearranged conferences.

LIMITATIONS AND GAINS IN CONTRACTS

Even in a sophisticated contract such as the one described above, there are omissions and weaknesses, for example, the provision of sabbatical leave in a profession where increasing emphasis is rightly placed on maintaining currency and stepping up the clinical component of practice.

It is certainly an indictment of nursing service administration as it is practiced that provision of time and space for the head nurse to do scheduling, evaluation, and other such duties must be included in an employment agreement. Similarly, the spelling out of a personnel evaluation system as an addendum to a contract, as above (or an actual gain, as in the case of the California settlement noted earlier) should be a cause for shame at this stage of professional nursing management. Such contract inclusions eloquently verify the need to update administrative practice, because they call for what should have long since been standard operating procedure.

Provision of a formalized grievance procedure is a considerable gain for nurses, because occasions of arbitrariness, vindictiveness, and unfairness on the part of nurse managers have been far from minimal over the years. This is not to say that complaining nurses have always been right, but only to note the absence of a course of redress when they have in fact been treated improperly and provide a procedure for them to be heard when they think they have been so treated.

Hepner and associates [pp. 271-272][8] list thirteen possible grievances. Seven of these (dealing with pay, holidays, and vacations; noncompensated temporary work; unequal weekend work; inadequate posting of time schedules; discharge without cause; absence of adequate locker facilities; and in-service programs) would be provided for by the above Seattle Area Hospital Council–Washington State Nurses' Association Employment agreement. The remainder (unfair shift assignment, unexplained or unconsulted transfer, minority group nurses passed over for promotion, nurses charged for breakage of equipment, and parking lot privileges) show areas of potential grievance not so obviated by the above contract.

Nurse retirement plans are not as advanced as are others in the economy, though the above contract calls for them to be reviewed and discussed. This provision for review and discussion gets the subject into the contract, from where it can be altered favorably at subsequent contractual deliberations. Cleland[19] speaks about the need for an industrywide retirement system comparable to that of institutions of learning, to avoid discrepancies and to allow for continuity in a highly mobile society.

Contractual arrangements contain the essential or highest priority elements of personnel policies. Where contracts do not exist, extant ones can serve as models, using prevailing salary ranges and related items in the area or region.

The advantages of contracts are thought to be staff stability, improved morale, and better communication: when issues are out in the open, the climate of the institution is healthier. There is a direct relationship between contracts and negotiations and sound administrative practices. The contract is actually a boon to managers, because it renders the personnel function more open and reciprocal as a result of precision and specificity. It is also a primary source of alleviation of long-standing oppression, bitterness, misunderstanding, and unfairness. Though history has shown hospital management to be resistant to contracts and negotiation, increased understanding of the personnel function and improved practice will facilitate contract negotiation on both sides of the desk, because the more sophisticated and precise the personnel function, the fewer points of contention there will be. For example, as the personnel function expands, it relies increasingly on records, as does negotiation and implementation of contracts. Improvement in one causes improvement in the other. In personnel evaluation, records should be kept of the date and nature of employee counseling, with subsequent evaluation dates and descriptions. If grievances arise, the record is clear on the appropriate notification and counseling of the employee relative to the grievance. The better the personnel practices within a hospital, the calmer and more receptive management personnel will be in negotiations with outside bodies. Business practices will be more straightforward and cordially conducted. The responsibility for sound business practices and cordiality also rests with the state nurses' associations and unions.

As contractual arrangements increase, the dimension of practice and the effects on patient care will be included in the deliberations. Quantitative and qualitative dimensions of nursing care are logical extensions of contractual arrangements and are in line with the growing sophistication of nursing services in measuring quantity and quality. Professional nursing practice committees are already a part of some nurse contracts. Time and specific committee membership is provided to deliberate about nursing practice in the specific hospital. These committees will provide the base for further deliberation and more intensive scrutiny of actual nursing practice. Nursing care ratios per patient and ratios of personnel to patients are among the many examples of specific considerations that could be dealt with in such committees.

Forerunners of these committees were the professional performance committees begun by efforts of the California State Nurses' Association [in Conta[20]] (though not tied to collective bargaining and representation by the Association). They were formed in response to requests from nurses, to deal with wide-ranging problems encountered by the nurses relative to economics, preparation, and practice. Though not part of the organizational structure of the nursing service, they were represented by all levels and categories in the service, and committee members were elected by the nurses. They always reported to the director of nursing, and sharing of agendas and minutes kept all informed. These seem to be the same professional performance committees opposed by Erickson (p. 216).

OTHER PERSONNEL POLICIES

There are personnel policies of a supportive nature, not important enough to be or as yet a part of a contract, but important enough to be stated formally. Regulations regarding parking lots and spaces, security measures provided, personnel recreation programs (bowling teams, seasonal or unit parties, and so forth), length of service awards, uniform requirements, child-care provisions on site or nearby, use of lounge, locker, and library facilities, and other employee services are spelled out in employee handbooks, which may also contain elaboration of personnel policies contained in contracts.

Health services

Health services illustrate use of contract or employee handbooks, because such services often consist of the minimum for which the contract provides. Health services can become quite comprehensive and sophisticated, providing initial and annual physical examinations, discounts on medication, home visits, health education, participation in surveys with national health organizations such as the American Heart Association and the American Cancer Society, and mental health services, including the services of a clinical psychologist. There is a strange incongruity here: one would think that hospitals would be in the vanguard of organizations providing such comprehensive health services, dedicated as they are or should be to the promotion of health. But it is naive to think that because workers are engaged in the health care industry they are somehow automatically possessed of optimum health resources and knowledge. Actually, our minimal personnel health services may parallel and be related to our minimal patient teaching services.

Merit pay

The question of compensation for performance of outstanding excellence remains unanswered. As contractual arrangements, with their precise salary schedules, become more common, individual remunerations for excellence will decrease. In times past, these individual remunerations resembled increments on an individual rather than uniform basis. As increments for satisfactory work become commonplace, there is less room and need for compensating individual excellence. However, acknowledgement of such excellence should be made in some form, not necessarily monetary, because there continue to be people who perform exceptionally well and their superlative performance should not go unnoted.

• • •

There seems little doubt but that there will be expansion of the role of professional associations and unions in salary and working condition determinations for hospital and nursing home personnel. Metzger and Pointer[6] speak of

a significant "pent-up" stimulus for higher wage levels in the hospital industry [p. 15]. . . . Today, employee organization activity in hospitals is now a reality. Approximately 11 per cent of all registered hospitals in the country are organized to some extent and the number is growing at a rate of about 30 per cent each day. Thus the need for enforceable, workable, uniform and equitable procedures of employee-employer relations in what is soon to be the nation's largest industry is critical. What is at stake is not only the internal viability of the health services industry, but the certain availability of good medical care to the citizenry [p. 248].

Administrators of nursing service can best participate in and facilitate this movement to a fair share of the health care industry dollar and pursuit of appropriate working conditions by an open attitude, respect for equity, and practice of modern personnel philosophy and methods.

The time is past when workers can be expected to subsidize the nation's health care. These workers are entitled to the same remuneration and congenial working conditions as people in other professions. Anything that will compensate them appropriately for the cruciality and pressure of the work situation should be done. It requires assertive workers and groups to penetrate the health care industry in efforts to achieve satisfactory salaries and working conditions. Openness to each other and the work world around us is also necessary. The convenient social virtue must end.

REFERENCES

1. Galbraith, J. K.: Economics and the public purpose, Boston, 1973, Houghton Mifflin Co., pp. 30-31.
2. Erickson, E.: Collective bargaining; an inappropriate technique for professionals, J. Nurs. Admin. 3(2):54-58, 1973.
3. News, Am. J. Nurs. 73(5):784, 1973.
4. Grand, N.: Nursing ideologies and collective bargaining, J. Nurs. Admin. 3(2):29-32, 1973.
5. PNHA to study feasibility of creating national union, Hospitals 48(22):91, 1974.
6. Metzger, N., and Pointer, D.: Labor-management relations in the health services industry, Washington, D.C., 1972, Science & Health Publications, Inc., pp. xxii, 12, 15, 34, 35-37, and 248.
7. ANA President's Message, Am. Nurse 6(1):4, 1974.
8. Hepner, J., Boyer, J., and Westerhaus, C.: Personnel administration and labor relations in health care facilities, St. Louis, 1969, The C. V. Mosby Co., pp. 271-272, 320-327, and 332-337.
9. Employment agreement between Vancouver Memorial Hospital and the Licensed Practical Nurses' Association of Washington State (termination date, September 30, 1974).
10. Baer, W.: Grievance handling, New York, 1970, American Management Associations.
11. The role of the director of an organized nursing service in collective bargaining, Am. J. Nurs. 70(3):554, 1970.
12. Driscoll, V.: The myth of two hats, Supervisor Nurse 5(6):24-27, 1974.
13. Zebrowski, D.: Collective bargaining and the director of nursing, Supervisor Nurse 5(6):16 and 21, 1974.
14. Rotkovitch, R.: The director of nursing and the

hat of administration, Supervisor Nurse **5**(6):31-36, 1974.
15. Schutt, B.: Collective action for professional security, Am. J. Nurs. **7**(11):1951, 1973.
16. Bowman, R., and Culpepper, R.: Power; Rx for change, Am. J. Nurs. **74**(6):1053-1056, 1974.
17. The philosophy, goals, policies and positions of the ANA Economic and General Welfare Program, New York, 1973, American Nurses' Association, p. 6.
18. Employment agreement by and between Seattle Area Hospital Council and Washington State Nurses' Association (October 29, 1974).
19. Cleland, V.: Role bargaining for working wives, Am. J. Nurs. **70**(6):1246, 1970.
20. Conta, A. L.: Professional committees, Am. J. Nurs. **68**(12):2601-2604, 1968.

CHAPTER 15
EQUIPMENT

Equipment is essential to the nursing staff because it contributes continuously to their efficient work or to frustration and impairment in the conduct of that work. It is, in effect, an extension of personnel. Materiel may constitute a hazard for nursing in that it permits preoccupation, of which we are often correctly accused, with things and procedures; however, it is the excessive rather than the proper preoccupation that evokes the criticism.

The last two to three decades have seen great advances in equipment used in hospitals. Machines, which have taken over manual duties, range from those for shaking down thermometers to sophisticated respiratory and drainage machines and monitoring devices. Moreover, the standard machines are continuously being improved to provide greater precision and facility in handling, for example, the sphygmomanometer, in which a light flashes when systolic sound comes in. There are sphygmomanometers available that produce print-outs of systolic, diastolic, and mean pressures.

Because of the tremendous complexity of machines, they cannot be serviced completely by in-house or company-connected engineers. This has given rise to a new health care worker: the biomedical engineer, a professional who works in the whole area of man and his relationship with machines, plans and conducts research, and manages the products of automation and the monitoring, diagnostic storage, and other uses of computers [Jackson[1]]. These engineers are paralleled by an electrical technician who assumes responsibility for maintenance, repairs, and safety testing of electrical equipment. The prevalent professional-technical relationship obtains here.

The tremendous increase in complicated and sophisticated equipment has been accompanied by, if not actually caused, the large-scale move to centralization of supplies, equipment, and transportation. Modern central supply rooms, though operating on the same principles as earlier ones, are a far cry from them in the range of materials, supplies, and equipment, and services they offer. The move to centralization in the interest of efficiency has been accompanied by a companion movement to apply job analysis and work simplification to procedures and techniques that utilize the vastly expanded services of central supply departments. Also accompanying centralization and job simplification are the structural changes that facilitate them. Piped oxygen and suction devices at bedsides, pneumatic tube deliveries, and mobile extensions of central supply rooms to patient units are examples. Moreover, there are multiple combinations of materials and equipment, such as the xerography machine for cancer detection, by which the breast can be visualized in considerable detail on special Xerox copy paper, with less radiation. The change in the traditional bath procedure by use of a specially cut and folded towel treated with a special solution (developed by Vestal Laboratories) is another example. There seems to be no end to the stream of products and machines produced to make hospital work more efficient and streamlined.

ECOLOGY MOVEMENT AND SYSTEMS THEORY

The last decades have seen the rise of the Ecology Movement and systems theory, whereby we view our world as a spaceship and our integral relationship to physical, biological, and other aspects of the environment as firm and ever-growing. Dubos [p. 67][2] illustrates the elusiveness of this relationship between man and his environment by pointing out the effect of weather on such physiologic activities as blood clotting and blood pressure. He cites the tremendous influence of the environment on our future anatomical structures, size, abilities, and behaviors as the environment interacts with the child in prenatal stages via the mother [p. 69]. Environment-person relationships in the health care facility can be seen in the effect of construction and decorating on patients. The contemporary use of glass to allow incorporation of the out of doors, various indoor and outdoor planting arrangements, indirect lighting, muted restful colors, and carpeting all contribute to the restful climate of patients' internal environment. Less apparent environment-person relationships were affected by the fuel shortage of 1974. Because fuel is used in the manufacture of plastics, thousands of pieces of equipment and devices in hospital use were threatened by the shortage. This situation illustrates the delicate balance of the environment-person relationship and the vigilance required to maintain that balance. It is certain that the future holds many other discoveries in this essential relationship. Jackson [p. 39][1] projects the excitement of such discoveries when she describes experimental units dominated by biomedical engineering, in which empiric observations yield to scientific ones in the care of both the ill and the healthy. She projects the fantastic possibilities of intervention by the use of transplants, circadian rhythms in air and space travel, and the like.

Disposable equipment

Disposables, which have revolutionized the modern hospital, are being reviewed because they contribute so greatly to the solid-waste disposal problem. It is increasingly clear that the earth cannot absorb nonbiodegradable products at the astronomical rate they are used. Their use will be curbed substantially to reduce the disposal problem in the hospital as elsewhere in our society.

Litsky and associates[3] propose that one should be sure before deciding to use disposables that they can be safely discarded and are used discriminately. They illustrate by defending the use of disposable diapers, but not the use of disposable kitchenware. Currently a disposable bedpan liner is widely advertised. One can imagine the boon it is to comfort and conservation of personnel time and energy; but can it really be flushed away? This liner is an excellent example of the advances in material and equipment that must be accompanied by enough skepticism to see that all alleged attributes are checked out.

From the cost viewpoint, management consultants for Battelle Northwest Systems Programs for Hospitals, sponsored by the Hospital Associations of Washington, Oregon, and Idaho, found in a study of thirty disposable nursing items that one third were justified for cost and benefit while two thirds were not, when judged on basic costs, labor costs, convenience, and infection control.[4]

Solid waste

In the matter of solid-waste disposal, Litsky and associates[3] provide astounding figures. The average American accounts for 5.5 pounds per day and the average hospital patient for 24.16 pounds! They propose the pneumatic chute as the safest means for collecting waste on site and use of appropriate incinerators for disposal of compact waste. Because of the high cost of such incinerators, they suggest that hospitals share this service.

SUPPLIERS

Suppliers of material are increasingly providing expertise in the use of their products, often citing scientific data to support the quality or effectiveness of these products. One supplier has a two-page advertisement for a departmental analysis program offered at no cost to the users.[5] The advertisement lists names and locations of twenty hospitals availing themselves of these services, with consequent efficiency and reduction in costs for such supplies. Another advertisement offers a broad educational service for primary and secondary use of its products, including such items as decontamination.[6] The growing sophistication and effectiveness of suppliers is increasingly accompanied by such knowledgeable and helpful services. Although such services are probably built into the cost of the product, they optimize the utilization of such products and thus get more value from them.

Comparison buying and checking out of claims made for products are in order, because the institution is ultimately responsible for the equipment and materials it uses. Also, reciprocal respect and consideration must pervade these relationships between hospitals and their suppliers. For example, respect for the time of the vendor is important. Setting up and keeping appointments helps both personnel and vendors.

Imaginative staff can often find cheaper equipment to satisfy a need, for example, a water or air mattress used for flotation purposes in summer recreation. The flotation concept has also given rise to many useful ways to reduce pressure on patients. Receptacles to hold clean and soapy water for bed bathing, in an effort to reduce the amount of soap left on the patient's body, is another such idea.

MAINTENANCE, CONSERVATION OF SUPPLIES, AND INVENTORY

Maintenance of equipment and conservation of supplies remain of major concern, so that their facile and complete utilization in nursing care and cost control can be maintained. Patency and cleanliness of all equipment are as essential as they ever were.

Inventory remains a time-consuming, monotonous task; however, as yet there is no replacement for it nor any respite from the conditions justifying it. Equipment and supplies disappear for many reasons, from carelessness to theft. These losses are so great that security guards check departing personnel in some institutions. There might have been a time when this kind of thievery from an employer could be construed to be occult compensation for inadequate wages, but it is doubtful that this obtains today. A staff must somehow be energized to conscientiously assist in inventory control, because it bears a serious indirect relationship to conscientious patient care. Inventory procedures require care to make certain that they remain current and are as streamlined as possible. Multiple participation is valuable in that it shares the task, thus reducing the onus as well as reminding the staff of the need for constant vigilance where supplies and equipment are concerned. There is also the possibility that hospitals, like businesses, can have inventory checking done by enterprises devoted exclusively to the task.

REFERENCES

1. Jackson, B.: The biomedical engineer; new member of the health team, Supervisor Nurse **5**(5):36-43, 1974.
2. Dubos, R.: A god within, New York, 1972, Charles Scribner's Sons, pp. 67 and 69.
3. Litsky, W., Martin, J., and Litsky, B.: Solid waste; a hospital dilemma, Am. J. Nurs. **72**(10):1841-1847, 1972.
4. A systems program for hospitals in Washington, Oregon, and Idaho; case studies in cost savings, Portland, Ore., Battelle Northwest Systems Programs for Hospitals, p. 3.
5. Advertisement, Supervisor Nurse **5**(5):1-2, 1974.
6. Advertisement, Inservice Training and Education **2**(5):43, 1973.

CHAPTER 16
LEGAL ASPECTS

MOVE TO GOVERNMENT CONTROLS

Squier[1] says that "The health care industry has entered the era of governmental control," and goes on to speak about the numbers of regulatory agencies limiting the freedom of the community hospital.

Medicare-Medicaid programs have had tremendous impact on the whole health industry. As landmark legislation in the history of health care, they brought multiple requirements of different varieties of an economic and professional nature, with all the attendant record keeping. However burdensome in many ways on the providers of health care, it is necessary that protective and regulatory measures be built in to assure that tax dollars supporting such large operations are spent judiciously and accountability is guaranteed.

Because Medicare-Medicaid have such far-reaching effects, it has taken time to reconcile reimbursement formulas with categories of levels of nursing care. It is incumbent on nurses as health care workers or as government appraisers to know comprehensive nursing care and its component parts intimately so that the greatest precision can be brought to bear on the Medicare-Medicaid operation. Moreover, such programs require nurses to determine whether comprehensive care is possible, as well as the nature and extent of rehabilitation therapy possible over and above custodial care in a given institution. Factual, measurable evaluations of what is attainable and being practiced in a given situation are necessary so that errors may be remedied, estimates reappraised, arithmetical precision achieved, and collaboration and coordination fostered.

The regulating operations of state health agencies that apply standards for licensure and certification also evaluate eligibility for use of federal funds for construction and renovation of hospitals and for the planning component of health care. Government regulation is beginning to have its effect on hospital empire building, though it is only recently that there is concrete evidence that new hospital construction is being bridled in favor of consideration of shared services or facilities, mergers, and consolidations. Hospitals simply do not have records for such cooperation and collaboration, making government regulation necessary so that total needs and services can be provided and distributed more economically and equitably. Increasing consumerism is also contributing to collaborative policies of hospitals. The frequent requirement to have a certain percentage of consumers in health care deliberating bodies opens the input and reduces the professional strength appropriately.

Nurse practice acts

The principal regulatory agents for nurses are state nurse practice acts, which have been evolving over the decades. Practical nurses are seeking the mandatory licensure that has long been a part of professional nursing. Nurse practice acts are undergoing changes to accommodate the expanded role of nurses in both institutional and public health nursing care. It is interesting to note that the Canadian decision to expand the role of the nurse to meet needs, rather than create new kinds of workers, simplifies procedures and consequent legislation.[2] Expansion is clearly in the direction of medical care. The need for legislation to protect nursing practice already moving into the medical field is accompanied by the need to review our already extended actions in this direction in terms of existing legislature. Creighton[3] points out that nurses who take over pharmacy duties in the absence of the pharmacist are violating pharmacist practice laws. There may be other areas of violation of which we are not aware. The inclusion of mandatory continuing education in nurse practice acts is another current consideration. The inclusion of consumers on state boards of nursing is contained in recent American Nurses' Association guidelines for composition of boards of nursing.[4]

Nurse practice laws are in need of constant surveillance and occasional change to maintain currency in the complex times in which we practice. However, altering existing nurse practice acts to meet the changing needs retains the current structure, which safeguards the public by providing individual licensure and accountability by every practitioner.

Threat of institutional licensure

Hershey's proposed challenge to individual licensure [in Kelly, pp. 566-572][5] would provide for licensure by employing agency, within the framework established by state institutional licensing bodies. Even with state guidelines, the specter of intermingled supervision and licensure by the employer evokes horror, benign superiors and institutions notwithstanding. Institutional licensure is one issue on which there is complete agreement within the profession: nursing organizations and physicians oppose it. Support for institutional licensure seems to come mainly from hospital associations. Experimental efforts toward institutional licensure are funded by the Department of Health, Education, and Welfare. Kelly [p. 572][5] calls on all nurses, along with their organizations, to involve themselves in this critical issue, because it is interwoven with other problems such as the increasing number of nurse auxiliaries and specialists, new classifications of health workers, upward mobility, clinical certification, mandatory continuing education, and opening up of all state boards of nursing. Relationships to such side factors abound in this issue, but nothing should be allowed to detract from or dissipate the central issue: continuance of individual licensure by objective policies and standards.

Kinkela and Kinkela[6] reiterate the need for vigilance and involvement. They dispose of the proffered reasons for institutional licensure expeditiously and lucidly, essentially within the framework of the protection of the public now afforded by individual licensure. They illumine the reversal of roles that would be brought about by institutional licensure, namely the decision regarding professional competency being placed with health care institutions of all kinds and sizes, while responsibility or guidelines for job descriptions and continuing education (for returning practitioners) would be the state's responsibility. Their arguments are so cogent and supportive of the general position of official and nonofficial nursing that one wonders how the movement toward institutional licensure survives.

Need for refined definition of nursing

Creighton points out the need to define the nurse's work. She reviews a common listing as:

1. Supervision of a total comprehensive nursing care plan for the patient
2. Observation, interpretation and evaluation of the patient's symptoms and needs (mental and physical)
3. Carrying out the legal orders of physicians for medication and treatment
4. Supervision of auxiliary help (practical nurses, student nurses, other health workers) who give patient care
5. Carrying out nursing procedures and techniques, especially those which require judgment, modification or calculations, based on technical information.
6. Giving health guidance and participating in health education
7. Accurately recording and reporting.*

---

*From Creighton, H.: Law every nurse should know, ed. 2, Philadelphia, 1970, W. B. Saunders Co., pp. 19-20.

At the least, broad definition is an essential concomitant of nurse practice legislation, as is precise delineation of successively added duties. An example is the Ohio Nurses' Association statement regarding intravenous therapy,[7] an eight-page description beginning with the preamble that includes reference to the Ohio Law Regulating the Practice of Nursing. The statement describes venipuncture and its administration and monitoring, and is divided into assessment, planning, implementation, and evaluation. It includes a nine-part outline for suggested content of intravenous therapy education programs.

Workmen's compensation laws

Personnel practices in health care institutions are affected by legislation to a considerable degree. Workmen's compensation laws provide a fixed schedule of benefits for work-related accident or disease. States vary as to whether these laws are elective or compulsory. Creighton [pp. 57-58][3] suggests that nurses check applicability in the states in which they work. In some states there is special provision for government workers, under the Federal Employees Compensation Act.

Social Security benefits

Nurses were not eligible for Social Security participation until 1950, when coverage was extended to hospitals where the employees favored it. This constitutes a 13-year deprivation of nurses in this retirement program that is now commonplace.

Civil rights legislation

We have mentioned the effect of labor relations legislation on nursing and the recent provision of the right to organize in nonprofit hospitals by revision of the Labor Management Relations Act (Taft-Hartley). Title VII of the Civil Rights Act of 1964, which forbids discrimination against any person on the grounds of race, color, or national origin, has had an important effect. Equal opportunity and affirmative action programs resulting from enforcement policies of the Equal Employment Opportunity Commission and the Office of Federal Contracts Compliance further secure the Civil Rights Act by insisting on figures and proof of attempts to recruit minorities aggressively where federal funds have been or are used, which in health care institutions is essentially universal as a result of Medicare-Medicaid and Hill-Burton legislation.

There are critics of government pressure in forcing this aggressive attempt to recruit minorities. These critics point out that this is tantamount to reverse discrimination in that equal opportunity is replaced by actual employment of minorities, without regard to equal opportunity. This in effect establishes a quota system [Ornstein[8]]. We have noted the large numbers of blacks in auxiliary nursing positions, especially in large cities, so such legislation will have its greatest impact at higher levels in the nursing service and in institutions in suburban or rural locations.

There are ways in which hospitals and nursing homes can adjust their practices to meet the law:

1. Review job application forms to comply with nondiscrimination rules as to sex, race, color, creed, national origin or age.
2. Place in writing the nondiscrimination policy of the institution stated and signed by the administrator.
3. Inform applicants as soon as possible of the decision made on employing them.
4. Keep employee applications for a longer period of time.
5. Establish management personnel audits to review actual practices within the institution.
6. Have current, complete job descriptions and specifications to support each selection.
7. Review all factors at the time of promotion of employees for compliance with the law. Place in writing the reasons used to justify the promotion.
8. Provide a definite and clearly understood probationary employment period, extendable only by explanation and definition in employee cases where needed.*

---

*From Hepner, J., and associates: Personnel administration and labor relations in health care facilities, St. Louis, 1969, The C. V. Mosby Co., pp. 235-236.

Compulsory health insurance

Currently there is serious consideration of compulsory health insurance. The American Nurses' Association endorses it in principle, without allying itself with any specific proposal. Nurses as citizens must participate in such deliberations individually or in the groups to which they belong, so that all ramifications of such plans can be compared and the best may be selected, insofar as this is possible considering the political and social polarizations surrounding these plans. Though 30 years have elapsed since compulsory health insurance plans have been drawn up, the time has come for the advanced ideas for national health insurance of such congressmen as Murray, Wagner, and Dingell, supported by unions and an occasional physician such as Henry Sigerist, a medical historian.

Enabling legislation for experimentation with health maintenance organizations is another current legislative position that has considerable implications for nursing.

Both compulsory health insurance and health maintenance organizations are directed to preventive practice and uniform accessibility of comprehensive health care by the general population. It is incumbent on nurses to prepare themselves for highly sophisticated practice, where all aspects of total nursing care are operative. Precision, clarity, and integration of such care are mandatory.

MALPRACTICE IN NURSING

Malpractice is an overriding potential legal consideration today. The growing professionalism of nursing is accompanied by, if not partially caused by, the accountability factor, which makes nurses responsible for their own acts. Seriously faulty acts constitute malpractice. The proper behavior of a reasonable person is assumed, and courts expect that all professionals or workers shall assume responsibility for their own acts. No longer is the employing agency or the physician held accountable for acts they permit or delegate, though the nurse, the hospital, and the physician frequently are prosecuted in combination.

Nurses must have sufficient knowledge about orders and instructions in order to know when to question them. They must refuse to comply unless satisfied that such orders and instructions are correct.

Nurses are increasingly likely to be prosecuted for malpractice acts, as a result of growth of a knowledgeable society in a litigious climate. These conditions are accompanied by, if indeed they do not cause, the loss of immunity to prosecution of nonprofit hospitals. Yet these conditions should not be lamented, because the public surely has a right to restitution where harm has been done by health care personnel. Consequently, malpractice insurance for nurses is steadily and increasingly utilized. It is wise to maintain individual coverage, even where there is hospital coverage.

In 1973 the Federal Commission on Medical Malpractice issued a report calling for inclusion of lay persons on state professional licensing boards; requirement of health professionals to stay abreast of changes in their fields for continuing licensure; formation of state offices for continuing health affairs and hospital-patient grievance committees; and formation of a central clearinghouse for malpractice information, research, education, and prophylaxis. The Commission defended the contingency basis for legal fees as the only means possible to many people. The report points out that very large sums are spent on malpractice insurance, which are passed on to patients in higher hospital and medical rates.[9]

Miller[10] corroborates the need for a central source for information on malpractice. She suggests that one of the national nursing organizations publish a magazine to keep nurses current about malpractice suits. She offers *The Citation*[11] as a model of a publication through which one can keep up on all recent court cases. Though directed to physicians, nurses also can benefit from it. Miller (citing Hershey) also points out that the great bulk of litigation results from negligent performance in quite ordinary nursing practice, because of the large volume of this kind of care.

The *American Journal of Nursing* and other nursing journals increasingly are carrying regular columns on legal matters and labor relations, because there is a persistent need for such information.

• • •

There is little doubt that a good deal of attention must be given all the legal aspects of nursing practice, because it parallels the complexity found in society and its institutions. Legal aspects embrace a wide range of activity within nursing and within its extensive coordinating and collaborating functions. Attention to legal ramifications of nursing attests to our growing sophistication and demands the precision and clarity we so often seem to lack.

REFERENCES

1. Squier, K.: Health care for the future (advertising supplement), Vancouver, Washington, The Columbian and East County News, May 12-18, 1974. p. 2.
2. News, Am. J. Nurs. **73**(6):964, 1973.
3. Creighton, H.: Law every nurse should know, ed. 2, Philadelphia, 1970, W. B. Saunders Co., pp. 20-21.
4. The American Nurse **6**(5):1, 1974.
5. Kelly, L.: Institutional licensure, Nurs. Outlook **21**(9):566-572, 1973.
6. Kinkela, G., and Kinkela, R.: Institutional licensure; cure-all or chaos? J. Nurs. Admin. **4**(3):16-19, 1974.
7. The registered nurse's role in intravenous therapy, Columbus, Ohio, 1973, Ohio Nurses' Association, pp. 3-10.
8. Ornstein, A.: Are quotas here to stay? National Review **26**(17):480-481, 1974.
9. News, Am. J. Nurs. **73**(6):165, 1973.
10. Miller, C.: The law and nursing education, Educational Horizons **49**(2):50-51, Winter 1970-71.
11. The Citation (biweekly issues), Chicago, American Medical Association.

CHAPTER 17
RESEARCH AND CREATIVITY

Research

Research in its broadest sense is an attempt to gain solutions to problems. More precisely, it is the collection of data in a rigorously controlled situation for the purpose of prediction or explanation [Treece and Treece[1]].

Research is closely related to the scientific method, which describes a way of stating, observing, analyzing, thinking, recording, and reporting. It demands strict and equal attention to objectivity, detail, and statement and must always be precise and exact. The scientific method assumes nothing, is skeptical until concrete evidence is available, tests hypotheses (tentative positions), and collects data systematically and logically within a controlled and circumscribed framework. Empiricism, or what is observable or experienced, is important in developing evidence and gathering data.

Leininger[2] speaks of the goals of science as consisting of the discovery of new knowledge. Nisbet[3] speaks of discovery and explanation as the overriding interrelating components of science, though discovery or observation always precede explanation. Chase[4] summarizes the scientific method as a problem about which the literature is examined, a theory is advanced in terms of probability, and a pattern is designed, accompanied by rigorous testing and examination, absence of emotion and bias, willingness to harbor doubt and admit error, concern for process, structure, and relationships, the possibility of emerging new or unexpected information, and openness of findings of, to, and from others [p. 17]. He illustrates the scientific method with an anecdote about two men who looked at sheep in a pasture. One remarked that the sheep had just been shorn. The other, a scientist, replied that it appeared to be so, at least on the side facing them [p. 11]. Nothing is taken for granted, and evidence is always required in the realm of science. Ellis[5] points out the need to analyze actions and develop theories about the actions, which can then be tested and made specific. Speculation and theorizing are in essential relationship to the scientific method.

Scholarship surrounds the scientific method of theorizing and testing and implies openness to experience and ideas in the search for truth, the involvement of the whole person, unconditional accuracy, and willingness to entertain and consider differing points of view, the habits of inquiry, and wonderment [Armiger[6]].

There is a clear obligation for scholars and scientists to criticize. Criticism is necessary for the refinement of the deliberations at hand. It may alter directions or reinforce them. Such criticism also strengthens the reality base of operation, because illusion can infiltrate even the work of the scholar and the scientist. To withhold criticism is to diminish personal integrity and that of the scientific and scholarly community. Criticism is directed to the issues and not to the person. It is always constructive, even when negative.

Fleming and Hayter[7] offer concrete guidance to nurses as critics in examining research studies. Such suggestions as looking for stated limitations, a hypothesis in an experimental study, the kinds of variables and their control, the relationship of findings and conclusions, and the quality of the summary are offered.

Stevens[8] is an insightful, efficient, and gracious critic of the Standards of Nursing Practice of the American Nurses' Association as representative of current nursing theory. In a detailed and careful analysis of the Standards, she points out apt and revealing discrepancies, for example, the inclusion of recording in the first standard dealing with data collection, but not in the second or third standards dealing with nursing diagnosis and goals, and in her evaluation of client/patient participation in the fifth standard. She is equally effective in her critique of name changes for nursing management personnel in the New Position Descriptions of the New York Nurses' Association.[9]

CLASSIFICATION OF RESEARCH

Research is usually classified as fundamental, implying that it is an end in itself, and applied, implying that it is to be used in some way. This distinction becomes decreasingly meaningful, because application is usually at least a remote possibility of fundamental research.

Mullane[10] speaks about action research identified by Corey as necessary for the improvement of practice and a means of testing ideas emanating from fundamental research. Both action and fundamental research are capable of generating new ideas and can be used in the considerable problems to be found and explorations to be made in nursing.

There are three main types of research: historical, descriptive, and experimental. Abdellah's[11] overview of 175 nursing research projects (funded in part by the U.S. Department of Health, Education, and Welfare, National Institutes of Health, Division of Nursing) during a 13-year period from 1955 to 1968 shows historical research. Surveys that provide examples of descriptive research are those done by ten hospitals in the United Kingdom and a Belgian consortium of five business and industrial firms [Wieland[12]]. They were based on the earlier work of Revans[13] in problem solving, communications, and morale in the hospital setting and were designed to help improve management effectiveness in the participating institutions. Experimental research is usually explanatory and requires strict controls. An illustration of experimental research is a large study of the effectiveness of the clinical specialist on nursing care, as judged by the quality of the card file (Kardex) as the focal point for carrying out the nursing care plan and medical orders. The study covered a 13-month period in which 764 patient card files were examined three times, in the pre-, mid-, and final experimental stages, on three experimental and three control units. Empirical evidence was gathered that supported the hypothesis that the presence of the clinical specialist did indeed alter the nursing care favorably, as demonstrated by the contents of the card files [Georgopoulos and Jackson[14]].

COLLABORATIVE AND COLLEGIAL RESEARCH

Research is usually collegial in that the work of others is used or considered where applicable, as in review of the literature that follows or even accompanies the inauguration of a study. Research is often collaborative, because even when one works alone (which is rare) there is usually an accessible advisory group. There is also the wider collaboration of collegiality by enjoining researchers, for the most part through the literature, which leads to much needed replication of research, that is, repeating it in comparable but different locations. This need for replication arising from collegiality is accompanied by the need to do related research for growth purposes. Growth upon growth is an inherent part of the research mentality.

Whether collegial relationships are one to one or remote, as in the case of written material, they are indispensable to researchers. Interdisciplinary research is also encouraged and enhanced by such collegial relationships. Nursing has always been open to being researched by various categories of social scientists, though we might be faulted for being more subject than collaborator. No less an authority than This[15] suggests the reverse movement of research, that is, from hospital personnel to social scientists. He specifically mentions such areas as TLC, extrasensory perception, the meaning of work, whispering, the validity of span of control, and equally exciting other possible hospital research projects that would contribute substantially to social science in the mutual constant search for ways to help people live more fully.

The need for collaboration and growth upon growth is indicated by Notter,[16] who proposes cluster studies in which people working together build on each others' work and consortia in which universities collaborate with each other on different parts of a study. Such arrangements provide the mutual support needed by researchers.

The report as the vehicle for dissemination of findings provides transmission of the work, not only for general interest, but particularized for those with similar or related interests or findings.

ETHICAL AND OTHER PHILOSOPHICAL COMPONENTS OF RESEARCH

There is a strong ethical component in research. In order to safeguard the rights of persons involved, informed consent, cessation of research if it interferes with therapeutic care, and protection for those unable to protect themselves (such as live fetuses or the recently dead) are required. The amount of government intervention necessary to protect these rights points up the need for greater care in discharging ethical responsibilities of researchers. Moreover, this is an increasingly crucial area of concern as a result of the great advances in science (for example, genetics) and the gradual eclipse of the study of ethics in the health professions. Indeed, attention to the whole of philosophy is important to researchers, because not only is ethics involved, but logic too. Other philosophical components, such as aesthetics, politics, and metaphysics, are important because an elegant, coherent research design is conceived and developed in a political arrangement of cooperating scholars in pursuit of truth with its metaphysical implications. Considering philosophy in the broad sense provides parallel safeguards, as does the systems approach to situations and problems.

DETERRENTS TO RESEARCH

Societal and professional deterrents to research in nursing include antiintellectualism, the pragmatic view that if it works it must be all right, and the national penchant for stockpiling rather than using studies in important areas such as urban and environmental planning. These societal restrictions are felt by nurses, too, as part of the larger community. There are the additional problems pertaining to the nursing profession, such as their being action rather than contemplation or analysis oriented, the inhibiting influence of the physician-nurse relationship, and the authoritarian past.

Dissipation of effort and resources also militates against research. There is at least some waste inherent in researching the obvious. Rational scrutiny and examination may be sufficient sometimes to establish the thesis. However, it must be admitted that stringent verification of the obvious may occasionally be necessary.

For example, in the above research that supported the hypothesis that the greater the clinical competence of the leader the better the nursing care, as demonstrated by card file entries, the question must be asked of whether this hypothesis did indeed require such a large-scale verification, or any verification beyond direct observation. If so, could it not have been done more economically by pre- and postexamination of the card files by the assignment of a more clinically competent leader in a unit (s) and with possible replication elsewhere? Economy of time and effort are to be safeguarded, and redundancy and overelaboration are to be avoided.

This matter of the relationship of obvious or obscure theses to the appropriate use of research resources and time suggests the need to keep research open-ended and multifaceted so that more refined or substantive evidence may be found. The classic example is the work of Dickson and Roethlisberger[17] at Western Electric. By testing variable after variable until they found the crucial one, they provided a research base for subsequent human relations theorists. Had they stopped at any of the earlier stages, the crucial finding—the influence of the work group on well-being and productivity—would have been missed or at least deferred.

RELATIONSHIP OF RESEARCH TO NURSING

Opinion is unanimous that research is an indispensable part of nursing. Research is needed to strengthen nursing's tenuous hold on professionalism, to mobilize its own resources and reduce its dependency on other disciplines, to determine its essence, to refine its historic and continuing relationship with medicine and newer health care professions, and to integrate or correlate its dual forms, art and science, whose interrelationship is cogently noted by Diers: "Science does not destroy art. It may focus, sharpen, delineate, deepen or shape art; but if the art of nursing is forever left closed to questions and evaluations, it will never move beyond its rituals and routines into greater service to man."[18] Boettinger[19] speaks of artists as possessing two essential qualities: competence in their special area and imagination, which they combine to transmit to those around them, whether they be master dancer or master manager.

There is unquestionably a dearth of researchers and research in nursing, despite the often expressed and acknowledged need. Somehow this knowledge has not been internalized by nurses sufficiently to make the significant difference. Nursing practice is replete with changes that never get tested for effectiveness. We are hurrying to primary assignment of care, without ever having systematically examined team nursing for its effectiveness or attributes. Sufficient followup and follow-through (see Chapter 8) would provide much needed impetus to testing innumerable nursing practices and measures and to releasing the latent scientific knowledge of practitioners that dates from preparatory days. We have never really plumbed the long-standing scientific bases for practice. We allude to the scientific principles, but rarely are comfortable using them. Moreover, the current reference to use of intuition in nursing practice may reflect collective failure to identify and apply long-standing scientific principles and concepts to practice more than it reflects the baseless, insightful judgment inherent in intuition. Identification and exteriorization of these scientific bases would help us become amenable to research and provide us with a sizeable, already researched scientific base, as well as aid our research pursuits and direction.

Some beginnings have been made in nursing research. The mid-1950s saw great impetus to research provided by the U.S. Department of Health, Education, and Welfare, National Institutes of Health, Division of Nursing, in the form of nurse training for research and a continuous and continuing flow of federal funds into nursing research projects [Gortner[20]]. Another significant compilation of research is the work of Aydelotte[21] on staffing, under the aegis of the Public Health Service, accompanied by the Report of the Conference on Research on Nurse Staffing in Hospitals [Levine[22]]. Aydelotte's compilation includes commentary on almost 200 studies and a bibliographical listing of over 1,000 studies. Because staffing is such a vast and multifaceted function, the research covered is quite diversified and comprehensive. The historical survey by Abdellah[11] attests further to the splendid contribution from this government source.

The journal *Nursing Research* was launched in 1952 and is devoted solely to research. The Spring 1960 issue, containing 200 abstracts substantially covering projects conducted between 1955 and 1958, is but one illustration of its contribution to nursing research.

In the 1950s nurses voluntarily assessed themselves to provide financial support for research. Since 1969 the Center for Health Research, Wayne State University, College of Nursing, Detroit, has carried out diversified research projects, including family planning, prevention of bacteriuria, and evaluation of the quality of care in nursing homes [Werley[23]]. The Center is working cooperatively with the Michigan Nurses' Association on research planning for that state.

Regular national research conferences have been held. The first meeting of the Council of Nurse Researchers of the American Nurses' Association was held in 1973; and in 1974 significant resolutions were passed by the House of Delegates of the American Nurses' Association in convention. Of the 41 resolutions passed, six are addressed to research and are concerned with the need for nurse representation on institutional research review committees, protection of the rights and safety of subjects, initiation of research in undergraduate nurse preparation, dissemination and implementation of research findings, and establishment of priorities in nursing research—development of systematic nursing practice information, development and testing of practice theory, and formation and selection of criteria to document nursing practice outcomes and effectiveness.[24] Nursing practice, service, and education are to embrace and be embraced by research.

The National Commission for the Study of Nursing and Nursing Education[25] listed research as the first of the three basic priorities, especially in the area of nursing practice, and noted that research is the means of discovering new ways to improve nursing practice and to measure the accruing benefits to patients. It corroborated the knowledgeable opinions of many who have noted the insufficiency of nursing research.

RESEARCH GOALS FOR THE FUTURE

There are three main goals of research efforts: to broaden the research base of practitioner and practice, to develop more trained researchers, and to rapidly multiply descriptive research. These goals are interdependent.

Concerted efforts are necessary to introduce research and research methods at all levels, among students and practitioners alike. It will be necessary to dissipate the mystique surrounding research by showing that the scientific method can be applied anywhere. Research constitutes a way of looking at things, from the simple to the complex. From this base, one can then structure, implement, and evaluate various investigative devices to study nursing and nursing problems.

A principal obstacle adding considerable reality to the mystique is the fear of and inability to cope with statistics. Jacox[26] addresses this difficulty forthrightly in considering the research component in master's degree programs in nursing service administration and suggests statistics courses of a nonparametric and applied type. The many nurses in management positions who do not have master's degree preparation can utilize statistics courses, consultants, and internal staff persons from computer or fiscal departments, as well as a wide range of possible research that does not require complicated statistics. Lack of education or aptitude for statistics should not deter research effort. Additionally, nurses should know as much as possible about computer usage; but, as in the use of statistics, there are knowledgeable people who are willing and able to work with nurses. Command of nursing and a scientific point of view are nurses' essential contributions to such joint effort. We must surmount the frustrations of limited time, the pressure of work, and the discouragement of working in uncharted areas. Doing the right thing is energizing, especially if everyone is in it together, providing moral and practical mutual support.

While not denying the frustrations and difficulties involved, Jackson[27] provides an exciting account of her work on a team where the staff was studying human energy exchange and metabolism in an experimental unit heavily dependent on electronics. She speaks of the new meaning taken on by commonplace things, such as temperature, rest, weight, and intake and output, when viewed as part of sophisticated experimental work. Such research is akin to breaking the physiological barrier where long-held empirical observations are tested. It seems almost like research behind the research.

Lindeman[28] describes a 4-year-old research program in a 300-bed hospital. Important and practical nursing procedures were improved, such as a nursing admission interview, an outpatient education program for diabetic patients and their families, judgmental rather than rigid catheterization routines in gynecological surgery, strengthened preoperative procedures, and parental participation on the pediatric unit. Involvement, support, and collaboration seem to characterize the effort.

If the base of nurses dedicated to and knowledgeable of the scientific method were expanded, the small number of qualified researchers would increase more naturally; they would come from wider numbers in lower echelons, rather than being recruited for this special work at the graduate level exclusively.

The plea from our research leaders is to do descriptive research, because we are in touch with patients in clinical settings—a primary requisite for such research. Ellis[5] and This[15] proposed the investigation of TLC; Guy[29] tells of surgical patients being discharged sooner because pain was relieved before the respiratory routine of turning, deep breathing, and coughing; and Lindeman[28] also offers cogent comments on the subject of postoperative respiratory routines. Norris[30] invites nurses everywhere to join and extend their research effort on the phenomenon, namely restlessness, as they meet it in their practice. We can substantiate the effectiveness of physician-nurse rounds as compared with physician-only rounds, determine the therapeutic effect of visitors, test the efficiency of a given procedure, ascertain the average nightly sleep range for patients, and learn what and how many deterrents there are to maximum respiratory function for patients. We must, however, instigate such investigations. Our clinical research has been described as primitive; let us accept the challenge.

ADJUNCTS TO RESEARCH

There are valuable adjuncts to research for nurse managers besides those that originate in our own past. These are often landmark research studies, from which we can learn and relearn (such as the experiments at Western Electric, with their implication for human relations).

We should not overlook the collateral research carried on in industries that serve hospitals and nursing (the revolutionary bath procedure mentioned earlier, antiembolism stockings, and the ultracare mattress for decubitus prevention). The effects and applications of research abound, and we must identify, test, and assimilate them into nursing practice.

Creativity

Research and creativity are interrelated. The quest, questioning, structure, dedication, and discipline of research partake of and generate creativity.

There has always been an aura of mystery about creativity. We have tended to think of it as inspiration or an indefinable something possessed by artists, composers, and the like. In the 1950s and 1960s there was intensive investigation of creativity. Characteristics of the quality, its nature, measurability, and application were made known in a general way. It became a concept by which to describe not only artists but people in more prosaic endeavors. Ghiselin[31] speaks of it as being as broad as life itself. Indeed, the discovery of its characteristics made prediction and assessment of its presence possible. The subject is far from exhausted, and the search continues; findings continue to be applied in industry, hospitals, and elsewhere.

Torrance[32] defines creativity as "the process of becoming sensitive to problems, deficiencies, gaps in knowledge, missing elements, disharmonies, and so on; identifying the difficulty, searching for solutions, making guesses, or formulating hypotheses about the deficiencies; testing and retesting them; and finally, communicating the results." Although Torrance's critics claim that his definition does not address the essential nature of creativity, his definition and work have helped considerably in getting creativity out of the rarified atmosphere of the Einsteins and Picassos and into the general stream of life.

Rogers's[33] definition has much in common with Torrance's. He says that "it is the emergence in action of a novel relational product, growing out of the uniqueness of the individual on the one hand, and the materials, events, people, or circumstances of his life on the other." This definition favors the wider point of view of the creative process, making it something to which every person may aspire.

FINDINGS OF STUDIES OF CREATIVE PERSONS

Getzels and Jackson[34] found a relationship, though not a strong one, between high I.Q. and high creativity scores in their study population. Motivation was undifferentiated. Teachers preferred students with high I.Q.s to highly creative pupils. In noting that the Getzels and Jackson findings on self-preferred personality traits demonstrated that highly creative children favored a sense of humor much more than did children with high I.Q.s, Eisner [pp. 20-21][35] points out the relationship of humor to creativity. Humorists are able to see relationships in the unrelated and can interplay these relationships. We noted elsewhere the humorous repartee that can be found among staff in nursing units. One wonders whether it is the particular individuals, the intimacy of the work relationship, a means of pressure relief, or what, that occasions it. Apparently, it is creative.

Exploratory work with creative individuals shows them to be flexible, sensitive, perceptive, expressive, open, independent, possessed of retentive memories for life experiences, concerned with meanings, relationships, theory, complex and unifying principles, and accepting of failure. The relationship of creativity to mental health remains obscure, perhaps because there is no unanimity on what precisely constitutes mental health [p. 24].[35]

CLASSIFICATION OF CREATIVITY

Eisner [pp. 30-35][35] proffers an interesting classification of creativity, consisting of aesthetic organizing, boundary pushing, inventing, and boundary breaking. Aesthetic organizing is the pleasing arrangement of things, work, and so forth. This quality is displayed increasingly in offices as managers grow in individuality, that is, where individuals have some choice other than mass-produced decoration. Some nursing stations display aesthetic organizing. Boundary pushing consists of new, original uses for articles. Plastic needle shields used as playroom equipment are an example. Inventing comprises new products that result from the combination of materials and ideas. Boundary breaking is reserved for the rare occasions when new assumptions are made or old ones are made problematic, as seen where promotion of health joins the care of the sick in nursing definition. A case could be made for the work of Bredenberg[36] and other early researchers in team nursing as qualifying for boundary breaking.

CREATIVITY IN MANAGEMENT

In speaking about management's need to be concerned about perpetuation and self-renewal, Drucker[37] suggests an organizational structure open to new ideas and ways of doing things. He speaks of innovative management where there is concern for the future state of the enterprise, supported by visionary, dynamic top management to supplement the operating management, which is responsible for present performance and output.

Roy[38] urges the encouragement of imagination and creativity, especially among staff personnel in fiscal, personnel, medical, and operations research departments, to enliven their more or less prosaic work. If achieved, enlivened figures can be used to help formulate policies, the personnel department will be able to diagnose and help handle conflict, and so on. Individual creativity is enriched by and enriches human relations, participation, planning, and controlling, because it is relational and interpenetrative. It cannot be measured by a clock, regulated at will, or surface in persons under constant pressure.

CREATIVITY AND WOMEN

Podeschi and Podeschi[39] tell of Maslow's interest in creativity as primary—inspirational and correlated with femininity—and secondary—hard work, striving, and evaluation correlated with masculinity. According to Maslow, the primary and secondary are synthesized in the truly creative person. However, he was concerned that men should encourage their primary creativeness and that women not negate secondary creativeness through tendencies toward dependency and passivity, lest the bisexual aspects of personality and creativity be stifled in both men and women.

Rudikoff[40] corroborates the need for nurturing Maslow's primary and secondary but coexisting components of creativity. She reviews the lives of a variety of successful women, such as Marie Curie, Rose Kennedy, Jane Addams, Helene Deutsch, and Margaret Mead, to counter or modify a current notion that women are afraid of success. She seems to wish to ameliorate this psychological dichotomy and establish the bisexual notion of success. The implications of a bisexual notion for creativity are relevant to nursing, a predominantly female profession.

CREATIVITY AND NURSES

Nurses are probably creative, innovative, and imaginative, though these traits may not be sufficiently developed. Such characteristics join the best in all people, and we should strive to achieve them. Neither pessimism nor optimism can prevail, because nurses have the same deficiencies as others and the same resources with which to correct them.

Donovan[41] notes creative activities among nurses and equates them with creative acts of others. The most revealing and pertinent is the instance of nurses who decide to abandon their starched, "bathing" efficiency and aid dying patients insofar as they can. Other examples of creativity, besides patented devices of various kinds, are nurses struggling to evolve a theory or philosophy of nursing, to care for children comprehensively with full attention to their psychological needs, to care for real and wide-ranging needs of patients in intensive care units, or head nurses who see that their staff can attend educational commitments with equanimity rather than harassment. Identification of such performance is a first step in unleashing our creative potential. Effort to carry it out can and should follow.

COMPREHENSIVE PROGRAM FOR CREATIVITY

Bennett's Employee Idea Program[42] describes a comprehensive program for maximizing employee contributions to achieving the goals of the enterprise and is also a methods-improvement program in which everyone can and is encouraged to participate. It consists of a highly structured program involving administration, in-service education, and management support. Because it is so structured, it provides guidance in how to manage and test ideas in order to eliminate randomness and vagueness. The program describes a point evaluation system for ideas and suggests possible awards, both nontangible such as a letter of commendation and tangible such as cash or gifts.

There have been suggestion boxes and such devices to encourage employees to submit their ideas. This program, however, is far more richly conceived and executed and represents tangible encouragement of employee idealism. There is reason to believe that we are only beginning to tap the creative potential of workers in all ways and at all levels.

REFERENCES

1. Treece, E., and Treece, J.: Elements of research in nursing, St. Louis, 1973, The C. V. Mosby Co., p. 3
2. Leininger, M.: Conference on the nature of science and nursing, Nurs. Res. **17**(6):484, 1968.
3. Nisbet, R.: Observing and explaining. In Rose, P., editor: Seeing ourselves, New York, 1972, Alfred A. Knopf, Inc., p. 4
4. Chase, S.: The proper study of mankind, New York, 1963, Harper & Row, Publishers, pp. 11 and 17.
5. Ellis, R.: The practitioner as theorist, Am. J. Nurs. **69**(7):1434-1438, 1969.
6. Armiger, Sr. B.: Scholarship in nursing, Nurs. Outlook **22**(3):160-164, 1974.
7. Fleming, J., and Hayter, J.: Reading research reports critically, Nurs. Outlook **22**(3): 172-175, 1974.
8. Stevens, B.: ANA's Standards of Nursing Practice; what they tell us about the state of the art (editorial), J. Nurs. Admin. **4**(5):16-18, 1974.
9. Stevens, B.: A second look at "New Positions Descriptions" in nursing, J. Nurs. Admin. **3**(6): 21-23, 1973.
10. Mullane, M.: Education for nursing service administration, Battle Creek, 1959, W. K. Kellogg Foundation, p. 164.
11. Abdellah, F.: Overview of nursing research, 1955-68, Nurs. Res. Part I, **19**(1):6-17, 1970; Part II, **19**(2):151-162, 1970; Part III, **19**(3): 239-252, 1970.
12. Wieland, G.: Manager-directed surveys for organizational improvement, J. Nurs. Admin. **2**(6):43-47, 1972.
13. Revans, R. W.: Standards for morale; cause and effect in hospitals, London, 1964, Oxford University Press.
14. Georgopoulos, B., and Jackson, M.: Nursing Kardex behavior in an experimental study of patient units with and without clinical nurse specialists, Nurs. Res. **19**(3):196-218, 1970.
15. This, L.: Why don't they . . .? Supervisor Nurse **2**(5):66-71, 1971.
16. Notter, L.: Nurse researchers hear plea to change research emphasis, Am. J. Nurs. **74**(6):1031, 1974.
17. Dickson, W., and Roethlisberger, F.: Management and the worker, Cambridge, Mass., 1939, Harvard University Press.
18. Diers, D.: This I believe . . . about nursing research, Nurs. Outlook **18**(11):52, 1970.
19. Boettinger, H.: Is management really an art? Harvard Business Review **53**(1):55, 1975.
20. Gortner, S.: Research in nursing; the federal interest and grant program, Am. J. Nurs. **73**(6): 1052-1055, 1973.
21. Aydelotte, M.: Nurse staffing methodology, Washington, D.C., 1973, U.S. Department of Health, Education, and Welfare, Division of Nursing, no. (NIH)73-433.
22. Levine, E.: Research on nurse staffing in hospitals, Washington, D.C., 1972, U.S. Department of Health, Education, and Welfare, Division of Nursing, no. (NIH)73-434.
23. Werley, H.: This I believe . . . about clinical research, Nurs. Outlook **20**(11):718-722, 1972.
24. Resolutions, The American Nurse **6**(8):5, 1974.
25. National Commission for the Study of Nursing and Nursing Education: Summary report and recommendations, Am. J. Nurs. **70**(2):285-286, 1970.
26. Jacox, A.: The research component in the nursing service administration master's degree program, J. Nurs. Admin. **4**(2):38-39, 1974.
27. Jackson, B.: The biomedical engineer, Supervisor Nurse **5**(5):41-43, 1974.
28. Lindeman, C.: Nursing research; a visible, viable component of nursing practice, J. Nurs. Admin. **3**(2):18-21, 1973.
29. Guy, J.: Letters, J. Nurs. Admin. **4**(2):5, 1974.
30. Norris, C.: Restlessness; a nursing phenomenon in search of meaning, Nurs. Outlook **22**(2):107.
31. Ghiselin, B.: The creative process, New York, 1952, The New American Library Inc., p. 24.
32. Torrance, E. P.: Scientific views of creativity and factors affecting its growth, Daedalus **94**(3): 663-664, 1965.
33. Rogers, G.: Toward a theory of creativity. In Parnes, S., and Harding, H., editors: A source book for creative thinking, New York, 1962, Charles Scribners' Sons, p. 65.
34. Getzels, J., and Jackson, P.: Creativity and intelligence, New York, 1962, John Wiley & Sons, Inc.
35. Eisner, E.: Think with me about creativity, Dansville, N.Y., 1964, F. A. Owen Publishing Co., pp. 20-21, 24, and 30-35.
36. Bredenberg, V.: Nursing service research, Philadelphia, 1951, J. B. Lippincott Co.
37. Drucker, P.: Management, tasks, responsibilities, practices, New York, 1974, Harper & Row, Publishers, p. 556.
38. Roy, R.: The administrative process, Baltimore, 1965, The Johns Hopkins University Press, p. 68.
39. Podeschi, R., and Podeschi, P.: Abraham Maslow; on the potential of women, Educational Horizons **52**(6):61-64, 1974.
40. Rudikoff, S.: Women and success, Commentary **58**(4):49-59, 1974.
41. Donovan, H.: Creativity and the nurse, Hospital Progress **45**(6):98-99, 1964.
42. Bennett, A.: An Employee Idea Program, New York, 1969, Preston Analearn.

CHAPTER 18
PUBLIC RELATIONS

Public relations has come recently to the hospital enterprise. The long-standing isolation of the hospital as a community resource has tended to separate it from the community it serves: it has never been an integrating and integrated part of the community. However, hospitals now are in many ways trying to compensate for past deficiencies and build a firm, two-way communication with the public they serve. Whether this opening up to the public is a result of the massive criticism of medicine and hospitals over the years or is completely voluntary is not so important as that it is happening. There is little doubt but that the fantastic increases in consumerism, communications, and hospital administration have all contributed to a growing public relations attitude on the part of hospitals.

In this chapter we shall view public relations within the hospital context. Certainly nursing is intimately woven into this larger picture. Indeed, the interweaving may be detrimental to nursing in that it camouflages or denies nursing's specific identity and tends to lump nursing with general services and costs.

In his monumental work on public relations and nursing 30 thirty years ago, Bernays[1] pointed out the need for strengthening the hospital administrator–nurse relationship by a give-and-take educational process. The same need exists today. We must not only strengthen this intercommunication but at the same time try to extricate nursing from the submerged status it has in the work of the hospital. The process of separating nursing's identity from that of the hospital may be the best means of fostering this necessary intercommunication and should bring clarification. The large part nursing plays in the operation of the hospital renders it culpable where it fails to keep hospital administration fulfilling its community obligations, that is, increasing reciprocal understanding of the hospital's mission.

Public relations is a well-communicated system of policies and actions designed to build and increase public confidence, understanding, and support and requires the essentials of good management. It consists of two-way communication for the purpose of appraising the dispositions of the public.[2] While this definition implies direct input on the part of the public, it is not stated precisely, which can be construed to be holding the public at length rather than incorporating it as part of this public service, that is, the care of the sick and the promotion of health.

Follett[3] spoke succinctly of the difference between two-way communication as an evaluative device and as a provider of direct input in discussing participating constituents. She sees the need to combine analyzed experience with that of the expert, in order to arrive at greater cooperation and efficiency. Melding of the experience of patients with the knowledge of professionals in the hospital situation contributes not only to Follett's participating constituents but to satisfactory public relations, because it renders both the consumer and the experts operative. Public opinion should arise from the combined experiences of the consumer and the expert. Direct input of consumers is necessary to effect this combined production, or public relations.

In his significant work for the American Nurses' Association, Bernays[4] pointed out some public relations essentials for nurses and hospital administration as the parent of the nursing enterprise. He speaks of good public relations as being dependent on mutual understanding, that is, of the experts, nurses, hospital administrators, and so forth, and the public they serve; and on meeting the real need of the public.

Two-way communication is present in the statements of the American Hospital Association[2] and Bernays, but the emphases are different. For Bernays they are directed to diagnosis, that is, finding out the nature of professional maladjustments on the one hand and the real needs of the public on the other; whereas the AHA statement is far less explicit. Bernay's statement is far more authentic and reciprocal and seems to cut through to the heart of the matter. It is far less likely to generate the stream of one-way communication that has dominated public relations. However, Bernay's statement is less likely to be acted on, because it is painful to face the opinions of people who experience our ministrations or lack of them. This painfulness may account for nursing's failure to take Bernay's findings seriously and for the late arrival of public relations on the hospital scene. While nursing continues to worry about its image, it fails to engage in the reality-based assessment of its maladjustment and the needs of its public. It is possible that concern for our image deflects us from concern for our reality. Image means a representation of something, yet the reality of the substance is more vital than is representation of substance.

Health personnel and institutions still have considerable reluctance to engage the public on its own terms: as partners or participants in decision making. The exclusion of the press (and so the public) from deliberations of physicians and trustees about the possible merger of two community hospitals occasioned the following response from the press:

> A lack of knowledge and understanding can best be remedied by more and better information. . . .
>
> The public deals quite well with "raw data" that emerges from meetings and discussions by public officials. Such formative information is a necessity if informed decisions are to be made.
>
> Those knowledgeable in health care risk a disservice to the community and to themselves whenever they thwart a clean flow of information.*

Another quote, addressed to a public school system, could just as easily be addressed to a hospital system, because the same obligations obtain, that is, accountability for a specific service to the community:

> Accountability means more than just publicizing the good news. . . . It means accepting responsibility for mistakes and following through with improvements.†

THE VARIOUS PUBLICS

In addition to hospital administrators, Bernays surveyed physicians, public opinion molders, and the public.[5-7] He found that, in general, physicians take nurses for granted. He proposed that the remedy lies in educating physicians individually and in groups. The public opinion molders saw a need for upgrading financial remuneration for nurses, to be accomplished by nurses themselves. Though it has taken many years, salaries have been upgraded, substantially through the efforts of the American Nurses' Association. They also saw the need to strengthen the education of nurses in psychology and culture. If culture means social factors, we are still struggling to enrich the psychosocial components of nursing, though we have come a long way in 30 years. Bernays found that there was not much understanding of the nursing problem by the public. The problem as he saw it was the conflict between the traditional role of the nurse and her need for

---

*From Van Nostrand, E.: Hospital concerns (editorial), Vancouver, Wash., The Columbian, October 8, 1974, p. 8

†From Maynard, R.: Accountability is more than just good news, Vancouver, Wash., The Columbian, November 12, 1974, p. 11.

professional status and adequate remuneration. Again he recommended educating the public. We have made some progress in these areas, but our professional status remains fragile and our increased compensation still marginal and strenuously fought for.

In his extensive and definitive work in public relations, Bernays[8] summarized nursing as technically a profession greatly in need of strengthening through increased prestige. He saw "demonstrable competence in nursing, higher salaries, evidence of greater interest in public affairs, and more independence" as possible avenues to the necessary increased prestige. This closely approximates our current status in securing professionalism.

Bernays did not address himself to nursing itself as a public. Whether one's own profession constitutes a public is debatable. It is not debatable, however, that we must bring more unity to nursing so that a cohesive message can be given and received. Conflicting opinion on directions we should take within the profession is not the sole problem, because much remains to be done to bring all nurses to a common view of nursing care. The concept of comprehensive nursing care does not have opponents so much as it has practitioners who are unaware of its ramifications. We have not universally interiorized the range of nursing care possible and available, yet until we do we cannot effectively educate others (physicians, hospital administrators, or the public). We need mass internal education so that there is a common denominator of knowledge and practice providing a base from which to launch educational efforts toward other publics. While we go about these wider educational efforts, we must direct them internally too, so that coherence, rather than fragmentation and tangents, can prevail.

PUBLIC RELATIONS RECORD IN NURSING

Nursing's public relations record is not impressive. Ignorance, disharmony, and conflicting views within the profession militate against sending messages to the various publics, but apathy is probably the biggest deterrent. We have not exploited the ethos of nursing or attuned ourselves to its nobility at any of its stages of formation. Moreover, apathy could have been dissipated more easily by the formidable base provided by Bernays under the aegis of the American Nurses' Association. It must have been expensive, because public relations specialists, unlike nurses, have always commanded high compensation.

Our official statements over the years have lacked a public relations component. There were occasional direct and some oblique references to public relations, as illustrated in the statements of the National League for Nursing.[9,10] Of the thirteen statements on the functions of a hospital department of nursing service (1964), only one refers directly to the public relations function and speaks of ways in which nursing can work with other groups to interpret the hospital and nursing service objectives to patients and community. The reciprocal nature of public relations is specific in this statement. However, in the 1965 statement on criteria for evaluation of a hospital department of nursing service, there is no reference to this function, though there is a patients' evaluation of the nursing care they received.

The statements of the ANA contain oblique references. Nursing's part in disaster plans is contained in Standards for Organized Nursing Services.[11] Hospital disaster plans have usually been correlated with community disaster plans, hence a community connection. The revised statement of 1973[12] recommends that nurses participate in health care organization and community committees. While neither of these statements really addresses public relations as such, they do recognize the need for nurses to be visible and operative in community health care programming. Sustained presence in these affairs contributes to community understanding of nursing. In the literature about head nurses there are references to their role in meeting the public, which raises the question of whether we have assumed that public relations rested with them rather than all nurse managers essentially because of accessibility of head nurses to the public.

There have been occasional abortive efforts to provide speakers' bureaus to carry nursing's message to community organizations, but by and large they have been too tentative and fragile to survive. However, this channel can still be exploited. Brock[13] urges nurses to interpret nursing needs knowledgeably, precisely, and as though we knew our business rather than petulantly declaring we are not understood. We are probably not understood because we have not made ourselves and our statements understandable.

Beletz[14] reinforces this need to represent ourselves specifically and with emphasis on our changed role. This suggests that we show nursing in its new and unique function. The work of nurses in coronary and intensive care units is an example we have not used sufficiently. In these sites nurses are practicing their original relationship of partnership with the physician, unobscured by other disciplines. Using these nurses as a model, we can define nursing work done elsewhere more lucidly and precisely, for example, in the extended-care location where the medical influence is felt less. The nurse's relationship to the phenomenally expanded chemotherapeutic component of medical care might yield specific descriptive data, because intensification of this therapy spans the years from the advent of antibiotics to the present. This chemotherapeutic emphasis demonstrates in some ways a quiescent period of nursing activity dating from the end of poultices, therapeutic immersion baths, and the like in preantibiotic days to the advent of the electronic activity of the coronary care units. Backrubs and massages were also eclipsed in the quiescent period, for related or different reasons. This proposition has obvious flaws and is proferred in its primitive state only for ideational purposes.

Amid the national surge of review, restatement, and reform of nurse practice laws,[15] we are cautioned to pay attention to criticism and try to rectify it before legislation mandates such correction. We have been oblivious and indifferent to the large amount of criticism contained in the popular press over the years. To be sure, such literature often addresses itself to the hospital and medical deficiencies in the health care system, but much is aimed directly at nursing. Harris[16] speaks to this flagrant disregard for and even combative attitude toward consumer (patient) opinion by noting professional reaction to his complaints that hospitals are run for the benefit of staff, not patients; the excessive restraints, rules, and procedures; and the little concern for patients as persons. He notes that on a successive hospitalization the pattern persisted, even though the staff was forewarned, and sees the necessity for overhauling the bureaucratic apparatus. We can persist in ignoring all such cogent criticism, or we can deliberate about it and make appropriate changes. The move is ours.

The August 1973 issue of *Ms* offered an excellent collection of articles about nurses and nursing. They are so comprehensive, pertinent, and penetrating that they could properly be on a required reading list for nurses. Such material encourages nurses to think about themselves and their profession in ways usually not open to them. Nursing journals should reprint such articles regularly. There are also little-known journals with insightful new approaches,[17] and underground newspapers carry important pertinent information, though in an offbeat or antiestablishment vein.[18]

Criticism occasionally penetrates professional journals. In one, Mauksch[19] provides insightful criticism of our treatment of the patient as a person. An abridged version of a frank and comprehensive view of consumer reaction and responses to the health care system is contained in *Nursing Digest* [Solomon[20]]. Dr. Cherkasky of Montefiore Hospital fame seems to reiterate the messages of Follett and Bernays when he recommends a team approach to health problems. Such a team would consist of professional people (to provide the expertise) and lay people who are socially aware.

On the positive side, there are beginnings of consumer representation where it will make a difference, such as the move to wider representation on hospital boards of various specific consumer publics, such as unions, and a movement to have nurse representation on them too. An exciting step in this direction is the formation of a lay advisory council for the New York State Nurses' Association, to advise nurses and provide consumer advocacy.[21] Schools of nursing have availed themselves of advisory committees over the years, but nursing service organizations have seldom done so. A nursing service department needs this kind of input, as do other nursing organizations—perhaps more so, because they serve such great numbers of people. Advisory committees serve the public relations interest well.

In convention in 1974, the American Nurses' Association passed a resolution that high priority be given to a broad public relations program, making maximum use of public media to show the involvement of well-educated, competent nurses in independent and interdependent practice of primary, long-term, and acute nursing.[22] The resolution is at least part of what Bernays proposed 30 years ago.

OPINION POLLS

Opinion polls are the prevalent means of gaining input from the public who use our services. Some valuable things are learned, but in general they elicit favorable responses. Though anonymity is provided, there may be the lingering fear of reprisal for negative criticism, should respondents require further hospitalization. This fear accompanies the frequently made and justified observation that patients are "good" and "cooperative" through fear of reprisal.

PUBLIC RELATIONS PERSONNEL

The number of public relations directors employed in hospitals is growing. They are often part of the personnel department or function independently as staff (advisory) personnel. They are knowledgeable about the various media and other community resources (service clubs and such). They have writing skill and synchronizing ability, because their work is frequently that of developing and helping others develop ideas. In general, public relations directors contribute substantially to the ever-widening social reporting component in the press and other media.

The collaboration of the public relations and nursing staffs is seen in a public service program on heart disease by St. Vincent Hospital and Medical Center, Portland, Oregon (Fig. 13). The idea originated with the nursing staff; then, in cooperation with public relations personnel, the program was planned, advertised, and executed. The blood pressure clinic attracted approximately 380 people not employed by the hospital, and physician referral cards were issued for 161 of them. The public information seminar attracted approximately 150 persons.[23]

More and more hospitals are offering similar community services either independently or in cooperation with local chapters of various health associations. The public relations director is largely responsible for the smoothness, integration, and coordination of such efforts.

PUBLIC RELATIONS AND THE EXPANDED ROLE OF THE HOSPITAL

The growing line of communication between the hospital and the community strengthens the public relations function substantially. Volunteerism is the major vehicle for this increased communication. Women's auxiliary groups not only provide great amounts of direct and indirect service to hospitals, but also provide invaluable liaison between the hospital and community, which enriches both. Volunteerism,

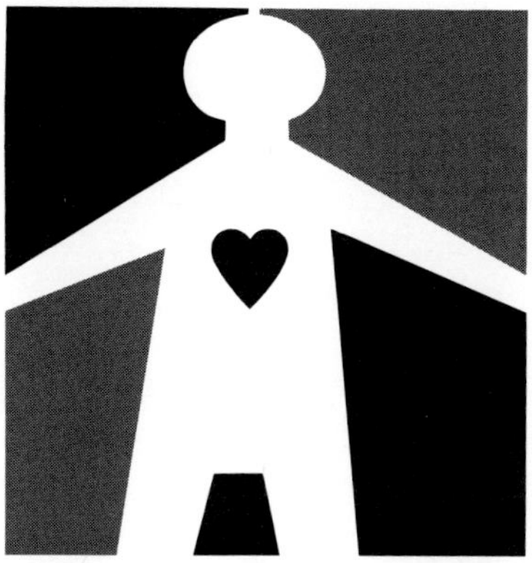

Heart Month

February is Heart Month. To further acquaint the public with the nation's number one killer, coronary artery disease, St. Vincent Hospital and Medical Center invites you to take part in several activities.

February 1 thru February 15 —	Display and pick-up material, courtesy of Oregon Heart Association, in the second floor lounge next to the elevators.
February 11 thru February 15 (Week of Valentine's Day) —	The Nursing Staff of the Cardiovascular Care Unit will conduct a blood pressure clinic for the public in the second floor lounge from 2 to 4 p.m. and from 7 to 8:30 p.m. daily. Where blood pressure levels indicate the need, referral cards will be issued and these persons will be urged to see their doctors.
February 23 (Saturday)	From 1 to 4 p.m., a public information seminar will be conducted in the East Dining Room, second floor, of the cafeteria. Herbert J. Semler, M.D., will speak on preventive cardiac medicine; Leonard B. Rose, M.D., will discuss what to do when a heart attack occurs in the home; and there will be cardiopulmonary resuscitation demonstrations and practice sessions.

Fig. 13

subsidized by the hospital and its staff, is making a growing contribution to community service, such as low-cost monthly service to senior citizens. Additionally, an eight-page newspaper supplement[24] describes a free comprehensive health education program geared to physical, mental, social, and spiritual aspects of people, with strong hospital support. Nutrition, weight-watching, exercise, and mental health instruction and a 5-day program to help people stop smoking, are offered, as well as a variety of health tests to detect proneness to heart attack, high blood pressure, and glaucoma.

Hospital personnel are often part of career education programs in high schools. Young people, including such groups as Future Nurse clubs, visit and work in hospitals, which substantially deepen hospital-community relations.

PUBLIC RELATIONS AND PUBLICATIONS

Hospitals often have house organs to keep personnel informed about the institution and its activities. They are very important for ongoing, in-house information for increased employee satisfaction. Such satisfaction is transmitted to patients in a wide variety of ways, not only as improved performance but as pride in the institution and willingness to communicate this pride to patients and others in an employee's sphere of influence. These house organs have a potential for achieving a high order of effectiveness in staff communications and understanding.

One such sophisticated effort contains a detailed statistical overview, with pictures of the central service department and a professional profile of its director [McGilvra, pp. 3-9].[25] The issue also contains a professional profile on the then new security chief. It almost reads as a community services profile, in that the work and preparation of this person runs a cohesive, coherent course of preparation for the post of security chief [p. 18]. The same issue contains a review of a book on medical ethics, providing the staff with up-to-date information on this important but obscure topic [back endpaper].

There is a three-way dimension to public relations, which integrates the numbers of two-way efforts in achieving mutual understanding and support. The variety of publications designed to improve the public's care of itself falls within this three-way dimension. Though intended for the public, or more precisely, the specifically affected public, they should be part of the professional's information service, so that the professional-patient relationship is enriched by the introduction of material from this third source. One such publication is *Focus,*[26] a quarterly of the Illinois Lung Association and addressed to people with emphysema. While it is possible that the professionals may know much of the material, they are not so familiar with publication formats and methods of getting professional information across to specific types of patients. We are more bound by our professional terminology and practice than we realize, and such publications can expand our professional versatility. Familiarity with these publications can enrich our practice by adding a resource in patient teaching as well as a reinforcement device.

The numbers of news stories about health and disease, the regular columns devoted to such subjects in newspapers and magazines, and the wealth of material available from the U.S. Government Printing Office also fall in this three-way category. For example, the October 1974 issue of *Consumer Report* carries an excellent nine-page detailed overview of hypertension, complete with descriptions of available sphygmomanometers for do-it-yourself use under medical supervision. The same issue carries a comprehensive report on health maintenance organizations. Of 64 pages in this issue, 16 are devoted to these two health topics. These figures give an idea of the great consumer interest we must satisfy if we are to deepen our public relations activity and enrich professional-public understanding.

Annual reports provide an excellent public relations resource for the various publics concerned, such as personnel within the organization, the public served, and the general public. These reports must be made more personally concerned with and comprehensive to the public, in the interest of wider readership and greater public relations impact in both directions.

We have something to learn from industrial public relations. For example, *The Sohioan* (magazine of the Standard Oil Company of Ohio)[27] is designed to reach the company's various publics, including employees, dealers, distributors, and stockholders. It contains an excellent account of tooth care (the connection to the company lies in the manufacture of needed supplies for tooth care by a subsidiary of the company). This issue also carries a detailed account of the changes in Social Security payment rates effective in June 1974.

Another widely distributed informational vehicle is a report of a conference that included representation from institutional stockholders on Progress in Areas of Public Concern (General Motors Corp.)[28] The conference offered presentations on a number of pertinent topics such as metal recycling, alternate power sources, mass transit systems, and an excellent article addressed to any manager anywhere, entitled "Employee Development and the Modern Work Force." The applicability of the content to the health care institution is amazing.

It can be countered that the public relations devices of industry are not applicable to the hospital situation because the latter are usually nonprofit enterprises and many of these devices are expensive productions. What can apply to our situation, however, is the imaginativeness, openness, and versatility that these publications display. They constitute models well worth our consideration.

• • •

There is a considerable intermingling of public relations efforts of the hospital and the nursing department, because it is important that a total picture precede a departmental one. Interrelationships abound. We must, though, as in every other phase of the hospital operation, try to isolate nursing's unique rather than diffuse contribution. It is possible that where the public relations function does not exist or is just emerging, the nursing department can lead the way. This is the way in-service education arrived on the hospital scene. To engage in the public relations function completely requires the continuing exploration of what we do, and how we do our work, along with the continuing exploration of how well it meets the needs of our patients.

In the actual mechanics of public relations as it exists today between hospitals and the various media, it is often the nurse supervisor, by dint of continuing presence, who is the hospital spokesperson to the media, especially after regular hours. For this reason, the nursing department can spur and contribute to the formulation of policies and procedures governing hospital-media relations. Where there are formalized disaster plans, there are usually provisions included for space and telephones for the press. These provisions can be expanded to cover all such encounters as they occur, so that both hospital and media personnel know precisely the details of their working relationships. The more definitively they are worked out mutually in advance, the smoother and more productive the encounters will be. The hospital's obligation to protect the privacy of patients and the media's obligation to provide news to the public can be reconciled only by careful, thoughtful attention to all the ramifications. The nursing department can contribute substantially to such a reconciliation.

REFERENCES
1. Bernays, E.: Hospitals and the nursing profession, Am. J. Nurs. **46**(2):112-113, 1946.
2. American Society for Hospital Public Relations of the American Hospital Association: A basic

guide to hospital public relations, Chicago, 1973, American Hospital Association, p. 2.
3. Follett, M.: Creative experience, New York, 1951, Peter Smith, pp. 212-213.
4. Bernays, E.: The nursing profession; a public relations viewpoint, Am. J. Nurs. **45**(5):351-353, 1945.
5. Bernays, E.: The medical profession and nursing, Am. J. Nurs. **45**(11):907-914, 1945.
6. Bernays, E.: Opinion molders appraise nursing, Am. J. Nurs. **45**(12):1005-1011, 1945.
7. Bernays, E.: What patients say about nursing, Am. J. Nurs. **47**(2):93-96, 1946.
8. Bernays, E.: Public relations, Norman, Okla., 1952, University of Oklahoma Press, p. 191.
9. Hospital Nursing Services: In pursuit of quality, New York, 1964, National League for Nursing, p. 8.
10. Criteria for evaluating a hospital department of nursing service, New York, 1965, National League for Nursing, p. 9.
11. Standards for organized nursing services, Kansas City, 1965, American Nurses' Association, p. 11.
12. Standards for nursing services, Kansas City, 1973, American Nurses' Association, p. 4.
13. Brock, M.: Bridging the gap between service and education, Supervisor Nurse **5**(7):31, 1974.
14. Beletz, E.: Is nursing's public image up to date? Nurs. Outlook **22**(7):432-435, 1974.
15. Nursing practice acts, Am. J. Nurse **74**(7):1316-1319, 1974.
16. Harris, S.: About hospital care, Vancouver, Wash., The Columbian, October 6, 1974, p. 30.
17. Nursing evolution, vol. 1, no. 1, Kansas City, Mo., October-November 1973, UB publications.
18. Donovan, H.: Can we work with the Black Panthers? Nurs. Outlook **18**(5):34-35, 1970.
19. Mauksch, H.: Patienthood as a criterion of quality in patient care, New York, 1965, National League for Nursing (no. 20-1184), pp. 54-55.
20. Solomon, J.: Health care; a buyer's market? Nursing Digest **1**(10):16-24, 1973.
21. News, Am. J. Nurs. **72**(12):2135, 1972.
22. Resolution on recognition of nurses during International Women's Year, The American Nurse **6**(8):3, 1974.
23. Personal correspondence, Mrs. Cathy Emms, March 5, 1974.
24. Century 21 Institute for Better Living (advertisement), Portland, Ore., The Oregonian, October 25, 1973.
25. McGilvra, M., editor: The voice of providence, Portland, Ore., June 1973, pp. 3-9 and 18.
26. Focus, Springfield, Ill., Office of Publication, Illinois Lung Association.
27. The Sohioan, **45**(4):8-9 and 16-17, 1973.
28. Report on progress in areas of public concern, Detroit, February 1973, General Motors Corp.

APPENDIX A
PERSONNEL EVALUATION FORMS*

REPORT: PROFESSIONAL PERFORMANCE

Name of
evaluatee _____ Date _____

School _____ Degree held _____ Years teaching experience _____

Position _____ Certificate _____ Years in Vancouver _____

Purposes of evaluation in order of priority:
    To improve the professional performance of the employee.
    Let the employee know how he is getting along on a regular basis not later than May 15 of each year.
    Specifically inform the employee of ways in which he can improve.
    Identify specific training needs of an employee.
    Establish a basis for contract renewal or nonrenewal, dismissal or any other disciplinary action against an employee. Normally, to be completed prior to February 1, if there is evidence of unsatisfactory service (Sec. II. Chapter 34, Laws of 1969 Ex. Session).

  I. During the period _____ to _____
                      (month) (day) (year)   (month) (day) (year)
    the professional services of the above named staff member *have been satisfactory* with the exceptions cited below.   ( )   No exceptions ( )
    A. Exceptions (or deficiencies):

    B. Recommendations for improvement and assistance offered to help the teacher to overcome the indicated deficiencies:

---
*Courtesy Vancouver Public Schools, School District No. 37, Vancouver, Wash.

II. Special commendations (citing specific strengths, talents or special activities that the evaluator would like to have made a part of the official record):

III. This report, including attachments as noted, is based on observations made (date, location, length of observation and comments) and compiled from notes on interview schedules of the current year.

Signature of evaluator _____ Date _____

I have read and discussed this evaluation with my evaluator. I do _____ do not _____ accept it as an accurate account of my services. An additional statement is _____ is not _____ attached, or will be submitted to the personnel office _____ within 10 working days with a copy to the evaluator.

_____ Date _____
Signature of evaluatee

Copies to: Evaluator, Evaluatee, Permanent File (Personnel Office)
                                            Received Personnel Office _____

PROFESSIONAL PERFORMANCE INTERVIEW SCHEDULE

Employee _____ Date _____

School _____ Degree held _____ Years teaching experience _____

Grade/subject _____ Certificate _____ Years in Vancouver _____

This interview covers professional service for time period _____ to
                                                          (month)   (year)

_____
(month)   (year)

Use of this interview schedule is optional with the supervisor or employee. It shall be utilized at the request of either party. A signed copy of the schedule is to be given to the employee at the conclusion of the evaluation conference. The schedule is not to become a part of the employee's permanent personnel file maintained in the district office. The supervisor may retain a copy for his personal file for use in future interviews and for reference in writing letters of reference for the employee for employment placement files in future years.

Space is provided following each evaluation criteria topic to record a brief summary of any discussion of the topic. If more space is needed use the reverse side of this interview schedule form.

I. Shows evidence of professional growth (college training, inservice, steering committees, classroom innovations and professional activities both in general and subject matter groups):

II. Shows evidence of competency in instructional skills:

   1. Provides for individual differences _____

   2. Seeks to understand the age group _____

   3. Uses classroom aids, field trips, resource people _____

   4. Carefully prepares and organizes his material _____

   5. Makes provision for class and individual activities _____

6. Has an adequate academic background _____
_____
_____

7. Shows competency in the area of assignment _____
_____
_____

8. Demonstrates creativity in instructional activity _____
_____
_____

9. Cooperatively works with others _____
_____
_____

10. Demonstrates ability to work at level of assignment ____
_____

III. Shows evidence of competency in guidance skills:

1. Understands and attends to emotional and social needs of pupils ____
_____
_____

2. Provides for teacher-pupil planning and evaluation _____
_____
_____

3. Seeks to understand the cause of pupil behavior _____
_____
_____

4. Has respect and confidence of his students _____
_____
_____

5. Is effective in group guidance _____
_____
_____

6. Is effective in individual guidance _____
_____
_____

7. Works effectively with parents _____
_____
_____

8. Shows respect for students _____
_____
_____

IV. Shows evidence of competency in classroom control and management:

    1. Plans work, long-range and daily _____
_____
_____

    2. Keeps room neat, interesting and attractive _____
_____
_____

    3. Shows ability to obtain courteous attention _____
_____
_____

    4. Is friendly but firm in discipline _____
_____
_____

    5. Is consistent and fair in dealing with children _____
_____
_____

    6. Knows his students and treats them as individuals _____
_____
_____

    7. Generates purposeful learning activities _____
_____
_____

V. Shows evidence of responsibility in general school service:

    1. Is punctual to school, class, meetings _____
_____
_____

    2. Accepts a fair share of out-of-class assignments _____
_____
_____

    3. Aids in developing and maintaining staff morale _____
_____
_____

258 Appendix A

4. Supervises pupils as needed in halls, grounds, etc. _____
   _____
   _____

5. Handles routine reports promptly and efficiently _____
   _____
   _____

_____   _____
Signature of evaluator   Signature of evaluatee
                                  Does not indicate concurrence with
                                  the comments—only that they have
                                  been seen and discussed with the
                                  evaluator.

_____
Date of Conference
Copies to: Evaluator and Evaluatee only

APPENDIX B
CASE STUDIES AND PATIENT INCIDENTS

CASE STUDIES
Mrs. Lindsay, patient*

Mrs. Lindsay called her physician to visit her at home after four days of illness, during which time her condition had become increasingly more acute. Dr. Bruce diagnosed her condition as acute gastroenteritis. He advised that she go to the hospital at once because of her weakened condition and dehydration, due to persistent vomiting. Dr. Bruce called the admitting office of the hospital and arranged for her admission to a semi-private room in the Sherman Pavillion.

On arriving at the hospital, the taxi driver said: "You must mean the Grant House." Being unfamiliar with the hospital, Mrs. Lindsay and her sister, who accompanied her, left the taxi and entered Grant House. Mrs. Lindsay sat in a barren waiting room in an uncomfortable chair while her sister went to the reception desk and informed the receptionist that she had brought Mrs. Lindsay for whom Dr. Bruce had arranged admission.

It was 7:10 in the evening and the receptionist appeared to have no knowledge of the patient's expected arrival. She called the admitting office which was located in another building, but received no answer. The call was repeated several times. Meanwhile, Mrs. Lindsay was becoming fatigued and appeared to her sister somewhat apprehensive. After waiting twenty minutes, the receptionist finally received an answer from the clerk in the admitting office, with instructions to take the patient to a room in the next building.

A wheelchair was secured in which Mrs. Lindsay was taken to the floor where she was met by a graduate nurse, Miss Everett.

*From Case studies in nursing service administration, vol 1, Boston, © 1954, Board of Trustees, Boston University Reprinted with permission from Boston University School of Nursing.

Miss Everett: "Good evening, are you Dr. Ives' patient?"
Mrs. Lindsay: "No, Dr. Bruce is my physician."
Miss Everett: "Oh, is he on the staff?"
Mrs. Lindsay: "I presume so. He made arrangements with the office for my coming here."
Miss Everett: (to receptionist) "She can go in private 341, the next to the last door on the left. I have to answer these lights."

Mrs. Lindsay's sister assisted her in getting into bed, unpacked her belongings, and, in observing their surroundings, became concerned that she was in a private rather than a semi-private room. She reasoned, from her general knowledge of hospitals, that there were probably no more semi-private rooms available.

Mrs. Lindsay complained of feeling too warm and her sister opened a window. The patient became restless and got her feet out from under the cover. After a time a student nurse entered the room.

Student: (in a brusque tone) "You will have to cover yourself or you will catch cold."

With no further consideration or identification, she closed the window and left the room. A moment later a second student entered the room with a clothes book in which, with the assistance of the patient's sister, she listed her clothing. At the same time she secured a thermometer from the dresser and after shaking down the mercury, placed it in Mrs. Lindsay's mouth and proceeded to count her pulse and respiration.

Within the next five minutes the clerk from the admitting office knocked and came into the room.

259

Clerk: I am sorry, but it is necessary for me to disturb you for some information. May I have your full name and residence? How old are you and what was the date of your birth? What is your present occupation? What was the occupation of your parents?"

After a few more questions, she said: "Would you kindly sign this?" handing a form to Mrs. Lindsay who signed and seemed agitated.

Mrs. Lindsay: "I had expected a semi-private room. It was my understanding that Dr. Bruce had made arrangements for it. I have Blue Cross Insurance, but I do not feel that I can afford a private room."

Clerk: I know nothing about the Blue Cross arrangements nor of any arrangement having been made for a semi-private room, but I will look into the matter and see if there is one available."

Student: "Well, I guess I won't go any further with this admitting procedure if she is going to be transferred."

The clerk and the nurse left. Thirty minutes went by without Mrs. Lindsay seeing anyone. She became restless. Since she understood Dr. Bruce had sent her to the hospital primarily for intravenous treatment to relieve her dehydration, she felt that it should have been started. Finally Miss Everett returned accompanied by a student nurse.

Miss Everett: "We have been notified to transfer you to a semi-private room in the Sherman Pavillion."

Exhausted, irritated, and on the verge of tears, Mrs. Lindsay exclaimed: "A patient might die here before anyone paid any attention to how she felt."

Miss Everett: "Oh, it wouldn't happen if you were really sick."

She helped Mrs. Lindsay into her dressing gown while her sister replaced her personal belongings. The student accompanied her to the Sherman Pavillion. After assisting her into bed, the student left and her sister again settled her, this time in a two-bed room which she shared with a white-haired woman. The other occupant was sitting up in bed surrounded with writing materials, boxes of cards, several vases of flowers, and a portable screen covered with greeting cards. She stopped her writing to observe the new patient and the activities in the room. No one spoke until the nurses had left the room. While Mrs. Lindsay's sister was arranging toilet articles, the patient said: "I am Jane Crowell. If you want anything you will have to get that cord hanging over there. You may have to wait some time for there are not many nurses after 7 o'clock."

Mrs. Lindsay thanked her and began to toss about restlessly. Her sister attempted to fix her pillows and arrange the bedclothes for greater comfort.

Mrs. Lindsay: I feel very nauseated."

Her sister put on the signal light and found a basin in the table. Before a nurse answered, Dr. Bruce arrived.

Dr. Bruce greeted Mrs. Lindsay in a friendly manner, drew the curtains between the patients, felt Mrs. Lindsay's pulse and asked her how she felt. He stated that he was sorry about the confusion relating to her admission, and that he would leave orders which would soon be carried out and which he believed would make her more comfortable. Dr. Bruce left, followed shortly by her sister, and Mrs. Lindsay resigned herself to waiting.

Just before 11 p.m., a young resident physician entered the room with a tray containing mysterious bottles, tubing, instruments, and towels. Placing them on the table, he said, "I am Dr. Smith. I am just going to prick your arm and give you some fluid which I think will make you feel much better."

Mrs. Lindsay: "Oh, I do hope so; I have waited so long. I am still nauseated and very warm and so tired. I have not slept much if any for four days."

Dr. Smith: "Well, we will try to help that."

A nurse entered with a flask and a gravity pole. Dr. Smith took Mrs. Lindsay's arm to find a vein for the injection, and with no further conversation, inserted the needle and started the intravenous. After splinting the arm in a comfortable position, he turned to the nurse and muttered something under his breath, and before leaving, said, "For three hours, and you watch it." This had no real meaning to Mrs.

Lindsay but it was obvious that she must lie quietly. Having a mysterious fluid running into her vein was a little frightening. The nurse made no attempt to make Mrs. Lindsay comfortable and said nothing to reassure her in any way. She gave her a pill, looked at Jane Crowell in the next bed who was breathing noisily, turned out the light and left the room. Mrs. Lindsay closed her eyes with the feeling that something was being done for her at last. She finally dozed.

About 2 AM Mrs. Lindsay was aroused by a strange nurse who entered the room briskly but said in a quiet voice, "This is finished and I will remove all this so you can sleep." After finishing, she said, "Is there anything you would like? Mrs. Lindsay was drowsy and upon moving found herself stiff, so merely shook her head. She was given a sip of water and her pillows and bed were made comfortable so that she dozed off shortly.

At about 5 AM Mrs. Lindsay was awakened by a strange nurse who entered her room rustling with starch, hair disheveled, a flashlight in one hand and thermometer in the other. With a crisp "good morning" to Mrs. Crowell, she drew back the curtains. Coming to Mrs. Lindsay's bed, she said, "Good morning, I hope you have slept enough to make you feel a little better." Mrs. Lindsay, feeling the night all too short, responded feebly that she guessed she had slept but that her mouth was very dry and she felt hot and her stomach unsettled and sore. The nurse took her temperature and bustled from the room.

There was more or less continuous activity outside Mrs. Lindsay's room. Some time later, breakfast was served. Mrs. Crowell would have been talkative if encouraged, but Mrs. Lindsay was in no mood for it. During this time a boy came in the room and called: "Paper?"

Mrs. Lindsay: "No thank you," and in an aside: "Oh why do I have to be bothered with such things now?"
Mrs. Crowell: "That is a service the hospital provides. You may appreciate it tomorrow. I'll have one, Johnny."

Soon after Johnny left the room a young man who stated that he was the hospital chaplain entered. To Mrs. Lindsay he appeared to lack composure and in response to his greeting, she declared: "I don't feel like talking to anyone."

Chaplain: "I quite understand and will not disturb you now but if any time I can be of service please call on me," and he left the room.

Some time passed before a nurse came in and said, "I'm going to fix you up now." She worked quickly and efficiently and made a few inconsequential pleasantries. During the process, to Mrs. Lindsay's surprise, she made her feel more comfortable than at any time since her admission to the hospital. She was hardly finished before Dr. Smith returned to give her another intravenous. This ran for three hours. Nurses came in and looked at it but did nothing. Mrs. Lindsay became restless and uncomfortable. Her signal cord was not within reach and she asked Mrs. Crowell, finally, as the fluid was nearly gone, if she would call a nurse. The needle was no more than removed when an aide came with a tray of liquids for her noon meal. It was left so far from her reach that she did not bother with it. The aide returned shortly with a tray for Mrs. Crowell.

Mrs. Crowell: "This food is so cold, how can anyone eat it? I would think they might have learned by this time that I can't eat cabbage."
Aide: "Well, I don't know anything about it. That is what I was told to bring you," and she turned abruptly and left the room.

Mrs. Crowell ate listlessly portions of her lunch and when finished tossed her napkin toward her tray. It fell to the floor. No one came into the room until Mrs. Lindsay's sister came to see her an hour later. Unfinished trays remained at both patients' beds. Mrs. Lindsay appeared flushed, her bed in the disorder of a restless patient, and the room generally untidy. Mrs. Lindsay's sister found words of encouragement difficult in this atmosphere.

Mrs. Lindsay's treatment continued for three days, after which time her acute symptoms subsided, she began to take nourishment and to feel somewhat stronger. When Dr. Smith visited her she asked him if she might go home. After examining her, he said it would depend on Dr. Bruce's judgment but that he would discuss it with him.

An hour before Mrs. Lindsay's sister's expected arrival, the head nurse came in to tell her she could go home that day after Dr. Bruce's visit. This was the first time she had seen the head nurse. A nurse whom she assumed to be supervisor had been in twice. Her interests appeared primarily concerned with housekeeping and the care of flowers.

Dr. Bruce confirmed her discharge on his one o'clock visit and gave her instructions for the next few days and an appointment at his office.

When Mrs. Lindsay's sister arrived and she assisted her in dressing and again packed her personal belongings, a nurse came to see that she had everything and said that the nursing aide would discharge her. As she went by the head nurse's station, the head nurse said that she hoped she was going home feeling much better. At the same time, the ward clerk handed her a stamped, self-addressed envelope saying the hospital would appreciate her filling out the enclosed questionnaire and returning it to them at her convenience.

A week later, at a morning conference, the hospital administrator gave Miss Gove, the Director of Nursing, three questionnaires, returned by patients, which he stated he thought she might wish to see and hoped she might be able to do something about. Two of them commented very favorably about the nursing care they had received. They were all signed and the third, written over Mrs. Lindsay's signature, was checked as follows:

Questionnaire*

1. Were you received by the admitting and information personnel in a friendly _____, formal __x__, cold or abrupt _____ manner?
2. In general, do you feel that you received good _____, average _____, poor __x__, nursing care?
3. Did you feel that you were treated as an individual _____, "just another case" __x__, or as a machine without personal feelings _____?
4. In general, were you very pleased _____, just satisfied _____, disappointed __x__?

Miss Gove, the Director of Nursing, had been in her position only a short time and this was her first experience as a Director. She was qualified by desirable academic preparation. The Head Nurse on the floor where Mrs. Lindsay was a patient had been in her position for a year. She was young and had been given the appointment immediately on graduation from this hospital school. She was quite confident of her ability and rather lenient with her staff. The nurse in charge on this floor in the evening was an older nurse forced to work for personal reasons during this period. She has been in her position for several years and appeared to resent questioning. Miss Gove returned to her office debating in her own mind what she should do.

Mrs. Johnson, patient

Mrs. Johnson called her neighbor and friend who was a nurse to come and see her. When Mary Brown arrived, she found Mrs. Johnson agitated and anxious. Mrs. Johnson told her that she had not had a bath since she had come into the home on Monday (this was Thursday). Moreover, they brought her into the TV room in a walker and just left her. Everyone said they were too busy to "walk" her and she must get used to the fact that this was a nursing home, not a hospital. She added that the therapist had worked with her legs and got some padding to make a pillow to elevate them. She explained to Mrs. Brown that she was not sure enough of herself in the walker and needed supervision and help with it. She wondered what she could do to get the care she needed so she could get strong enough to go home.

Mrs. Brown suggested that she ask to see the director of nursing, Mrs. Baldwin. Mrs. Johnson wondered how she would get through to her. Mrs. Brown offered to call Mrs. Baldwin, as she had met her at a nursing meeting. Mrs. Brown also offered to call the nurse at Dr. Smith's office. Mrs. Johnson seemed most grateful. The next morning Mary Brown called Mrs. Baldwin, identified herself, and asked if she would check into Mrs. Johnson's care, because she was upset and dissatisfied. Mrs. Brown also called Dr. Smith's office and told the story to the nurse, adding that Mrs. Johnson was not asking Dr. Smith to see her but just wanted him to know.

A week later, after the family vacation, Mrs. Brown went to see Mrs. Johnson. She was anxious to know if things had improved for her. Mrs. Johnson was resting but was glad to see Mrs. Brown. She had many things to tell her. First of all, she had five stitches and a bruise over one eye. She had fallen getting into the bathtub. The nurse assisting her had said she did not need another person helping when Mrs. Johnson had asked if she (the nurse) could get her into the tub by herself. They had taken her

---

*Questions relative to dietary and housekeeping service in this questionnaire have been omitted from this case as they appear to be of little significance.

to the physician's office to have the stitches put in, and she was to go back the next day to have them removed. She also told her that she was fearful in the toilet, because the seat was low and she had great difficulty pulling herself up and the hand bars were out of reach. However, her roommate, who had a broken arm, was helpful about keeping an eye on her and calling the nurses. Mrs. Brown asked if Mrs. Baldwin had been in. "Oh yes," replied Mrs. Johnson. She went on to tell Mrs. Brown that she had asked if Mrs. Johnson were trying to make trouble between the home and the physician, because his office had been deluged with calls about Mrs. Johnson's care at the home. Mrs. Johnson said there had been only two calls—one from her daughter-in-law and one from her neighbor, a nurse named Mrs. Brown.

Some time later Mrs. Brown again visited Mrs. Johnson and found her alone with the door closed. She was crying. It was a gray day, and neither her son nor any of her family had been in. She was worried about him, as he had had what was thought to be a slight stroke and was having tests done. Her other son and family had moved away only recently and had not been in since. Mrs. Brown asked Mrs. Johnson if she would like to play solitaire (she had been a daily player prior to her accident). Mrs. Johnson replied that she might. Mrs. Brown asked at the desk about cards, but the reply was vague. Mrs. Johnson said that she would have her grandson bring some from home when he went up for the mail sometime. Two workers came in and inquired how she was, praised the piece of apple pie Mrs. Brown had brought for her supper, and left.

Some days later Mrs. Brown again visited Mrs. Johnson. She was fully dressed, even to stockings, and looked better. She was walking without a walker, and Dr. Smith had been to see her. Because she was nervous and her hands were shaking, he had prescribed medicine and suggested she do some of the things she used to do. She said she would be going home in a week or two, but her family and the physician told her not to hurry because she had Medicare. She had gotten a housekeeper to stay with her after she went home and seemed quite relieved about finding someone.

She told her she had had another bad experience in the bathtub. The nurse had forgotten her, and an hour had elapsed when her roommate made inquiries to the nurse about her. The nurse hurried in, but Mrs. Johnson was quite upset by then. She was also cold but had managed to reach a towel and put it around her shoulders. She said that she had tried to put hot water into the tub, but it was very difficult to reach, and when she got cold water, she was afraid she might get burned if she tried to adjust it.

Mrs. Brown suggested that she drive Mrs. Johnson home so that she could get some of the knitting she was doing for the fall bazaar. Mrs. Johnson enjoyed the ride and visiting and got the sweater she had been knitting, as well as wool and needles to knit bedroom slippers for the bazaar. They then returned to the home. Upon returning to the room, Mrs. Johnson said how glad she was to be by the window now, since her roommate was gone. She explained how she pulled one curtain right across the room and her own part way and left the door open at night. She hoped the other bed would remain empty. As she reached for something in her drawer she pulled out a little flower made from a flattened pill cup and bearing the signatures of the nurses at the hospital.

She told Mrs. Brown how they had brought it into her on an individual cake the day she had left the hospital to go to the home. She seemed pleased to remember their kindness. Mrs. Johnson and Mrs. Brown walked to the nurses' station with the cane Mrs. Johnson had brought from home. The rubber tip was worn through. The nurse took adhesive and put it over the end. Mrs. Johnson said it no longer slid on the floor. She smiled as she told Mrs. Brown how Dr. Smith had said that three legs are better than two. As she walked with Mrs. Brown to the door, they passed a cart of cleaning materials; a maid was mopping nearby. Mrs. Johnson remarked how they were always cleaning somewhere.

A few days later Mrs. Johnson was moved back to her first room and, because her roommate seemed odd and she was walking so well, she called the physician and asked to go home. She observed that a flashily dressed woman with lots of makeup had been given the room by herself that she had vacated.

She was happy to get home and liked her housekeeper very much.

PATIENT INCIDENTS
Visiting

1. "My brother got in the wheelchair and came down to the first floor to see the children (aged 5 and 2). He only stayed about 5 minutes

though. He was pretty tired. He is also worried about how he looks to them, because he is losing so much weight. He tried not to take any shots just before visiting hours so he can talk to us. If there are more than two of us, he comes out into the hall in the wheelchair. Sometimes if the other patient in the room has no visitors my brother asks if he will count us as his visitors in case the nurses come in.

"He'd like to go home for a while, but he needs intravenous therapy every day or so. I'm going to ask Mrs. Jones up the street if she will give it to him at home if he needs it and it is OK with the doctor."

Mrs. Jones agreed to do so as needed. (She works 2 nights a week at this hospital.) The pain was so severe, the patient returned to the hospital the very night he went home. He had his brother drive him up the highway awhile before returning to the hospital. He died within 10 days.

2. A 75-year-old mother said she was hurrying to the hospital to see her daughter before visiting hours ended. "I used to go anytime when she was in a private room. It was a lot easier then."

3. "Do not waken him, he needs his rest," said the nurse to the mother of a hospitalized 2-year-old at 1 PM.

The mother had waited in the hall 30 minutes for permission of the supervisor to see the child outside regular visiting hours. She was there at that time because a friend had volunteered to keep her other children while she went to the hospital for a quick visit. The child had been admitted the evening before with pneumonia.

Surgery

1. "They need more men to do the turning. The only one who turned me without hurting me was an orderly who came from another floor. The nurses turn back the covers, but not off my toes. This is enough to hold me back." (Patient had had a spinal fusion.)

2. "Don't they ever shave women's armpits in the hospital?" asked a woman as she told a nurse about her friend who, after 3 weeks of extreme pain, had had surgery on her spine. When the friend returned home, the woman had gone over to ask if there was anything she could do. The friend said, "Oh, yes, please shave my armpits; they feel so uncomfortable."

3. The patient asked her visitor for some chewing gum to freshen her mouth after having had an anesthetic that day while a broken arm was set.

4. "I waited from 9 to 10 PM for them to bring Mary's suppository for sleep. (Mary, age 4, had had her tonsils and adenoids removed that morning.) It had been a long day for us. I was exhausted. Mary was getting restless. She had taken water, sherbet and Jell-O fine. The practical nurse who was assigned to us kept checking to see if the medicine nurse was coming yet."

5. A visitor reported that her friend had had surgery of the gastrointestinal tract and was allowed only fluids and Jell-O. The Jell-O, she said, was too rubbery, so she was having her family bring some thinner Jell-O to her. The nurses thought it was a good idea.

6. A young man who had had surgery on his knee complained that it took the nurses 45 minutes to bring his pain pill, so he started to ask for it sooner, hoping to get it before the throbbing started. No one told him whether he was to exercise the leg.

7. A patient's husband complained that he had been told his wife's operation would be at 7 AM. When he got there, a little before 7, she had already been taken to the operating room. He could get no report about her for 3 hours.

His wife told him later that she had become anxious when she heard nurses talk with some alarm about her blood pressure. She was unable to speak or open her eyes.

Miscellaneous

1. "The woman in the corner bed was delirious for 3 nights. We were frightened. We helped her back to bed several times."

2. "The dietitian will come up tomorrow and talk to him when he is discharged," the head nurse told the patient's wife when she inquired about diet the day before her husband's anticipated discharge. (Her husband had angina pectoris.)

The next morning when his wife arrived, her husband had a diet outline consisting of ten pages—three of instructions and seven of recipes. The dietitian had waited to see if he had any questions.

3. The wife of an 83-year-old patient who was to have a gastrointestinal tract x-ray series reported to her friend that he had gotten break-

fast by mistake that morning, so there would be a day's delay in the tests. Two daughters had come from Seattle and San Francisco to be with their parents at this time because they were worried about their father. They feared cancer, because he was so sick and had lost weight.

4. "They never washed my glasses all the time I was there, although they were always cleaning the halls," reported a patient who had been hospitalized for pelvic surgery.

5. "There's only one who leaves the stool with my slippers on it beside the bed instead of under it."

6. "There's only one who warms the stethoscope when she takes my blood pressure after I've been put to bed."

NURSING HOME INCIDENTS

1. Mrs. Lamphier thanked Mrs. Ogden when she finished filing her nails and applying cream to her hands. She asked if Mrs. Ogden would trim her toenails. She replied that she would be glad to and went to the nurses' station to get a pair of scissors. When she returned, the nurse told her that no one cut toenails there. The podiatrist came regularly and did this service.

Mrs. Lamphier died not long after. Mrs. Ogden wondered if her toenails had ever gotten trimmed.

2. "Mrs. Knapp was very annoyed that I had Doris take everything off her table and clean it. She said she was going to have her children take her out of this home," said Mrs. Allen, the relief RN. "I must phone Mrs. Camp so she will be ready for the complaints when she comes back," she continued. "They sure do hate to have anything touched," replied the aide, Doris.

3. "The odor hits you when you come in the door, but soon you don't notice it," the volunteer said to the volunteer group at their meeting. "I wish we could spray a deodorant around without offending Mrs. Green," added another volunteer. (Mrs. Green was the RN in the home.)

4. "The 3 to 11 o'clock shift leaves things for us to do! Why don't they do them themselves. Just the other day they left a note asking us to cut Mr. Yaeger's toenails. They could do it as well as us." (Mrs. White was complaining about the 3 to 11 o'clock shift to another RN at lunchtime.)

5. "Couldn't someone have phoned for absentee ballots?" asked the volunteer. "I can't, I'm so busy giving the medicines and 'shots' and checking all the medicine supply," replied Mrs. Gould, the RN.

"How about an aide then?" continued the volunteer.

"They can't either; there are only two of them today and we've got fifty patients," Mrs. Gould replied.

Note: The volunteer had previously arranged for registering four of the patients to vote. This nursing home does not have bedridden or seriously ill patients.

6. "Mrs. Hill says quite often that she hasn't been walked since the last time I did it," reported one volunteer to another as they were talking about their activities.

"I wish they'd set up a craft corner so the people could work with things in between our visits," replied the other volunteer. "You just can't do it and get the things put away in 2 hours."

7. While talking to a volunteer Mr. Jones said, "I'm so glad to be home again," as he stood, with his newly shortened cane and a lady's apron protecting his shirt and trousers. "My cane was too long," he continued, "and I fell." (Mr. Jones is 84 years old and has had periodic strokes over the last 10 years. He had fallen and was taken to the hospital, then to an acute care nursing home, and finally back to the home.)

INDEX

A

Accountability
  of clinical specialists, 71
  and organization structure, 66-67
  in personnel evaluation, 122
  and position in organization, 70-71
Accreditation procedures, 160
Accuracy in reporting, 186
Ad hoc committees, 75-76, 177
Adjuncts to nursing care plans, 147, 150-151
Adjuncts to nursing service administration, 199-252
Adjuncts to research 240
Administration in nursing, 1-46
Advantages of budgeting, 197-198
Advantages and disadvantages of committees, 177
Annual report, 189-190
Attitudes toward pain, 20
Audit system in nursing services (JCAH), 11-12
Autocratic-democratic leadership, 8

B

Battelle Northwest Systems Programs for Hospitals, 136, 137
Benedikter audit, 168
Benefits of planning, 50
Bennett's Employee Idea Program, 242
Budget, 194-195
Budgeting, 193-198
Bureaucracy, 7-8

C

Calculation of nursing hours, 112-113
Care-cure-coordination view of nursing, 18
Case studies, 259-263
Case studies in in-service education, 212; *see also* Case studies
CASH; *see* Commission for Administrative Services in Hospitals
Categories of workers, 88-94
Centralized and decentralized in-service education, 206
Challenges to nursing practice, 20-21
Change and its management, 38-39
Change of shift reports, 188-189
Changing titles and terms in the health field, 94-95
Characteristics of organizational structure, 65-66
Checklists of patient discharge needs, 61
Circulation and storage of reports, 187-188
City of Hope Medical Center, philosophy of nursing department, 52-54
Civil rights legislation, 232
Classification of creativity, 241

Classification of nursing diagnoses, 150-151
Classification of research, 236
Classification of workers, 88-94
Clinical competence of supervisors, 129-130
Clinical enrichment in staffing, 116
Clinical specialists, 70-71
Clinical specialists, duties and responsibilities of, 91-93
Clinically directed organization schema, 78, 80
Code of Ethics (ANA), 44
Collaboration, departmental–personnel department, 87
Collaborative and collegial research, 236-237
Collegiality in staffing, 88
Commission for Administrative Services in Hospitals (CASH), 136, 137, 142
Committees, 75-76
  nursing representation on, 76
  in coordination, 177-178
Communication
  and confused thought, 36-37
  and easy concensus, 36
  with the dying, 35
  and human relations, 33-37, 48-49
  indirect, 35-36
  precision and clarity in, 35
  in staffing, 118-119
  stereotyping and, danger of, 35
Community resources for patients, 20, 61-62
Community services in discharge planning, 61
Complemental nurse, 114
Compulsory health insurance, 233
Computerized nursing care, 175-176
Conceptualization, ability of leaders in, 8-9
Conferences, 151-152
Conflict, logic in resolution of, 41
Conflict between staff and patients, 20
Confrontation-negotiation leadership, 9
Conscientious objectors, 94
Conservation of nurse time, 101-103
Consultant services, 136-137
Consultants, 160
Continuing education and in-service education, 201-202
Contract negotiating procedure, 219-221
Contracts, limitations and gains in, 223-224
Controlling, 155-169
  and coordination, 174-176
  mechanisms, 160-168
  need for standards in, 157-158
Conventional staffing pattern, 110-111
Coordinating, 170-184

266

Index

Coordination
  within coordination, 176-177
  and departmentalization, 172
  interdepartmental, 178-181
  intradepartmental, 178
  lateral, 181
  and medical records department, 180-181
  in nursing, 170-171
  physician-nurse, 180
Council of Nursing Service Facilitators, 3, 39, 94
Creative persons, findings of studies of, 241
Creativity
  classification of, 241
  comprehensive program for, 242-243
  in management, 241-242
  and nurses, 242
  and women, 242
Criteria for selection and placement of personnel, 99-101
Cyclical staffing pattern, 110

D

Decentralized organization schema, 78, 79
Decision making
  in planning, 51
  and organization structure, 68-69
Deficiencies in nursing care, 19-20
Definition of nursing service administration, 7, 47
Definitions of nursing care, 17-19
Delegation of responsibility, 67-68
Delegation-responsibility-accountability triad, 67, 69
Deterrents to nursing service administration, 4-5
Deterrents to research, 237-238
Development of personnel, 48
Diagnoses, classification of nursing, 150-151
Dignity and worth of the individual, 29-32
Directing, 128-154
Directing and coordination, 174
Discharge planning and referral, 20
  evaluation of, 62-63
  Program Evaluation and Review Technique (PERT), 63
Disposable equipment, 228
Duties and responsibilities
  of licensed practical nurses, 90-91
  of nurses' aides, 88-89
  of orderlies, 89
  of professional nurses, 91
  of technicians, 89
  of ward clerks, 89
Dying Person's Bill of Rights, 35

E

Early nursing study, innovations in nursing from, 135
Ecology Movement and systems theory, 227-228
Economic and General Welfare Program of ANA, 5, 44
Economic position of nursing, 4, 5
Economic waste in budgeting, 197

Education
  continuing and in-service, 201-202
  equal opportunity for, 206-207
  patient, 20, 210
Equipment, 227-229
Equipment and inventory maintenance, 196
Establishment-maintenance view of leadership, 9
Esthetics in nursing philosophy, 44
Ethical codes for nurses, 43-44
Ethical considerations in humanization 43-44
Ethical and other philosophical components of research, 237
Evaluation
  behavior in, common understanding of, 120-124
  devices, 160-162
  of discharge planning and referral, 62-63
  Flanagan critical-incident technique in, 121
  nonchecklist form for, 123, 255-258
  objectivity in, 120
  of organization structure, 80-82
  by peers, 124
Examination of nursing care, 17-26
Example of hospital planning, 63-64
Execution of the budget, 195
Executive committee, 75
Executive development, 209-210
Expanded role of nursing, 24-25
External nursing service reports and records, 190
Extrainstitutional coordination, 181-183

F

Feminist Movement, effect on nurses, 118
Financial incentives and budgeting, 196-197
Flanagan critical-incident technique in evaluating, 121
Float personnel, 97
Flow process chart, 140, 141
Fluidity in nursing, 101
Forecasting in planning, 58
Forecasting in staffing, 85-86
Formalization of nursing service administration, beginning of, 5
Forty-hour, 4-day work week, 110-111
Framework for study of nursing service administration, 47-198
Friesen plan, 152-153

G

"Games People Play," 118
General periodic reports, 189
Goals of the enterprise, effect of, 28-29
Goals of nursing service, long- and short-range, 60-62, 63-64
Goals of workers and organization, 58-59
Good writing techniques in reporting, 186-187
Government control of health care industry, move to, 230-233

H

Head nurse, status of in nursing service administration, 3-4, 73

268 Index

Health educators, 93-94
Health services for personnel, 224-225
Hill-Burton Act, 31
Hospital Administration Services of AHA, 136
Hospital annual report, 189-90
Hospital planning, example of, 63-64
Human relations
  openness and, 29
  research in industry, 30
  and society, 30
  theory in administration, 13-14
Humanizing the enterprise, 27-46
  consideration of stress in, 41-43
  metaphysics in, 45
  moral attributes in, 45

I

Incentives, financial and budgeting, 196-197
Incidental teaching, 210
Increased nurse responsibility, 103-106
Indirect communication, 35-36
Innovations in nursing from early study, 135
In-service education
  continuing education and, 201-202
  determining worker needs, 204-206
  equal opportunity for, 206-207
  evaluation of, 213-215
  involvement of professional organizations in, 202-203
  methods of, 211-213
  on-the-job training, 207-208
  place in the enterprise, 203-204
  types of, 207-210
In-service programs, elements of, 206-210
In-service programs and budgeting, 196
Inspection programs, systematic and routinized, 165
Institutional licensure, threat of, 231
Instructing patients in self-care, 20
Insurance, malpractice, for nurses, 66
Interdepartmental coordination, 178-181
Interdependent-dependent-independent aspects of nursing care, 18
Internal movement of plans, 59-60
Internal nursing service reports and records, 188-189
Internalization of nursing care, 17
Interviewing, 119
Intradepartmental coordination, 178
Inventory, maintenance of, 229

J

Job analysis, 137-138
Job descriptions, 138-139
Job evaluation, 139-140
Job simplification, 140-143
Joint Commission on Accreditation of Hospitals (JCAH)
  audit system in nursing services, 11-12
  nursing audit, 169

Joint Commission—cont'd
  standard for evaluation, 75

K

W. K. Kellogg Foundation, 5

L

Lateral coordination, 181
Leadership, 8-9
Legal aspects of health care industry, 230-234
Liaison nurse, 114, 173-174
Licensed practical nurses, duties and responsibilities of, 90-91
Licensure, threat of institutional, 231
Licensure of nurses, 88
Line-staff concept of organization structure, 69-71
List of 21 nursing problems, 23-24
Logic in resolution of conflict, 41
Long- and short-range goals of nursing service, 60-62, 63-64

M

Maintenance, conservation of supplies, and inventory, 229
Malpractice in nursing, 233-234
Malpractice insurance for nurses, 66
Management, kinds of, 7-9
Management by exception, 13, 158
Management by objectives, 10-12, 123
Manpower, concept of, 88
Manuals as direction, 132-134
McGregor theory, 14, 123
Medical records department and coordination, 180-181
Medicare-Medicaid, 230
Merit pay, 225
Methods of in-service education, 211-213
Montefiore Hospital home health program, 20
Morale, 37-39

N

National Association for Practical Nurse Education and Service, Inc., 91
National Commission for the Study of Nursing and Nursing Education, 95, 104, 239
National Federation of Practical Nurses, 91
National Labor Relations Act, 218, 219, 232; *see also* Taft-Hartley Act
Negativism, 117-118
Nurse-patient relationship, 19
Nurse practice acts, 25, 230-231
Nurse practitioners, 25, 92, 101
Nurse therapists, 114
Nurses
  in the emergency room, 104
  in extended-care facilities, 105
  as extenders of patient care, 104-105
  in utilization-evaluation programs, 105-106
  as women, 118
Nurses for Political Action, 118

Nurses' rights, 32
Nursing
  economic position of, 4, 5
  expanded role of, 24-25
  fluidity in, 101
Nursing audit, 165-169
  essential characteristics of, 166
  Nursing Audit Criteria, 157
Nursing care
  deficiencies in, 19-20
  direction, 143-152
  examination of, 17-26
  internalization of, 17
  need for standards of, 130-132
  self-pacing process of, 24
  SOAP process of, 24, 191-192
Nursing care plans, 143-147
Nursing home incidents, 265
Nursing philosophy
  City of Hope Medical Center, 52-54
  esthetics in, 44
Nursing process, 21-23
Nursing representation on committees, 76
Nursing service
  ANA *Standards for Nursing Services* (1973), 21
  internal reports and records, 188-189
  long- and short-range goals, 60-62, 63-64
  objectives of, 21-26
Nursing service administration
  definition of, 7, 47
  deterrents to, 4-5
  formalization, beginning of, 5
  framework for study of, 47-198
  status of, 3-6
Nursing Service Administration Project (1950-51), 5

O

Objectives of nursing service, 21-26
Objectives in planning, 55-57
Objectivity in evaluation, 120
Objectivity in reporting, 186
Office management, 7
On-the-job training, 207-208
One-to-one nurses, 114
Ongoing education, 208-209
Operations analysis, 134-137
Operations analysis, derivatives of, 137-143
Opinion polls, 248
Orderlies, duties and responsibilities of, 89
Organization chart, 66
Organization structure
  decision making and, 68-69
  evaluation of, 80-82
  line-staff concept of, 69-71
  and personnel evaluation system, 66
Organizational behavior, 116-118
Organizational effectiveness, checklist of, 81-82
Organizational schemas, 76-80
Organizing, 65-83
Organizing in coordination, 172-173

Orientation for new personnel, 207
Outside learning experiences, 210-211
Overcommunication, 36
Overlapping supervision, 72

P

Patient assignment, methods of, 113-116
Patient chart, 190-191
Patient distribution in direction, 153-154
Patient education, 20, 210
Patient incidents, 263-265
Patient's rights, 30-33
Pediatric Bill of Rights, 31
Peer evaluation, 124
Personhood, 27-28
Personnel
  administration, 86-87
  criteria for selection and placement of, 99-101
  development of, 48
  evaluation of, 119-125
  evaluation forms, 122-123, 253-258
  evaluation system and organizational structure, 66
  health services for, 224-225
  for in-service education, 206
  optimal utilization of, 101-106
  orientation, 207
  personal preferences and aptitude of, 100
  policies and contracts, 216-226
    history and trends in, 216-217
    supportive, 224
  portion of the budget, 195
  in position, 95-125
  selection interview, 99
  testing in selection and placement of, 100
  turnover rate, 113
Personnel department
  functions of, 86
  and recruiting, 98
PERT; *see* Professional Evaluation and Review Technique
Phaneuf audit, 166
Philosophy
  of City of Hope Medical Center, 52-54
  of Harper Hospital, 56-57
  of Illinois State Psychiatric Institute, 54-55
  in planning, 51-55
  in public versus private institutions, 51-52
Physical plant in directing, 152-153
Physician-nurse coordination, 180
Planning for the nursing service, 50-64
  comprehensiveness of, 63
  in coordination, 171-172
  decision making in, 51
  forecasting in, 58
  objectives in, 55-57
Policy manuals, 133-134
Politics in nursing, 44-45
  activities of, 118
  Nurses for Political Action, 118
POSDCORB, 47-48

Preventive medicine, 20-21
Primary care nurses, 114
Problem-oriented medical record, 191-192
Problem-solving approach to nursing process, 22
Procedures manuals, 132-133
Professional associations and unions, efforts of, 217-219
Professional nurses, duties and responsibilities of, 91
Professional Performance Interview Schedule, 123, 255-258
Professional performance report, 253-254
Professional Standards and Review Organization (PSRO), 105, 118
Program Evaluation and Review Technique (PERT), 63
PSRO; see Professional Standards and Review Organization
Psychological needs of patients, 19-20
Public relations
 and the expanded role of the hospital, 248, 250
 personnel, 248
 and publications, 250-251
 record in nursing, 246-248

Q

Quality Patient Care Scale, 161, 166
Quantifying nursing staff, 108-110
Quantifying patients' nursing needs, 107-108

R

Recruitment of personnel, 95-99
Recruitment and function of personnel department, 86
Relationship
 of controlling to other parts of the administrative process, 158-160
 of coordination to other elements of administration, 171-176
 between direction and supervision, 128-129
 of guidelines and standards, 132
 of morale and quality of leadership, 38
 of reporting to the administrative process, 185-186
 of research to nursing, 238-239
Reporting
 general attributes of, 186-188
 good writing techniques in, 186-187
 objectivity in, 186
 timeliness in, 186
Reports
 circulation and storage of, 187-188
 in controlling, 164-165
 general periodic, 189
 Professional performance, 253-254
 regulatory or accrediting agency, 190
 Report of the National Commission on Health Manpower, 164
Research
 classification of, 236
 and creativity, 235-243
 deterrents to, 237-238

Research—cont'd
 ethical and other philosophical components of, 237
 goals for the future, 239-240
Resolution of conflict, 39-41
Responsibility, delegation of, 67-68
Rounds, 162-164

S

Self-actualization of workers, 116-117
Self-care, instructing patients in, 20
Self-evaluation, 123-124
Self-pacing process of nursing care, 24
Service Unit Management (SUM), 90
Seven-days-on, 7-days-off staffing pattern, 111
Slater Nursing Competencies Rating Scale, 121, 161, 166
SOAP process of nursing care, 24, 191-192
Social Security benefits for nurses, 232
Solid waste disposal, 228
Span of control or supervision, 71-72
Specialization, 73-75
Spiritual needs of patients, 20
Staff communication, 75-76
Staffing the enterprise, 84-127
 and coordination, 173-174
 forecasting in, 85-86
 need for clinical enrichment in, 116
Staffing patterns, 106-116
 and budgeting, 195
 determinants of, 106-107
 types of, 110, 111
Standards as base for direction and control, 131-132
Standards of Nursing Service (ANA), 21, 130, 131, 220
Standing committees, 75, 177
Status of nursing service administration, 3-6
Stress, consideration of in humanizing the enterprise, 41-43
Strikes against hospitals, 221
Supervisors, 129
Supervisory management, 7
Supplies, conservation of, 229
Suppliers, 228-229
Supportive personnel policies, 224
SUM; see Service Unit Management
Survey of Hospital Nursing Services, 130, 143
Systems analysis, 49
Systems approach to the nursing process, 23
Systems approach to staffing the enterprise, 84, 85, 86
Systems structure, 77-78
Systems theory and the Ecology Movement, 227-228

T

Taft-Hartley Act, 221; see also National Labor Relations Act
Team nursing, 114-115
Technical-professional dilemma, 25-26
Technicians, duties and responsibilities of, 89
Tentative List of Nursing Diagnoses, 150-151
Terminology associated with administration, 7-9

Terminology in controlling, 156-157
Testing in selection and placement of personnel, 100
Theories of administration, 9-16
Traditional administration, 9, 10
Traditional organization schema, 76-77
Types of in-service education, 207-210
Types of staffing patterns, 110-111

U

Unions, 218-219
Unity of command, 72-73

V

Variations on theories of administration, 14-16

Various publics, 245-246
Visiting Nurse Association, 20, 61
Volunteers, 93

W

Wage and salary administration and budgeting, 195-196
Ward clerks, duties and responsibilities of, 89
Ward manager, 71, 90
Wedge organization schema, 77
Work of executives, 7
Workers
 classification of, 88-94
 as individuals, 116-117
Workmen's Compensation laws, 232